Long-Term Health Effects of COVID-19

Disability and Function Following SARS-CoV-2 Infection

Paul A. Volberding, Bernice X. Chu, and Carol Mason Spicer, *Editors*

Committee on the Long-Term Health Effects Stemming from COVID-19 and Implications for the Social Security Administration

Board on Health Care Services

Health and Medicine Division

Consensus Study Report

NATIONAL ACADEMIES PRESS 500 Fifth Street, NW Washington, DC 20001

This activity was supported by Contract No. 28321318D00060015 between the National Academy of Sciences and U.S. Social Security Administration. Any opinions, findings, conclusions, or recommendations expressed in this publication do not necessarily reflect the views of any organization or agency that provided support for the project.

International Standard Book Number-13: 978-0-309-71860-8
International Standard Book Number-10: 0-309-71860-0
Digital Object Identifier: https://doi.org/10.17226/27756
Library of Congress Control Number: 2024939460

This publication is available from the National Academies Press, 500 Fifth Street, NW, Keck 360, Washington, DC 20001; (800) 624-6242 or (202) 334-3313; http://www.nap.edu.

Suggested citation: National Academies of Sciences, Engineering, and Medicine. 2024. *Long-term health effects of COVID-19: Disability and function following SARS-CoV-2 infection.* Washington, DC: The National Academies Press. https://doi.org/10.17226/27756.

Reviewers

This Consensus Study Report was reviewed in draft form by individuals chosen for their diverse perspectives and technical expertise. The purpose of this independent review is to provide candid and critical comments that will assist the National Academies of Sciences, Engineering, and Medicine in making each published report as sound as possible and to ensure that it meets the institutional standards for quality, objectivity, evidence, and responsiveness to the study charge. The review comments and draft manuscript remain confidential to protect the integrity of the deliberative process.

We thank the following individuals for their review of this report:

STEPHEN B. BAYLIN, Sidney Kimmel Comprehensive Cancer Center at Johns Hopkins Medicine
TAE HWAN CHUNG, Johns Hopkins University
TODD E. DAVENPORT, University of the Pacific & Workwell Foundation
ALLEN W. HEINEMANN, Northwestern University
ANTHONY L. KOMAROFF, Harvard Medical School and Brigham and Women's Hospital
MONICA KURYLO, University of Kansas Medical Center
SINDHU MOHANDAS, Children's Hospital Los Angeles, Keck School of Medicine, University of Southern California
SHARON SAYDAH, U.S. Centers for Disease Control and Prevention
AMANDA VERMA, Washington University School of Medicine in St. Louis
JUAN WISNIVESKY, Icahn School of Medicine at Mount Sinai
YONGKANG ZHANG, Weill Cornell Medical College

Although the reviewers listed above provided many constructive comments and suggestions, they were not asked to endorse the conclusions or recommendations of this report nor did they see the final draft before its release. The review of this report was overseen by **ROBERT S. LAWRENCE**, Johns Hopkins Bloomberg School of Public Health, and **ERIC B. LARSON**, University of Washington School of Public Health. They were responsible for making certain that an independent examination of this report was carried out in accordance with the standards of the National Academies and that all review comments were carefully considered. Responsibility for the final content rests entirely with the authoring committee and the National Academies.

Contents

Boxes, Figures, and Tables

BOXES

FIGURES

TABLES

ANNEX TABLES

Preface

Infection with SARS-CoV-2 can trigger health effects that can continue well after resolution of the initial COVID-19 illness. These effects have protean manifestations, often involving numerous organ systems, that can persist for months or years and may, in some cases, be disabling. Children and adolescents are affected as well as adults. While most aspects of these conditions are poorly understood, concern is real that they may result in an increase in applications for disability received by the Social Security Administration (SSA). Accordingly, SSA commissioned a consensus report from the National Academies of Sciences, Engineering, and Medicine reviewing the long-term health effects of COVID-19 and potential implications for SSA disability. To this end, the National Academies convened an ad hoc committee of experts to provide an overview of this persisting clinical condition, its effects and natural history in a variety of affected populations, and the current status of treatment and management and of ongoing research efforts. The committee was also charged with reviewing the spectrum of health effects associated with this new condition and their impact on function in both adults and children.

Given that the long-term health effects of COVID-19 are complex and that knowledge of those effects is rapidly evolving, the committee convened by the National Academies included experts in the epidemiology, diagnosis, and clinical management of what has come to be called Long COVID. This committee, including researchers and clinicians, some themselves affected, collected evidence, heard presentations from invited speakers, and deliberated in response to a statement of task from SSA.

This consensus report was prepared with a sense of urgency in light of the rapid evolution of knowledge about the diagnosis of SARS-CoV-2 infection and the long-term health effects and disordered function that may follow COVID-19, against the backdrop of what has been learned about other complex chronic conditions, such as myalgic encephalitis/chronic fatigue syndrome and fibromyalgia, themselves potentially triggered by infections. The committee identified ways in which the diagnosis and management of Long COVID represent unique challenges and raise many remaining questions for the SSA disability program. The committee and I are grateful for the opportunity to point out that the symptoms experienced by these patients are real and should be taken seriously.

The committee extends its sincere thanks to the many individuals who shared their time and expertise to support its work and inform its deliberations. The study was sponsored by SSA, and we thank Brendan Rogak, Vincent Nibali, Megan Butson, and Steve Rollins for their guidance and support. The committee acknowledges Vincent Nibali at SSA for verifying the accuracy of relevant technical content pertaining to the disability determination process. The committee also benefited greatly from discussions with individuals who presented at the committee's open sessions: Karin Denault, Lucas Denault, Robert Holman, Akiko Iwasaki, Anthony Komaroff, Avindra Nath, Vincent Nibali, David Putrino, Steve Rollins, Eric Van Gieson, Angela Meriquez Vázquez, and Alexandra Yonts. In addition, the committee's work benefited from presentations during two concurrent National Academies activities: *Symposium on Long COVID: Examining the Working Definition* (June 2023), hosted by the Committee on Examining the Working Definition for Long COVID, and *Toward a Common Research Agenda in Infection-Associated Chronic Illnesses: A Workshop to Examine Common, Overlapping Clinical and Biological Factors* (June 2023), hosted by the Forum on Microbial Threats and the Forum on Neuroscience and Nervous System Disorders. Appreciation goes as well to Sonya Marshall-Gradisnik and Natalie Eaton-Fitch for their work on a paper commissioned by the committee to review chronic conditions similar to Long COVID.

The committee thanks the reviewers of this report for their invaluable feedback on an earlier draft and the monitor and coordinator who oversaw the report review.

The committee also acknowledges the many staff within the Health and Medicine Division (HMD) who provided support in various ways to this project, including Carol Mason Spicer (study director), Bernice Chu (program officer), Elizabeth Ferré (research associate), Violet Bishop (research assistant), Burgess Manobah (research associate), Joe Goodman (senior program assistant), Karen Helsing (senior program officer), and Hoda Soltani (former program officer). The committee extends great thanks and appreciation to Sharyl Nass, senior director, Board on Health Care Services, who oversaw the project. Greysi Patton (finance business partner), Arzoo Tayyeb (finance business partner), Julie Wiltshire (senior finance business partner), and Ron Brown (deputy director, HMD program finance) oversaw finances for the project; Rebecca Morgan (senior research librarian) provided research assistance, and Anne Marie Houppert (senior librarian) assisted with fact checking; and the report review, production, and communications staff all provided valuable guidance to ensure the success of the final product. Rona Briere and her staff provided superb editorial assistance in preparing the final report.

Paul A. Volberding, *Chair*
Committee on the Long-Term Health Effects Stemming from COVID-19
and Implications for the Social Security Administration

Acronyms and Abbreviations

AAPRM	American Academy of Physical Medicine and Rehabilitation
ADL	activity of daily living
aHR	adjusted hazard ratio
ARDS	acute respiratory distress syndrome
BUN	blood urea nitrogen
CBT	cognitive-behavioral therapy
CDC	U.S. Centers for Disease Control and Prevention
CFQ	Cognitive Failures Questionnaire
CI	confidence interval
CLIA	chemiluminescent immunoassays
CMR	cardio magnetic resonance
COMPASS 31	31-question Composite Autonomic Symptom Score
COVID-19	coronavirus disease 2019
CPET	cardiopulmonary exercise testing
CRISPR	clustered regularly interspaced short palindromic repeats
CRP	c-reactive protein
CT	computed tomography
CTPA	computed tomography pulmonary angiography
CXR	chest x-ray
DALY	disability-adjusted life year
DLCO	diffusing capacity of the lungs for carbon monoxide

DM	diabetes mellitus
DMS-5-TR	*Diagnostic and Statistical Manual of Mental Disorders, Fifth Edition*
DSQ	DePaul Symptom Questionnaire
EBV	Epstein-Barr virus
ECG	electrocardiogram
ECog	Everyday Cognition Scale
EECP	enhanced external counterpulsation
ELISA	enzyme-linked immunosorbent assays
ESR	erythrocyte sedimentation rate
FDA	Food and Drug Administration
FM	fibromyalgia
g-AChR	ganglionic neuronal nicotinic acetylcholine receptor
GET	graded exercise therapy
GPCR	G-protein-coupled receptor
GWAS	genomic-wide association studies
HADS	Hospital Anxiety and Depression Scale
HIV	human immunodeficiency virus
IACC	infection-associated chronic conditions
IADLs	instrumental activities of daily living
ICD-11	*International Classification of Diseases and Related Health Problems, 11th Revision*
IADL	instrumental activity of daily living
ICF	*International Classification of Function, Disability and Health*
ICU	intensive care unit
IGRA	interferon-γ (IFN-γ) release assay
IRR	incidence rate ratio
LAMP	loop-mediated isothermal amplification
LFIA	lateral flow immunoassays
LQBTQI+	lesbian, gay, bisexual, transgender, queer, intersex, or other
MCAS	mast cell activation syndrome
MCI	mild cognitive impairment
ME/CFS	myalgic encephalomyelitis/chronic fatigue syndrome
MFI	Multidimensional Fatigue Inventory
MFIS	Modified Fatigue Impact Scale

miRNA	microRNA
MIS-C	multisystem inflammatory syndrome in children
NAAT	nucleic acid amplification test
NASA	National Aeronautics and Space Administration
NCS	neurocardiogenic syncope
NICE	National Institute for Health and Care Excellence
NIH	National Institutes of Health
OH	orthostatic hypotension
PAOFI	Patient's Assessment of Own Functioning Inventory
PASC	post-acute sequelae of COVID-19
PCCI	post-COVID-19 cognitive impairment
PCR	polymerase chain reaction
PedsQL	Pediatric Quality of Life
PEM	post-exertional malaise
PICS	post-intensive care syndrome
POTS	postural orthostatic tachycardia syndrome
PROMIS	Patient-Reported Outcomes Measurement Information System
PTSD	posttraumatic stress disorder
RECOVER	Researching COVID to Enhance Recovery
ROS	reactive oxygen species
RT-PCR	real-time reverse transcription PCR
SARS-CoV-2	severe acute respiratory syndrome coronavirus 2
SD	standard deviation
SF-36	36-Item Short Form Survey
SSA	Social Security Administration
SSDI	Social Security Disability Insurance
SSI	Supplemental Security Income
SSRI	selective serotonin reuptake inhibitor
TSH	thyroid-stimulating hormone
VA	U.S Department of Veteran Affairs
$\dot{V}O_2$	volume of oxygen consumption
VQ	ventilation perfusion
WHO	World Health Organization

Summary[1]

Since the onset of the coronavirus disease 2019 (COVID-19) pandemic in early 2020, many individuals infected with the virus that causes COVID-19, severe acute respiratory syndrome coronavirus 2 (SARS-CoV-2), have continued to experience lingering symptoms for months or even years following acute infection. The COVID-19 pandemic is a complex event that has changed over time with mutations in the virus and the development of and access to vaccines and antiviral treatments. Knowledge about COVID-19, the virus, and lingering new or worsening health effects following acute infection is still embryonic, and available information will evolve as more is understood about the virus and its sequelae.

Long COVID is one of many terms used to refer to persistent symptoms and new or worsening health effects following acute infection with SARS-CoV-2. There currently is no consensus definition of Long COVID. Among other terms used to describe the long-term health effects of SARS-CoV-2 are post-acute sequelae of SARS-CoV-2 or post-acute sequelae of COVID-19, Post-COVID Syndrome, Post-acute COVID Syndrome, Post-Covid Condition, Post-Covid Conditions (condition is pluralized), and Long Haulers Syndrome. The term "Long COVID" is used in this report not only because it was the first, most inclusive, and most widely used term denoting the long-term health effects of SARS-CoV-2 infection, but also because it recognizes the voices of patients who first alerted the world and the medical and scientific communities that SARS-CoV-2 can lead to long-term health consequences.

---

[1]This summary does not include references. Citations to support the text and conclusions herein are provided in the body of the report.

The definition of Long COVID continues to evolve, and numerous definitions are used in the literature, with varying lengths of time after infection. A separate National Academies of Sciences, Engineering, and Medicine committee concurrently examined the working definition of Long COVID.

Data from the U.S. Centers for Disease Control and Prevention's (CDC's) National Health Interview Survey show that in 2022, 6.9 percent of U.S. adults and 1.3 percent of children had Long COVID at some point, while 3.4 percent of adults and 0.5 percent of children had Long COVID at the time of interview. Based on these surveys, it is estimated that approximately 8.9 million adults and 362,000 children reported Long COVID symptoms in the United States in 2022. Among U.S. adults, data from the CDC's Household Pulse Survey show that the prevalence of Long COVID declined from 7.5 percent in June 2022 to 5.9 percent in January 2023, then increased to 6.8 percent in January 2024, reflecting a complex event that has changed over time and continues to evolve. Despite the recent overall decline in prevalence since June 2022, Long COVID's disease burden remains substantial.

CONTEXT FOR THIS STUDY

The population of individuals with Long COVID is of special interest to the Social Security Administration (SSA) as their condition may cause them to meet or contribute to their meeting SSA's criteria for disability. For many individuals with Long COVID, symptoms resolve within 6 months; for some, however, symptoms persist for 12 months or more. Some health effects of Long COVID, such as chronic fatigue and post-exertional malaise, post-COVID-19 cognitive impairment (sometimes referred to as brain fog), and autonomic dysfunction, can impair an individual's ability to work or attend school for an extended period of time. Even individuals with a mild initial course of illness can develop Long COVID with severe health effects.

Diagnosis, measurement, and treatment of Long COVID are complicated by the relative novelty of the condition, as well as its heterogeneous presentation and symptomology and the episodic nature of many of the associated health effects. SSA therefore seeks the most current information available on the long-term health and functional effects of COVID-19 as related to SSA's disability programs.

STUDY CHARGE AND SCOPE

In August 2022, SSA requested that the Health and Medicine Division of the National Academies convene an ad hoc committee of relevant experts[2]

---

[2]The committee included experts in cardiology; epidemiology; family, internal, and pediatric medicine; health metrics; health policy; immunology; infectious disease; neuropsychology; occupational medicine; occupational therapy; pediatric neurology; and rehabilitation medicine.

to investigate and provide an overview of the current status of the diagnosis, treatment, and prognosis of long-term health effects related to prior SARS-CoV-2 infection. The committee's work was to be based on published evidence (to the extent possible) and professional judgment (where evidence is lacking). Box S-1 contains the committee's full statement of task. SSA requested that the committee's report include conclusions, but no recommendations.

BOX S-1
Statement of Task

An ad hoc committee of the National Academies of Sciences, Engineering, and Medicine will review the evidence regarding long-term disability that may result from COVID-19 illness and produce a report addressing the current status of the diagnosis, treatment, and prognosis of related disabilities based on published evidence (to the extent possible) and professional judgement (where evidence is lacking). In regards to the long-term health effects stemming from COVID-19 infection, the committee's report will:

1. Identify the committee's preferred terminology (e.g. Long COVID, PASC, PACS, Post-COVID Syndrome, Long Hauler's Syndrome);
2. Describe commonly reported and observed long-term health effects and describe what is known about:
   a. The frequency and distribution of their severity and duration in the general population, as well as any differences along racial, ethnic, sex, gender, geographic, or socioeconomic dimensions, or differences specific to populations with particular pre-existing or comorbid conditions;
   b. Clinical standards for diagnosis and measurement of the specific health effects or identified patterns or clusters of health effects;
   c. Any special considerations regarding the health effects' identification and management in special populations, including pregnant people and those with underlying health conditions;
   d. Best practices to quantify the functional impacts of those health effects; and
   e. Identified challenges for clinicians in evaluating persons with those health effects;
3. Identify and describe the tests, findings, and signs currently clinically accepted to establish a history of COVID-19 in the following three categories:
   a. Tests for SARS-CoV-2;
   b. Findings from antibody tests or other diagnostic tests; and
   c. Signs consistent with COVID-19;

continued

BOX S-1 Continued

4. Identify any methods generally accepted by the medical community to establish a history of COVID-19 in patients that are not covered by the following three categories:
   a. A report of a positive viral test for SARS-CoV-2,
   b. A diagnostic test with findings consistent with COVID-19 (e.g., chest x-ray with lung abnormalities, etc.), or
   c. A diagnosis of COVID-19 based on signs consistent with COVID-19 (e.g., fever, cough, etc.);
5. Identify patterns of long-term, work-related functional decline observed in adults and the frequency, severity, duration, risk factors, and associated signs or laboratory findings;
6. Identify distinct patterns of long-term functional decline observed in children and the frequency, severity, duration, risk factors, and associated signs or laboratory findings;
7. Identify any trends in the frequency, severity, and duration of functional decline, including those specific to different racial, ethnic, sex, gender, geographic, or socioeconomic groups and those specific to populations with particular pre-existing or comorbid conditions;
8. Describe any variations in functional or long-term effects based on initial infection with the various identified strains of the virus or based on vaccination status, both at the time of initial infection and illness or that are long-lasting; and
9. Summarize completed, on-going, or planned research, and any resultant medical knowledge, regarding similarities between this condition and impairments such as fibromyalgia or myalgic encephalomyelitis (chronic fatigue syndrome), including mechanisms of action, effective testing regimes, prognosis and progression, and potential treatments.
10. Summarize the committee's conclusions regarding best practices for assessing disability in these populations.

The report will include findings and conclusions but not recommendations.

STUDY APPROACH AND SCOPE

The committee conducted a review of the literature pertaining to (1) methods for establishing a history of COVID-19, (2) commonly reported and disabling health effects of COVID-19 in adults and children, and (3) functional trajectories related to those health effects. Given the newness of the disease and the insufficiency of high-quality prospective studies in the

United States, the committee performed a global literature search instead of limiting its search to U.S. studies. The committee did not conduct a systematic review; rather, the committee developed criteria for determining relevance to the statement of task by focusing on studies involving relatively large populations followed for at least 6 months and including significant symptoms and functional outcomes. Throughout the study, recognizing that literature on Long COVID is rapidly evolving, the committee members applied their expertise to identify other studies in progress and perspectives not yet represented in publications. The committee also used a variety of resources to supplement its review of the literature. Meeting seven times, the committee held three public information-gathering workshops with invited speakers, including several people having lived experience with Long COVID.

THE COMMITTEE'S CONCLUSIONS

The committee formulated nine conclusions about Long COVID in the following areas: (1) diagnosis, (2) epidemiology, (3) health effects, (4) functional impact and risk factors, (5) Long COVID in children and adolescents, (6) management, (7) disease course and prognosis, (8) health equity, and (9) similar chronic conditions.

Diagnosis of Long COVID

Long COVID is associated with a wide range of new or worsening health conditions and encompasses more than 200 symptoms involving nearly every organ system. There currently are no consensus-based diagnostic criteria for the condition; criteria for diagnosis are evolving as experience and research findings develop. Diagnosis of Long COVID is generally based on a known or presumed history of acute SARS-CoV-2 infection (as indicated by a positive viral test or patient self-report; as of this writing, no diagnostic test for Long COVID is available), the presence of Long COVID health effects and symptoms, and consideration of other conditions and etiologies that could be causing the symptoms.

Testing to diagnose acute SARS-CoV-2 infection, as well as testing capacity and behaviors, has changed dramatically over the course of the COVID-19 pandemic. Testing was constrained during the early phase of the pandemic, although it subsequently became increasingly available, and the introduction of at-home testing meant that many people may not have reported their positive results to health care systems. As a result of these two drivers, many individuals infected with SARS-CoV-2 never received formal documentation of their diagnosis. Sole reliance on a documented history of SARS-CoV-2 infection when diagnosing Long COVID will miss these individuals. Therefore, the presence of signs and symptoms and self-reported prior infection are generally considered sufficient to establish a diagnosis of SARS-CoV-2 infection. Continued research on and discussion of Long COVID will help inform a case definition and standardized diagnosis.

Based on its review of the literature, the committee reached the following conclusion:

1. *Long COVID is a complex chronic condition caused by SARS-CoV-2 infection that affects multiple body systems. Because of wide variability in testing practices over the course of the pandemic, many people experiencing Long COVID have not received a formal diagnosis of prior SARS-CoV-2 infection. A positive test for SARS-CoV-2 is not necessary to consider a diagnosis of Long COVID.*

Epidemiology

Long COVID can impact people across the lifespan, from children to older adults, as well as across sex, gender, racial, ethnic, and other demographic groups. Women are twice as likely as men to experience Long COVID. Population surveys suggest that, as noted above, in 2022 the overall prevalence of Long COVID was around 3.4 percent in U.S. adults and 0.5 percent in children. Estimates of the prevalence of specific long-term health effects of SARS-CoV-2 vary in the literature. This variation reflects the dynamic nature of the pandemic itself, as the virus has evolved and spawned many variants and subvariants (likely with different propensities to cause Long COVID), as well as the introduction of vaccines and treatments for acute infection (e.g., antivirals, steroids), both of which have been shown to reduce the risk of long-term health effects. Variation in incidence and prevalence estimates also stems from the heterogeneity of study designs, including choice of control groups, methods used to account for the effect of baseline health, specification of outcomes, and other methodological differences.

In addition, the broad multisystem nature of Long COVID and the fact that the associated health effects are expressed differently by age group and sex and by baseline health compound the challenge of identifying and quantifying affected populations. Symptoms of SARS-CoV-2 infection range in severity from mild to severe, and the literature suggests that the severity of acute SARS-CoV-2 infection is a risk factor for Long COVID. For example, a large Scottish population-based study found that 5 percent of those with mild infection had not recovered at least 6 months following infection, compared with 16 percent of those who required hospitalization—a ratio of approximately 1:3.

Based on its review of the literature, the committee reached the following conclusion:

2.   *The risk of Long COVID increases with the severity of acute infection. By the committee's best estimate, people whose infection was sufficiently severe to necessitate hospitalization are 2–3 times more likely to experience Long COVID than are those who were not hospitalized, and among those who were hospitalized, individuals requiring life support in the intensive care unit may be twice as likely to experience Long COVID. However, people with mild disease can also develop Long COVID, and given the much higher number of people with mild versus severe disease, they make up the great majority of people with Long COVID.*

Health Effects

Long COVID is associated with hundreds of symptoms and new or worsening health effects that manifest in many different body systems. In keeping with the three domains of functioning in the *International Classification of Functioning, Disability and Health* model of disability, health effects experienced in Long COVID may manifest as impairments in body structures and physical and psychological functions, with resulting activity limitations and restrictions on participation. Evidence on clustering of the post-acute and long-term health effects of SARS-CoV-2 infection remains inconsistent across studies. Consensus is needed on terms, definitions, and methodological approaches for generating better-quality and more consistent evidence.

Based on its review of the literature, the committee reached the following conclusion:

3.   *Long COVID is associated with a wide range of new or worsening health conditions impacting multiple organ systems. Long COVID can cause more than 200 symptoms and affects each person differently. Attempts to cluster symptoms have yielded heterogeneous results.*

Functional Impact and Risk Factors

Some of the symptoms and health effects associated with Long COVID can be severe enough to interfere with an individual's day-to-day functioning, including participation in work and school activities. Functional disability associated with Long COVID has been characterized as the inability to return to work, poor quality of life, diminished ability to perform activities of daily living, decreased physical and cognitive function, and overall disability. The severity of acute COVID-19 is a major risk factor for poor functional outcomes, but even people with mild initial illness can experience long-term functional impairments. Increased number and severity of long-term symptoms correlates with decreased quality of life, physical functioning, and ability to work or perform in school. Other risk factors for poor functional outcomes include female sex, lack of vaccination against SARS-CoV-2, baseline disability or comorbidities, and smoking.

There is some overlap between SSA's current Listing of Impairments (Listings) and health effects associated with Long COVID, such as impaired lung and heart function. However, it is likely that most individuals with Long COVID applying for Social Security disability benefits will do so based on health effects not covered in the Listings. Three frequently reported health effects that can significantly interfere with the ability to perform work or school activities and may not be captured in the SSA Listings are chronic fatigue and post-exertional malaise, post-COVID-19 cognitive impairment, and autonomic dysfunction, all of which can be difficult to assess clinically in terms of their severity and effects on a person's functioning.

Based on its review of the literature, the committee reached the following conclusion:

> 4. *Long COVID can result in the inability to return to work (or school for children and adolescents), poor quality of life, diminished ability to perform activities of daily living, and decreased physical and cognitive function for 6 months to 2 years or longer after the resolution of acute infection with SARS-CoV-2. Increased number and severity of long-term health effects correlates with decreased quality of life, physical and mental functioning, and ability to participate in work and school. Health effects that may not be captured in SSA's Listing of Impairments yet may significantly affect an individual's ability to participate in work or school include, but are not limited to, post-exertional malaise and chronic fatigue, post-COVID-19 cognitive impairment, and autonomic dysfunction.*

Long COVID in Children and Adolescents

While there are various definitions of children, adolescents, and young people, for the purposes of this report, "children" or "pediatrics" refers to the entire pediatric age range, and "adolescents" to children at the older end of the spectrum (i.e., ages ~11 to 18 years). Even though most children experience mild acute COVID-19 illness, they can experience Long COVID regardless of the severity of their acute infection. As with adults, they may experience health effects across many body systems. Commonly reported symptoms include fatigue, weakness, headache, sleep disturbance, muscle and joint pain, respiratory problems, palpitations, altered sense of smell or taste, dizziness, and dysautonomia. Although pediatric presentations and intervention options may overlap with those in adults—particularly among adolescents, who may be more likely than children to mimic the adult presentation and trajectory—pediatric management of Long COVID entails specific considerations related to developmental age and/or disabilities and history gathering. In general, children have fewer preexisting chronic health conditions compared with adults; thus, Long COVID may represent a substantial change from their baseline, particularly for those that were previously healthy.

Limited data are available on long-term outcomes in children. Some youth with persistent symptoms experience difficulties that affect their quality of life and result in increased school absences, as well as decreased participation and performance in school, sports, and other activities. Risk factors for the development of Long COVID include acute-phase hospitalization, preexisting comorbidity, and infection with pre-Omicron variants. Most children with Long COVID recover slowly over time, but not all. In one prospective cohort study of 1,243 children (ages 4–10) with Long COVID, for example, 48 percent remained symptomatic at 6 months, 13 percent at 12 months, and 5 percent at 18 months after infection. Importantly, severity of symptoms and functional impairment from Long COVID symptoms were not correlated with traditional clinical testing (e.g., lung ultrasound, standard systolic and diastolic function on echocardiogram).

It is important to note that in pediatrics, because of typical development, the baseline for performance of skills is constantly changing, especially among young children. This can make deviations in their performance during Long COVID challenging to assess, and there may be a delay in recognition of any deviations (e.g., lack of developing a skill at the appropriate age). Additionally, the duration of symptoms (e.g., 1 or 3 months) can feel very different to and have a greater impact on children compared with adults. Currently, there is a dearth of prospective and cross-sectional studies on the prevalence, risk factors, and time course and pattern of Long COVID in children. More research is needed to identify the long-term functional implications of Long COVID in children, because information from adult studies may not be directly applicable to the pediatric population.

Based on its review of the literature, the committee reached the following conclusion:

> 5. *Although the large majority of children recover fully from SARS-CoV-2 infection, some develop Long COVID and experience persistent or intermittent symptoms that can reduce their quality of life and result in increased school absences, as well as decreased participation and performance in school, sports, and other activities. Overall, the trajectory for recovery is better among children compared with adults. More research is needed to understand the long-term functional implications of Long COVID in children, as information from adult studies may not be directly applicable.*

Disease Management

Currently there are no Food and Drug Administration (FDA)–approved drugs or disease-modifying treatments for Long COVID. As with other complex multisystem conditions, management of Long COVID relies on techniques for controlling symptoms and improving functional ability, such as pacing (i.e., balancing periods of activity and rest in daily life), mobility support, social support, diet modulation, pharmacological treatment of secondary health effects, cognitive-behavioral therapy, and rehabilitation. Management often requires a multidisciplinary team. Because of the multisystem nature of the condition, different approaches may be needed to address the variety of clinical presentations and environmental factors (e.g., living situation, work requirements, family support) among individuals. Numerous randomized controlled trials are currently being undertaken to determine the efficacy of a number of identified pharmacological agents; however, limited data have been published, and trials are yet to be finalized.

Based on its review of the literature, the committee reached the following conclusion:

> 6. *There currently is no curative treatment for Long COVID itself. Management of the condition is based on current knowledge about treating the associated health effects and other sequelae. As with other complex multisystem chronic conditions, treatment focuses on symptom management and optimization of function and quality of life.*

Disease Course and Prognosis

Recovery from Long COVID varies among individuals, and data on recovery trajectories are rapidly evolving. Initial data suggest that people with persistent Long COVID symptoms generally improve over time, although preliminary studies suggest that recovery can plateau 6–12 months after acute infection. Studies have shown that only 18–22 percent of those who have persistent symptoms at 5–6 months following infection have fully recovered by 1 year. Among those who do not improve, most remain stable, but some worsen. More information on recovery trajectories at 1 year or longer may become available in the next few years. Rehabilitation and symptom management, including pacing, may improve function in some people with Long COVID, regardless of the severity of disease or duration of symptoms, although the benefits are greater for those who are younger and who have had Long COVID for a shorter period of time.

Based on its review of the literature, the committee reached the following conclusion:

7. *Recovery from Long COVID varies among individuals, and data on recovery trajectories are rapidly evolving. There is some evidence that many people with persistent Long COVID symptoms at 3 months following acute infection, including children and adolescents, have improved by 12 months. Data for durations longer than 12 months are limited, but preliminary data suggest that recovery may plateau or progress at a slower rate after 12 months.*

Health Equity

The burden of seeking care and finding adequate services for Long COVID is challenging and can impact the potential for recovery. Patients with Long COVID may encounter skepticism about their symptoms when they present in medical settings, which discourages care seeking. This is particularly true for individuals disadvantaged by their social or economic status, geographic location, or environment, and can result in preventable disparities in the burden of disease and opportunities to achieve optimal health. Disadvantaged groups include members of some racial and ethnic minorities, people with disabilities, women, LGBTQI+ (lesbian, gay, bisexual, transgender, queer, intersex, or other) individuals, people with limited English proficiency, and others.

Individuals with Long COVID have increased health care utilization and financial burden, which may be exacerbated if they are unable to work to gain income and or receive health insurance coverage. Members of disadvantaged groups, especially early in the pandemic, were more likely to contract SARS-CoV-2, more likely to be hospitalized with acute COVID-19, more likely to have adverse clinical outcomes, and less likely to be vaccinated, potentially increasing their risk of developing Long COVID. In addition, these groups are more likely to be uninsured or underinsured. Even for those with insurance coverage, some of the services that have been shown to improve function may not be covered by their benefits. Moreover, the availability of specialized Long COVID services is limited, and capacity does not match the demand for rehabilitation specialists. Limited transportation, distance from clinics, and the inability to take time away from work or school are known barriers to care. The availability issue is particularly problematic for individuals living in medically underserved areas.

Information about COVID is rapidly evolving, and this dynamic nature of the science may contribute to some patient hesitancy regarding prophylactic and therapeutic management for acute infection or Long COVID. Low levels of health literacy may also place some individuals at increased risk for misinformation, which may prevent them from fully taking advantage of health care resources to protect and improve their health. Low health literacy may also impact individual self-management of the symptoms and conditions associated with Long COVID.

Based on its review of the literature, the committee reached the following conclusion:

> 8. *Social determinants of health, such as socioeconomic status, geographic location, health literacy, and race and ethnicity, affect access to health care. With respect to acute SARS-CoV-2 infection and Long COVID, adverse social determinants of health have contributed to disparities in access to SARS-CoV-2 testing; vaccination; and therapeutics, including treatments for acute infection and specialized rehabilitation clinics for Long COVID. In addition, the demand for specialty care exceeds capacity, resulting in waitlists for the receipt of services.*

Similar Chronic Conditions

Long COVID shares many features with other complex multisystem conditions, including myalgic encephalomyelitis/chronic fatigue syndrome (ME/CFS), fibromyalgia, and postural orthostatic tachycardia syndrome (POTS). The mechanism of action for infection-associated chronic illnesses remains unclear, and further investigation is needed. Current theories regarding potential mechanisms of action include viral persistence, immune dysregulation (including cytokine dysregulation or mast cell activation), neurological disturbances (e.g., neuroinflammation), cardiovascular damage (e.g., endothelial dysfunction, coagulation issues, orthostatic intolerance), gastrointestinal dysfunction (e.g., secondary to gut microbiome dysbiosis), metabolic issues (energy insufficiency, reactive oxygen species production, mitochrondrial dysfunction), and genetic variations.

Currently, there are no specific laboratory-based diagnostic tests for Long COVID or ME/CFS, and diagnosis involves consideration of other potential causes of the symptoms. In general, Long COVID (especially that which does not meet criteria for ME/CFS) has a better prognosis than ME/CFS. Some manifestations of Long COVID are similar to those of ME/CFS, and like ME/CFS, Long COVID appears to be a chronic illness, with few patients achieving full remission. Studies comparing Long COVID and ME/CFS have several limitations, however. Because Long COVID is a new disease, study participants are usually newly diagnosed, while ME/CFS study participants often have had the condition for longer and so are less likely to improve. Moreover, the definition of ME/CFS requires that symptoms be ongoing for 6 months or more, whereas the duration criteria for Long COVID vary in the literature from 2 to 6 months, making the two conditions difficult to compare.

Based on its review of the literature, the committee reached the following conclusion:

9. *Complex, infection-associated chronic conditions affecting multiple body systems are not new, and Long COVID shares many features with such conditions as myalgic encephalomyelitis/chronic fatigue syndrome, fibromyalgia, and postural orthostatic tachycardia syndrome. Current theories about the pathophysiology of these conditions include immune dysregulation, neurological disturbances, cardiovascular damage, gastrointestinal dysfunction, metabolic issues, and mitochondrial dysfunction. More research is needed to understand the natural history and management of complex multisystem chronic conditions, including Long COVID.*

1

Introduction

The Social Security Administration (SSA) provides disability benefits to people living with disabilities through two programs: Social Security Disability Insurance (SSDI) and Supplemental Security Income (SSI). Established in 1956, the SSDI program provides benefits to eligible adults with disabilities who have paid into the Disability Insurance Trust Fund, as well as to their spouses and adult children who are unable to work because of severe long-term disabilities. Enacted in 1972, SSI is a means-tested program based on income and financial assets that provides income assistance from U.S. Treasury general funds to adults aged 65 and older, individuals who are blind, and adults and children with disabilities. As of December 2023, 8.5 million individuals in the United States received benefits through SSDI, and 7.4 million individuals received benefits through SSI (SSA, 2023b).

Since the onset of the coronavirus disease 2019 (COVID-19) pandemic in early 2020, many individuals infected with the virus that causes COVID-19, severe acute respiratory syndrome coronavirus 2 (SARS-CoV-2), have continued to experience lingering symptoms for months or even years after acute infection. Data from the U.S. Centers for Disease Control and Prevention's (CDC's) National Health Interview Survey show that in 2022, 6.9 percent of U.S. adults and 1.3 percent of children had Long COVID at some point, while 3.4 percent of adults and 0.5 percent of children had Long COVID at the time of the interview (Adjaye-Gbewonyo et al., 2023; Vahratian et al., 2023). Based on these surveys, it is estimated that approximately 8.9 million adults and 362,000 children reported Long COVID symptoms in the United States in 2022 (Adjaye-Gbewonyo et al., 2023; Vahratian et al., 2023). Among U.S. adults, data from the CDC's Household Pulse Survey show that the prevalence of Long COVID declined from 7.5 percent in June 2022 to 5.9 percent in January 2023, then increased to 6.8 percent in January 2024 (NCHS, 2024), reflecting a complex event that has changed over time and continues to evolve.

The epidemiology of Long COVID is affected by many drivers, including different variants of the virus, vaccination status, and potentially treatments for acute COVID-19 (e.g., steroids, antivirals). Evidence suggests that individuals infected with the Omicron variant are less likely to develop Long COVID than those infected with earlier variants (Antonelli et al., 2022; Fernandez-de-Las-Penas et al., 2022; Hedberg and Nauclér, 2024), and that vaccination lowers the risk of developing Long COVID (Catala et al., 2024; Lundberg-Morris et al., 2023; Marra et al., 2023; Notarte et al., 2022; Watanabe et al., 2023). Although an area of research interest, evidence is less clear about the effect of treatments for SARS-CoV-2 infection on the risk of developing Long COVID. While some studies have found a reduction in the risk of Long COVID following treatment with antivirals (Bajema et al., 2023; Fung et al., 2023; Xie et al., 2023), others have not (Congdon et al., 2023; Durstenfeld et al., 2024). There is limited evidence that the use of steroids in the treatment of acute COVID-19 illness appears to reduce the risk of Long COVID (Davelaar et al., 2023).

Despite the overall decline in prevalence since June 2022, the most recently reported figure of 6.8 percent of all U.S. adults represents a large disease burden. Additionally, symptoms of Long COVID such as autonomic dysfunction, brain fog, and post-exertional malaise can impair an individual's ability to work or attend school for an extended period of time. Even individuals with a mild initial course of illness can develop Long COVID with severe health effects. In January of 2024, approximately 22 percent of adults with Long COVID reported significant activity limitations (NCHS, 2024). It is interesting to note that, although rates of self-reported disability in the U.S. population have increased since the onset of the pandemic, applications for SSA disability benefits have remained flat (SSA, n.d.b).

CONTEXT FOR THIS STUDY

The population of individuals with Long COVID is of special interest to SSA as their condition may cause them to meet or contribute to their meeting SSA's criteria for disability. For many individuals with Long COVID, symptoms resolve within 6 months; for some, however, symptoms persist for 12 months or more. Diagnosis, measurement, and treatment of Long COVID are complicated by the relative novelty of the condition, as well as its heterogeneous presentation and symptomology and the episodic nature of many of the associated health effects.

SSA has continuously been monitoring disability cases involving Long COVID symptoms. Symptoms reported include, but are not limited to, difficulty breathing, shortness of breath, persistent cough, fatigue, post-exertional malaise, difficulty thinking or concentrating, headache, and joint or muscle pain. SSA has issued guidance for disability adjudicators in evaluating cases of reported Long COVID symptoms and is in the process of expanding that guidance (SSA, 2022; 2023c). The agency therefore seeks the most current information available on the long-term health and functional effects of COVID-19 as related to SSA's disability programs.

STUDY CHARGE AND SCOPE

In August 2022, SSA requested that the National Academies of Sciences, Engineering, and Medicine (NASEM) convene an ad hoc consensus study committee to investigate the state of medical knowledge surrounding persistent functional limitations related to a past SARS-CoV-2 infection. The committee included experts in in cardiology; epidemiology; family, internal, and pediatric medicine; health metrics; health policy; immunology; infectious disease; neuropsychology; occupational medicine; occupational therapy; pediatric neurology; and rehabilitation medicine. The committee's statement of task (SOT) is presented in Box 1-1.

BOX 1-1
Statement of Task

An ad hoc committee of the National Academies of Sciences, Engineering, and Medicine will review the evidence regarding long-term disability that may result from COVID-19 illness and produce a report addressing the current status of the diagnosis, treatment, and prognosis of related disabilities based on published evidence (to the extent possible) and professional judgement (where evidence is lacking). In regards to the long-term health effects stemming from COVID-19 infection, the committee's report will:

1. Identify the committee's preferred terminology (e.g. Long COVID, PASC, PACS, Post-COVID Syndrome, Long Hauler's Syndrome);
2. Describe commonly reported and observed long-term health effects and describe what is known about:
   a. The frequency and distribution of their severity and duration in the general population, as well as any differences along racial, ethnic, sex, gender, geographic, or socioeconomic dimensions, or differences specific to populations with particular pre-existing or comorbid conditions;
   b. Clinical standards for diagnosis and measurement of the specific health effects or identified patterns or clusters of health effects;
   c. Any special considerations regarding the health effects' identification and management in special populations, including pregnant people and those with underlying health conditions;

continued

BOX 1-1 Continued

    d. Best practices to quantify the functional impacts of those health effects; and

    e. Identified challenges for clinicians in evaluating persons with those health effects;

3. Identify and describe the tests, findings, and signs currently clinically accepted to establish a history of COVID-19 in the following three categories:

    a. Tests for SARS-CoV-2;

    b. Findings from antibody tests or other diagnostic tests; and

    c. Signs consistent with COVID-19;

4. Identify any methods generally accepted by the medical community to establish a history of COVID-19 in patients that are not covered by the following three categories:

    a. A report of a positive viral test for SARS-CoV-2,

    b. A diagnostic test with findings consistent with COVID-19 (e.g., chest x-ray with lung abnormalities, etc.), or

    c. A diagnosis of COVID-19 based on signs consistent with COVID-19 (e.g., fever, cough, etc.);

5. Identify patterns of long-term, work-related functional decline observed in adults and the frequency, severity, duration, risk factors, and associated signs or laboratory findings;

6. Identify distinct patterns of long-term functional decline observed in children and the frequency, severity, duration, risk factors, and associated signs or laboratory findings;

7. Identify any trends in the frequency, severity, and duration of functional decline, including those specific to different racial, ethnic, sex, gender, geographic, or socioeconomic groups and those specific to populations with particular pre-existing or co-morbid conditions;

8. Describe any variations in functional or long-term effects based on initial infection with the various identified strains of the virus or based on vaccination status, both at the time of initial infection and illness or that are long-lasting; and

9. Summarize completed, on-going, or planned research, and any resultant medical knowledge, regarding similarities between this condition and impairments such as fibromyalgia or myalgic encephalomyelitis (chronic fatigue syndrome), including mechanisms of action, effective testing regimes, prognosis and progression, and potential treatments.

10. Summarize the committee's conclusions regarding best practices for assessing disability in these populations.

The report will include findings and conclusions but not recommendations.

STUDY APPROACH

The committee's statement of task included many individual questions regarding Long COVID. The committee chose to aggregate those questions into three major groupings to facilitate its review of the relevant literature: (1) methods for establishing a history of COVID-19, (2) commonly reported and disabling health effects of COVID-19 in adults and children, and (3) functional trajectories related to those health effects. The committee limited its literature search to articles published in English, but examined many studies conducted outside the United States that otherwise met its inclusion criteria. Initial searches were conducted on PubMed, Embase, and Scopus, yielding more than 1,300 articles selected from the tens of thousands published since the pandemic began in early 2020 (Appendix B). This large volume of source material precluded conducting formal systematic reviews that would meet standards published by the Institute of Medicine in 2011 (IOM, 2011), and the committee did not find systematic reviews on these three topics published by other investigators. Instead, the committee developed criteria for determining relevance to the statement of task by focusing on larger populations followed for at least 6 months and including significant symptoms and functional outcomes. In general, studies with very small numbers of subjects, short durations, and particular study designs (e.g., case control studies) were excluded, but occasionally referenced during the committee's discussions. Recognizing that literature on Long COVID is rapidly evolving, members of the committee used their expertise throughout the study to identify other studies in progress and perspectives not yet represented in publications. It is important to recognize that results from studies conducted at the height of the pandemic will need to be interpreted in light of new information, new SARS-CoV-2 variants, and other shifts in the epidemiology of COVID-19.

The committee discussed at length which health effects to include in this report, balancing usefulness to SSA with inclusiveness that might inform a larger audience. It decided to focus on health effects that appear to impact function most significantly and that result in visits to Long COVID clinics, finding that many of these health effects are not well understood and are challenging to treat. The committee also reviewed other issues known to be relevant to Long COVID, such as in hospital and intensive care unit (ICU) settings, rehabilitation strategies, selected populations, and pediatrics. Ultimately, the literature selection was made by consensus judgment of the committee members based on population, study design, measurement, and clinical and functional outcomes relevant to the statement of task.

In addition to examining the published literature, the committee commissioned a paper on chronic conditions similar to Long COVID, such as myalgic encephalomyelitis/chronic fatigue syndrome (ME/CFS), fibromyalgia, and hypermobile Ehlers-Danlos syndrome. The committee supplemented the paper's findings with systematic reviews on the same topics.

The committee met seven times; three of these meetings included public sessions with invited speakers. Topics at the public workshops included

- the natural history of Long COVID and potential mechanisms of action;
- current practices in defining and diagnosing Long COVID;
- research advances under way in COVID-19 diagnosis;
- similarities between Long COVID and ME/CFS;
- experiences of Long COVID patients and their caregivers; and
- experiences of clinicians who treat Long COVID.

Finally and importantly, the committee's work was informed by presentations from individuals with lived experience of Long COVID, made at a concurrent NASEM workshop titled *Symposium on Long COVID: Examining the Working Definition,* hosted by the Committee on Examining the Working Definition for Long COVID (NASEM, 2023b);[1] by follow-up presentations from two individuals with lived experience who originally spoke at a 2022 SSA-sponsored workshop titled *Long COVID: Examining Long-Term Health Effects of COVID-19 and Implications for the Social Security Administration* (NASEM, 2022a); and by two committee members with lived experience. The committee also used materials from previous NASEM reports: *Long COVID: Examining Long-Term Health Effects of COVID-19 and Implications for the Social Security Administration* (NASEM, 2022a); *Selected Heritable Disorders of Connective Tissue and Disability* (NASEM, 2022b); *Functional Assessment for Adults with Disability* (NASEM, 2019); and *Beyond Myalgic Encephalomyelitis/Chronic Fatigue Syndrome* (IOM, 2015), in addition to a workshop examining overlap in Long COVID and other chronic conditions. Finally, the committee reviewed the proceedings of a workshop titled *Toward a Common Research Agenda in Infection-Associated Chronic Illnesses: A Workshop to Examine Common, Overlapping Clinical and Biological Factors* (NASEM, 2024).

TERMINOLOGY AND DEFINITIONS

Long COVID

In May 2020, shortly after the beginning of the COVID-19 global pandemic, several accounts by patients in online forums (Twitter, Reddit,

---

[1] A recording of the workshop can be viewed at this link: https://www.nationalacademies.org/event/06-22-2023/examining-the-working-definition-for-long-covid-workshop (accessed January 17, 2024).

and others) and mainstream media (OpEd pieces) started to emerge, reporting that many previously healthy individuals had not fully recovered from COVID-19 and were experiencing lingering health problems. These patients leveraged social media platforms to share their experiences with these lingering health effects. They started to refer to themselves as "long haulers" and coined the term "Long COVID" (Callard and Perego, 2021).

The first known use of the term "Long COVID" dates back to a tweet by Eliza Perego (an Italian archeologist) and a previously healthy individual who had COVID-19 in early 2020 but continued to have lingering health effects. Semantically, the term is meant to describe the multitude of persistent health problems experienced after acute SARS-CoV-2 infection. The term has since gained momentum, evolving to become an umbrella term encompassing all the (initially reported and subsequently discovered) long-term health effects of SARS-CoV-2 infection. It is the most commonly used term by patients, health care providers, public health officials, governments, and the public at large.

In this report, the committee opted to use the term "Long COVID" not only because it is the first, most inclusive, and most widely used term denoting the long-term health effects of SARS-CoV-2 infection, but also because it recognizes the voices of patients who first alerted the world and the medical and scientific communities that SARS-CoV-2 infection can lead to long-term health consequences. Other terms used to describe the long-term health effects of SARS-CoV-2 include post-acute sequelae of SARS-CoV-2 or post-acute sequelae of COVID-19, Post-COVID Syndrome, Post-acute COVID Syndrome, Post-COVID Condition, Post-COVID Conditions (condition is pluralized), Long Haulers Syndrome, and many others. Annex Table 1-1 at the end of this chapter lists the most common terms and their definitions. The *International Classification of Diseases and Related Health Problems, 11th Revision* (ICD-11) code for Long COVID is "Post COVID-19 condition" (WHO, 2023). Given the evolving terminology, many of the other terms found in Annex Table 1-1 may also appear in the medical record.

The definition of Long COVID continues to evolve as well; numerous definitions are used in the literature, along with varying lengths of time after infection. A separate National Academies committee concurrently examined the working definition of Long COVID (EnSpark Consulting, 2023; NASEM, 2023a). The current federal working definition is as follows:

> Long COVID is broadly defined as signs, symptoms, and conditions that continue or develop after initial COVID-19 or SARS-CoV-2 infection. The signs, symptoms, and conditions are present four weeks or more after the initial phase of infection; may be multisystemic; and may present with a relapsing-remitting pattern and progression or worsening over time,

with the possibility of severe and life-threatening events even months or years after infection. Long COVID is not one condition. It represents many potentially overlapping entities, likely with different biological causes and different sets of risk factors and outcomes. (HHS, 2022)

A challenge in defining Long COVID is that that the definition needs to be broad enough to be inclusive but specific enough to be useful.

Disability

Recent reports of the National Academies have provided detailed background on the evolution of concepts of disability over the past several decades (NASEM, 2019, 2020, 2021). One relevant conclusion from those reports is the growing recognition that the effects of a given medical condition on functioning, activities, and participation are mediated by an individual's physical and social environments, as well as a variety of personal factors. This recognition has been embodied in the framework for disability developed by the World Health Organization (WHO) in the *International Classification of Functioning, Disability and Health* (ICF) and illustrated in Figure 1-1.

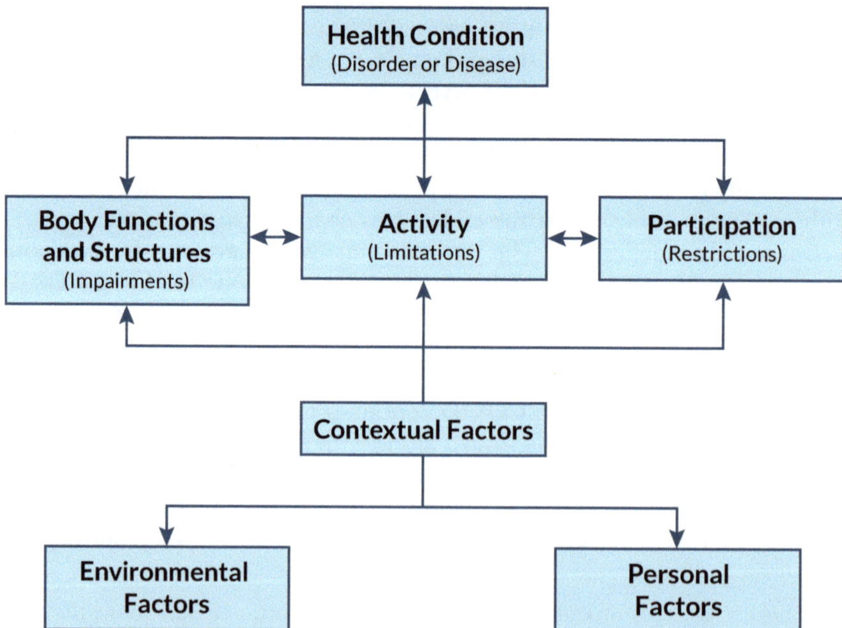

FIGURE 1-1 *International Classification of Functioning, Disability and Health* framework
SOURCE: WHO, 2001, p. 18.

This framework shows the interactions among health conditions, body functions and structures (i.e., physiological functions of the body, including psychological functions, and functioning of body structures), activity (i.e., actions or tasks), and participation (i.e., performance of tasks in a social context, such as school or work), all of which are elements of the conceptualization of disability, and all of which are mediated by contextual factors, including environmental and personal factors (WHO, 2001). Note that the arrows in the diagram are bidrectional since the relationships can involve feedback.

Different agencies and organizations have defined disability in various ways. However, most definitions include the concept of a physical or mental impairment combined with the inability to fulfill social roles or expectations. SSA's definition of disability for adults incorporates a length of time and whether a person can perform work. Specifically, to receive disability benefits (SSDI or SSI) from SSA, an individual must meet the statutory definition of disability, which, for adults, is the "inability to engage in any substantial gainful activity by reason of any medically determinable physical or mental impairment which can be expected to result in death or which has lasted or can be expected to last for a continuous period of not less than 12 months."[2] Substantial gainful activity is defined via an earnings threshold. In short, for an adult to be deemed disabled, a medical condition must lead to limitations that themselves affect the ability to engage in substantial gainful activity in the labor market. A child under age 18 is considered disabled if he or she "has a medically determinable physical or mental impairment, which results in marked and severe functional limitations, and which can be expected to result in death or which has lasted or can be expected to last for a continuous period of not less than 12 months."[3] A finding of disability in both adults and children depends on the severity of functional limitations arising from the claimant's impairment or combination of impairments.

When SSA evaluates a disability claim based on a physical or mental impairment, it requires sufficient evidence to (1) establish the presence of a medically determinable physical or mental impairment or impairments, (2) assess the degree of functional limitation imposed by the impairment(s), and (3) establish the expected duration of the impairment(s). Once SSA has established the presence of a severe medically determinable physical or mental impairment(s), it determines whether the impairment(s) meets or medically equals (is equivalent in severity to) the criteria in the

---

[2]C.F.R. § 404.1505.
[3]42 USC § 1382(c).

Listing of Impairments (Listings).[4] The Listings are applied in step 3 of the sequential evaluation processes for adults and children. For adults, the Listings describe, for each of the major body systems, impairments SSA considers to be severe enough to prevent a person from engaging in *any gainful activity*, regardless of his or her age, education, or work experience, and serve as a "screen-in" step. When an impairment is severe but does not meet or medically equal any of the Listings, SSA assesses in step 4 whether the applicant's physical or mental residual functional capacity allows her or him to perform past relevant work. Applicants who are able to perform past relevant work are denied benefits, while those who are unable to do so proceed to step 5. At step 5, SSA considers, in combination with the applicant's residual functional capacity, such vocational factors as age, education, and work experience, including transferable skills, in determining whether the individual can perform other work in the national economy. Applicants determined to be unable to adjust to performing other work are allowed benefits, while those determined able to adjust are denied.

For children, SSA determines at step 3 whether the impairment(s) meets, medically equals (is equivalent in severity to), or functionally equals (i.e., the impairment[s] results in functional limitations equivalent in severity to) the criteria in SSA's Childhood Listings (SSA, n.d.a).[5] If a child's impairment or combination of impairments "does not meet or medically equal any listing, [SSA] will decide whether it results in limitations that functionally equal the listings."[6] Functional equivalence refers to functionally equaling the Listings: SSA's technique for determining functional equivalence is a "whole child" approach that "accounts for all of the effects of a child's impairments singly and in combination—the interactive and cumulative effects of the impairments—because it starts with a consideration of actual functioning in all settings" (SSA, 2009).

Figures 1-2 and 1-3 depict SSA's adjudication process for adults and children, respectively, in greater detail.

Currently, there is no Listing for Long COVID, nor are there Listings for similar chronic conditions, such as ME/CFS and fibromyalgia. However, disability can be established for these conditions with documentation of a medically determinable impairment of sufficient duration and severity of functional limitation. SSA provides formal guidance

---

[4]The Adult Listings are available at http://www.ssa.gov/disability/professionals/bluebook/ AdultListings.htm. The Childhood Listings are available at http://www.ssa.gov/disability/ professionals/bluebook/ChildhoodListings.htm. Also see 20 Code of Federal Regulations (CFR) 404.1525, 404.1526, 416.925, and 416.926.

[5]20 CFR 416.926; 20 CFR 416.926a.

[6]20 CFR 416.926a.

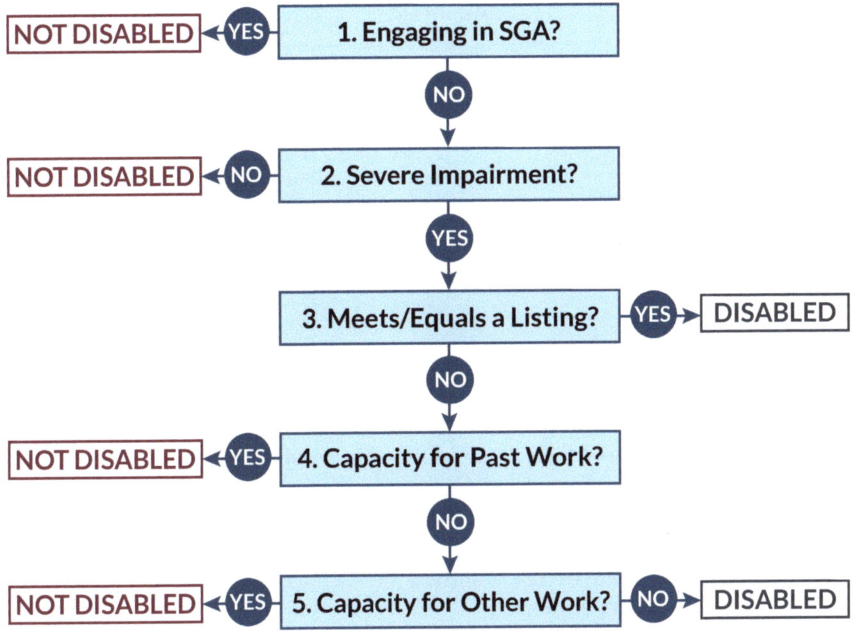

FIGURE 1-2 Social Security Administration's adjudication process for adults.
SOURCES: NASEM, 2020, p. 18, based on 20 CFR § 404.1520 and 416.920.

for evaluating these conditions.[7] In the guidance for providing medical evidence for claims involving Long COVID, SSA notes that the claimant should provide medical records that include "a thorough description of the individual's medical history, with information on the diagnosis, onset, duration, and prognosis of the individual's COVID-19; Long COVID; conditions that might be associated with, exacerbated by, or consistent with Long COVID; and any other conditions," as well as treatments prescribed and the response to those treatments. SSA explicitly states that "a positive viral test result for SARS-CoV-2 is not necessary for a diagnosis of COVID-19 or Long COVID." It considers all findings related to the claimant's condition, including those that relate to another disorder or establish that the claimant has a co-occurring condition. In addition,

---

[7]See *Long COVID: A Guide for Health Professionals on Providing Medical Evidence for Social Security Disability Claims (SSA, 2023a), Providing Medical Evidence for Individuals with Myalgic Encephalomyelitis/Chronic Fatigue Syndrome (ME/CFS) (SSA, 2018), and SSR 12-2p: Titles II and XVI: Evaluation of Fibromyalgia (SSA, 2012).*

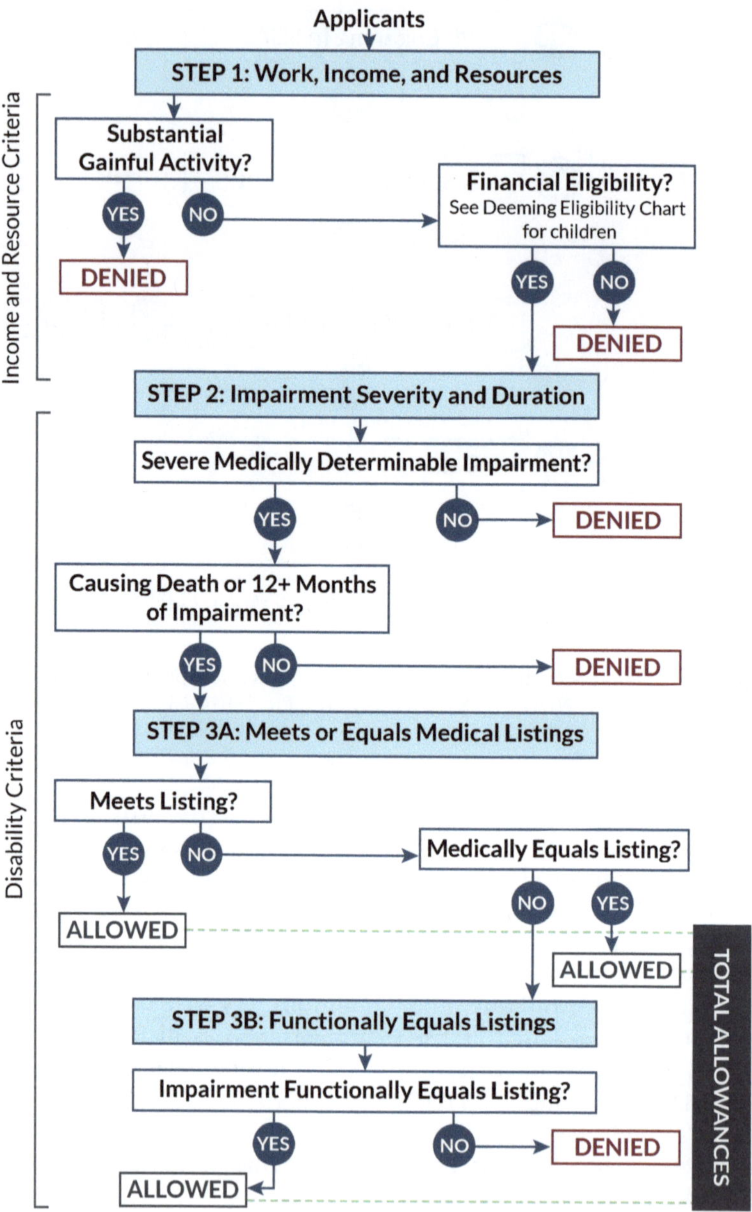

FIGURE 1-3 Social Security Administration's adjudication process for children. NOTE: Substantial Gainful Activity (SGA) is a term "used to describe a level of work activity and earnings. Work is 'substantial' if it involves doing significant physical or mental activities or a combination of both." More information on SGA can be found at https://www.ssa.gov/oact/cola/sga.html (accessed April 15, 2024). SOURCE: Wixon and Strand, 2013.

it asks for a report of signs and symptoms consistent with Long COVID, including, but not limited to,

- persistent or relapsing fatigue resulting in reduction or impairment of the ability to carry out daily or work-related activities;
- post-exertional malaise (worsening of symptoms after physical, cognitive, or emotional effort);
- exercise intolerance;
- respiratory difficulties, such as labored breathing or sudden breathlessness;
- muscle or joint pain or tenderness;
- weakness;
- chest tightness, pain, or tenderness;
- cognitive impairment(s) such as difficulty with information processing, memory, or concentration and attention;
- headaches of a new type, pattern, or severity;
- changes in taste or smell;
- gastrointestinal disturbances or discomfort, diarrhea, or constipation;
- dizziness when standing up;
- paresthesia (numbness, tingling, or pins-and-needles sensation); and/or
- sleep problems (SSA, 2023a).

Finally, SSA considers descriptions of functional limitations, including the following:

- physical functions—the ability to walk, stand, sit, lift, push, pull, reach, carry, and handle; and/or
- mental functions—the ability to understand, remember, and carry out simple instructions; the ability to use appropriate judgment; and the ability to respond appropriately to supervision, coworkers, and usual work situations, including changes in a routine work setting (SSA, 2023a).

The committee notes that while this preliminary guidance may be helpful in determining whether a disability is related to Long COVID, it does not provide sufficient guidance for assessing functional status or weighing severity.

HEALTH EQUITY

The burden of seeking care and finding adequate services for Long COVID is challenging and can impact the potential for recovery. Although Long COVID may manifest as impairments in body structures and physical and psychological functioning, it is not psychological in origin. Nevertheless, patients with Long COVID may encounter skepticism about their symptoms when they present in medical settings, which discourages care seeking. This is particularly true for individuals disadvantaged by their social or economic status, geographic location, or environment, and can result in preventable disparities in the burden of disease and opportunities to achieve optimal health (CDC, 2017). Disadvantaged groups include women, members of some racial and ethnic minorities, people with disabilities, LGBTQI+ (lesbian, gay, bisexual, transgender, queer, intersex, or other) individuals, people with limited English proficiency, and others. For example, one study found that Black and Hispanic Americans appear to experience more symptoms and health problems related to Long COVID compared with White people but are less likely to be diagnosed with the condition (Khullar et al., 2023).

Individuals with Long COVID have increased health care utilization and financial burden, which may be exacerbated if they are unable to work to gain income. Members of disadvantaged groups, especially early in the pandemic, were more likely to contract SARS-CoV-2, more likely to be hospitalized with acute COVID-19, more likely to have adverse clinical outcomes, and less likely to be vaccinated, potentially increasing their risk of developing Long COVID. In addition, these groups are more likely to be uninsured or underinsured (Berger et al., 2021). Even for those with insurance coverage, some of the services that have been shown to improve function may not be covered by their benefits. Moreover, the availability of specialized Long COVID services is limited, and capacity does not match the demand for rehabilitation specialists (Berger et al., 2021). Limited transportation, distance from clinics, and the inability to take time away from work or school are known barriers to care (Berger et al., 2021). The availability issue is particularly problematic for individuals living in medically underserved areas.

In addition, as a complex, chronic condition, Long COVID requires a multidisciplinary approach. Individuals disadvantaged by their social or economic status, geographic location, or environment may find navigating the health care system especially challenging without adequate social and financial resources. Inadequate access to interpreter services may also limit the ability of some with Long COVID to benefit fully from care.

Information about COVID-19 is rapidly evolving, and this dynamic nature of the science may contribute to some patient hesitancy regarding prophylactic and therapeutic management for acute infection or Long COVID. Low levels of health literacy may also place some individuals at increased risk for misinformation, which may prevent them from fully taking advantage of health care resources to protect and improve their health. Low health literacy may also impact individual self-management of the symptoms and conditions associated with Long COVID.

REPORT ORGANIZATION

Chapter 2 describes established methods of diagnosing acute COVID-19, as well as methods that may become available in the near future, and touches on how to determine whether a person has Long COVID in the absence of immunological confirmation (PCR/antibody test). Chapter 3 reviews common and disabling long-term health effects associated with COVID-19 and how their functional impacts can be assessed. Chapter 4 reviews the literature on the functional trajectories of those long-term health effects, and includes discussion of differences among hospitalized, nonhospitalized, post-ICU, and pediatric patients. It also comments on how rehabilitation affects functional outcomes. Chapter 5 summarizes research on the similarities between Long COVID and other chronic conditions, such as ME/CFS and fibromyalgia. Chapter 6 provides the committee's overall conclusions based on the evidence presented throughout the report.

REFERENCES

AAPMR (American Academy of Physical Medicine and Rehabilitation). 2023. *PASC consensus guidance*. Rosemont, IL. https://www.aapmr.org/members-publications/covid-19/pasc-guidance (accessed October 13, 2023).

Adjaye-Gbewonyo, D., A. Vahratian, C. G. Perrine, and J. Bertolli. 2023. Long COVID in adults: United States, 2022. *NCHS Data Brief* (480):1–8.

Antonelli, M., J. C. Pujol, T. D. Spector, S. Ourselin, and C. J. Steves. 2022. Risk of Long COVID associated with Delta versus Omicron variants of SARS-CoV-2. *The Lancet* 399(10343):2263–2264.

ATS (American Thoracic Society). 2022. *Long COVID patient fact sheet*. New York: ATS. https://www.thoracic.org/patients/patient-resources/resources/long-covid.pdf (accessed October 13, 2023).

Bajema, K. L., K. Berry, E. Streja, N. Rajeevan, Y. Li, P. Mutalik, L. Yan, F. Cunningham, D. M. Hynes, M. Rowneki, A. Bohnert, E. J. Boyko, T. J. Iwashyna, M. L. Maciejewski, T. F. Osborne, E. M. Viglianti, M. Aslan, G. D. Huang, and G. N. Ioannou. 2023. Effectiveness of COVID-19 treatment with nirmatrelvir-ritonavir or molnupiravir among U.S. veterans: Target trial emulation studies with one-month and six-month outcomes. *Annuals of Internal Medicine* 176(6):807–816.

Behnood, S. A., R. Shafran, S. D. Bennett, A. X. D. Zhang, L. L. O'Mahoney, T. J. Stephenson, S. N. Ladhani, B. L. De Stavola, R. M. Viner, and O. V. Swann. 2022. Persistent symptoms following SARS-CoV-2 infection amongst children and young people: A meta-analysis of controlled and uncontrolled studies. *Journal of Infection* 84(2):158–170.

Berger, Z., D. E. J. V. Altiery, S. A. Assoumou, and T. Greenhalgh. 2021. Long COVID and health inequities: The role of primary care. *Milbank Quarterly* 99(2):519–541.

Callard, F., and E. Perego. 2021. How and why patients made Long COVID. *Social Science & Medicine* 268:113426.

Catala, M., N. Mercade-Besora, R. Kolde, N. T. H. Trinh, E. Roel, E. Burn, T. Rathod-Mistry, K. Kostka, W. Y. Man, A. Delmestri, H. M. E. Nordeng, A. Uuskula, T. Duarte-Salles, D. Prieto-Alhambra, and A. M. Jodicke. 2024. The effectiveness of COVID-19 vaccines to prevent Long COVID symptoms: Staggered cohort study of data from the UK, Spain, and Estonia. *The Lancet Respiratory Medicine* 12(3):225–236

CDC (U.S. Centers for Disease Control and Prevention). 2017. *Health disparities.* https://www.cdc.gov/aging/disparities/index.htm (accessed January 11, 2024).

CDC. 2023. *Long COVID or post-COVID conditions.* https://www.cdc.gov/coronavirus/2019-ncov/long-term-effects/ (accessed October 23, 2023).

Congdon, S., Z. Narrowe, N. Yone, J. Gunn, Y. Deng, P. Nori, K. Cowman, M. Islam, S. Rikin, and J. Starrels. 2023. Nirmatrelvir/ritonavir and risk of Long COVID symptoms: A retrospective cohort study. *Scientific Reports* 13(1):19688.

Davelaar, J., N. Jessurun, G. Schaap, C. Bode, and H. Vonkeman. 2023. The effect of corticosteroids, antibiotics, and anticoagulants on the development of post-COVID-19 syndrome in COVID-19 hospitalized patients 6 months after discharge: A retrospective follow up study. *Clinical and Experimental Medicine* 23(8):4881–4888.

Durstenfeld, M. S., M. J. Peluso, F. Lin, N. D. Peyser, C. Isasi, T. W. Carton, T. J. Henrich, S. G. Deeks, J. E. Olgin, M. J. Pletcher, A. L. Beatty, G. M. Marcus, and P. Y. Hsue. 2024. Association of nirmatrelvir for acute SARS-CoV-2 infection with subsequent Long COVID symptoms in an observational cohort study. *Journal of Medical Virology* 96(1):e29333.

EnSpark Consulting. 2023. *What we heard: Engagement report on the Working Definition for Long COVID.* Washington, DC.

FDA (U.S. Food and Drug Administration). 2021. *FDA CERSI lecture on Long COVID: Risk factors, symptomology and patient reported outcomes captured through a novel digital platform by Dr. Erica Spatz & Dr. Kelli O'Laughlin.* https://www.fda.gov/science-research/advancing-regulatory-science/fda-cersi-lecture-long-covid-risk-factors-symptomology-and-patient-reported-outcomes-captured (accessed October 13, 2023).

Fernandez-de-Las-Penas, C., K. I. Notarte, P. J. Peligro, J. V. Velasco, M. J. Ocampo, B. M. Henry, L. Arendt-Nielsen, J. Torres-Macho, and G. Plaza-Manzano. 2022. Long-COVID symptoms in individuals infected with different SARS-CoV-2 variants of concern: A systematic review of the literature. *Viruses* 14(12):2629.

Fung, K. W., F. Baye, S. H. Baik, and C. J. McDonald. 2023. Nirmatrelvir and molnupiravir and post-COVID-19 condition in older patients. *JAMA Internal Medicine* 183(12):1404–1406.

Gluckman, T. J., N. M. Bhave, L. A. Allen, E. H. Chung, E. S. Spatz, E. Ammirati, A. L. Baggish, B. Bozkurt, W. K. Cornwell, K. G. Harmon, J. H. Kim, A. Lala, B. D. Levine, M. W. Martinez, O. Onuma, D. Phelan, V. O. Puntmann, S. Rajpal, P. R. Taub, and A. K. Verma. 2022. 2022 ACC expert consensus decision pathway on cardiovascular sequelae of COVID-19 in adults: Myocarditis and other myocardial involvement, post-acute sequelae of SARS-CoV-2 infection, and return to play. *Journal of the American College of Cardiology* 79(17):1717–1756.

Hedberg, P., and P. Nauclér. 2024. Post–COVID-19 condition after SARS-CoV-2 infections during the Omicron surge vs the Delta, Alpha, and wild type periods in Stockholm, Sweden. *Journal of Infectious Diseases* 229(1):133–136.

HHS (U.S. Department of Health and Human Services). 2022. *National research action plan on Long COVID.* Washington, DC: Office of the Assistant Secretary for Health. https://www.covid.gov/assets/files/National-Research-Action-Plan-on-Long-COVID-08012022.pdf (accessed April 22, 2024).

Humana. n.d. *COVID-19: Long COVID resource guide.* Louisville, KY: Humana. https://docushare-web.apps.external.pioneer.humana.com/Marketing/docushare-app?file=4676399 (accessed October 13, 2023).

ICD10 Data. 2023. *ICD-10-CM codes.* https://www.icd10data.com/ICD10CM/Codes/U00-U85/U00-U49/U09-/U09.9 (accessed October 13, 2023).

IDSA (The Infectious Diseases Society of America). n.d. *COVID-19 real time learning network.* https://www.idsociety.org/covid-19-real-time-learning-network/ (accessed October 13, 2023).

IOM (Institute of Medicine). 2011. *Finding what works in healthcare.* Washington, DC: The National Academies Press.

IOM. 2015. *Beyond myalgic encephalomyelitis/chronic fatigue syndrome: Redefining an illness.* Washington, DC: The National Academies Press.

Khullar, D., Y. Zhang, C. Zang, Z. Xu, F. Wang, M. G. Weiner, T. W. Carton, R. L. Rothman, J. P. Block, and R. Kaushal. 2023. Racial/ethnic disparities in post-acute sequelae of SARS-CoV-2 infection in New York: An EHR-based cohort study from the RECOVER program. *Journal of General Internal Medicine* 38(5):1127–1136.

Lundberg-Morris, L., S. Leach, Y. Xu, J. Martikainen, A. Santosa, M. Gisslen, H. Li, F. Nyberg, and M. Bygdell. 2023. COVID-19 vaccine effectiveness against post-COVID-19 condition among 589 722 individuals in Sweden: Population based cohort study. *BMJ* 383:e076990.

Marra, A. R., T. Kobayashi, G. Y. Callado, I. Pardo, M. C. Gutfreund, M. K. Hsieh, V. Lin, M. Alsuhaibani, S. Hasegawa, J. Tholany, E. N. Perencevich, J. L. Salinas, M. B. Edmond, and L. V. Rizzo. 2023. The effectiveness of COVID-19 vaccine in the prevention of post-COVID conditions: A systematic literature review and meta-analysis of the latest research. *Antimicrobial Stewardship and Healthcare Epidemiology* 3(1):e168.

NASEM (National Academies of Sciences, Engineering, and Medicine). 2019. *Functional assessment for adults with disabilities.* Edited by P. A. Volberding, C. M. Spicer, and J. L. Flaubert. Washington, DC: The National Academies Press.

NASEM. 2020. *Selected health conditions and likelihood of improvement with treatment.* Washington, DC: The National Academies Press.

NASEM. 2021. *Childhood cancer and functional impacts across the care continuum.* Edited by P. A. Volberding, C. M. Spicer, T. Cartaxo and L. Aiuppa. Washington, DC: The National Academies Press.

NASEM. 2022a. *Long COVID: Examining long-term health effects of COVID-19 and implications for the Social Security Administration: Proceedings of a workshop.* Edited by L. A. Denning and E. H. Forstag. Washington, DC: The National Academies Press.

NASEM. 2022b. *Selected heritable disorders of connective tissue and disability.* Edited by P. A. Volberding, C. M. Spicer, T. Cartaxo, and R. A. Wedge. Washington, DC: The National Academies Press.

NASEM. 2023a. *Examining the working definition for Long COVID.* https://www.national academies.org/our-work/examining-the-working-definition-for-long-covid (accessed April 22, 2024).

NASEM. 2023b. *Symposium on Long COVID: Examining the working definition.* https://www.nationalacademies.org/event/06-22-2023/examining-the-working-definition-for-long-covid-workshop (accessed April 22, 2024).

NASEM. 2024. *Toward a common research agenda in infection-associated chronic illnesses: Proceedings of a workshop.* Washington, DC: The National Academies Press.

NCHS (National Center for Health Statistics). 2024. *Long COVID household pulse survey.* Atlanta, GA: U.S. Centers for Disease Control and Prevention. https://www.cdc.gov/nchs/covid19/pulse/long-covid.htm (accessed March 14, 2024).

NICE (National Institute for Health and Care Excellence). 2020. *COVID-19 rapid guideline: Managing the long-term effects of COVID-19.* London, UK: NICE.

Notarte, K. I., J. A. Catahay, J. V. Velasco, A. Pastrana, A. T. Ver, F. C. Pangilinan, P. J. Peligro, M. Casimiro, J. J. Guerrero, M. M. L. Gellaco, G. Lippi, B. M. Henry, and C. Fernandez-de-Las-Penas. 2022. Impact of COVID-19 vaccination on the risk of developing Long-COVID and on existing Long-COVID symptoms: A systematic review. *EClinicalMedicine* 53:101624.

RECOVER (Researching COVID to Enhance Recovery). 2023. *RECOVER: Researching COVID to enhance recovery.* Bethesda, MD: National Institutes of Health. https://recovercovid.org/ (accessed October 13, 2023).

Soriano, J. B., S. Murthy, J. C. Marshall, P. Relan, and J. V. Diaz. 2022. A clinical case definition of post-COVID-19 condition by a delphi consensus. *The Lancet Infectious Diseases* 22(4):e102–e107.

SSA (Social Security Administration). 2009. *SSR 09-1p: Title XVI: Determining childhood disability under the functional equivalence rule—The "whole child" approach*. https://www.ssa.gov/OP_Home/rulings/ssi/02/SSR2009-01-ssi-02.html#fn4 (accessed April 22, 2024).

SSA. 2012. *SSR 12-2p: Titles II and XVI: Evaluation of fibromyalgia*. https://www.ssa.gov/OP_Home/rulings/di/01/SSR2012-02-di-01.html (accessed April 22, 2024).

SSA. 2018. *Providing medical evidence for individuals with myalgic encephalomyelitis/chronic fatigue syndrome (ME/CFS)*. https://www.ssa.gov/disability/professionals/documents/64-063.pdf (accessed February 13, 2024).

SSA. 2022. *Evaluating cases with coronavirus disease 2019 (COVID-19)*. EM-21032 REV. https://secure.ssa.gov/apps10/reference.nsf/links/08092022072836AM (accessed February 13, 2024).

SSA. 2023a. *Long COVID: A guide for health professionals on providing medical evidence for Social Security disability claims*. https://www.ssa.gov/disability/professionals/documents/EN-64-128.pdf (accessed February 13, 2024).

SSA. 2023b. *Monthly statistical snapshot, July 2023*. https://www.ssa.gov/policy/docs/quickfacts/stat_snapshot/ (accessed August 31, 2023).

SSA. 2023c. Presentation to the Committee on the Long-Term Health Effects Stemming from COVID-19 and Implications for the Social Security Administration, January 26, 2023. Washington, DC.

SSA. n.d.a. *Disability evaluation under Social Security—Listing of impairments—Childhood listings (Part B)*. https://www.ssa.gov/disability/professionals/bluebook/ChildhoodListings.htm (accessed October 12, 2023).

SSA. n.d.b. *Selected data from Social Security's disability program*. https://www.ssa.gov/oact/STATS/dibStat.html (accessed January 31, 2024).

VA (U.S. Department of Veterans Affairs). n.d. *Long COVID*. https://www.veteranshealthlibrary.va.gov/142,41528_VA (accessed October 13, 2023).

Vahratian, A., D. Adjaye-Gbewonyo, J.-M. S. Lin, and S. Saydah. 2023. Long COVID in children: United States, 2022. *NCHS Data Brief* 479:1–6.

Watanabe, A., M. Iwagami, J. Yasuhara, H. Takagi, and T. Kuno. 2023. Protective effect of COVID-19 vaccination against Long COVID syndrome: A systematic review and meta-analysis. *Vaccine* 41(11):1783–1790.

WHO (World Health Organization). 2001. *International classification of functioning, disability and health*. Geneva, Switzerland: WHO.

WHO. 2023. *International statistical classification of diseases and related health problems, 11th revision*. Geneva, Switzerland: WHO.

Wikipedia. 2023. *Long COVID*. https://en.wikipedia.org/wiki/Long_COVID (accessed October 13, 2023).

Wixon, B., and A. Strand. 2013. Identifying SSA's sequential disability determination steps using administrative data. Research and Statistics Note No. 2013-01. Social Security Administration, Office of Retirement and Disability Policy. http://www.ssa.gov/policy/docs/rsnotes/rsn2013-01.html (accessed January 29, 2024).

Xie, Y., T. Choi, and Z. Al-Aly. 2023. Association of treatment with nirmatrelvir and the risk of post-COVID-19 condition. *JAMA Internal Medicine* 183(6):554–564.

ANNEX TABLE 1-1 Terminology and Definitions for "Long COVID"

Source	Term	Definition	Reference
Patients and people with lived experience; patient-researchers	**Long COVID**	Can be broadly defined as signs, symptoms, and sequelae that continue or develop after acute COVID-19 or SARS-CoV-2 infection for any period of time; are generally multisystemic; might present with a relapsing–remitting pattern and a progression or worsening over time, with the possibility of severe and life-threatening events even months or years after infection	(Callard and Perego, 2021)
Centers for Disease Control and Prevention (CDC)	**Post-COVID 19 conditions (plural)**	Umbrella term for the wide range of physical and mental health consequences experienced by some patients that are present four or more weeks after SARS-CoV-2 infection, including by patients who had initial mild or asymptomatic acute infection; equivalent to the lay term, "Long COVID"	(CDC, 2023)
Department of Veterans Affairs (VA)	**Post-COVID conditions**	Post-COVID conditions are symptoms that last or start weeks or months after a person was infected with the SARS-CoV-2 virus. This is the virus that causes COVID-19. This can happen even if you didn't know you had the virus. You may hear these conditions called long COVID, post-acute COVID, chronic COVID, or other terms. The symptoms can include tiredness, headaches, loss of taste and smell, trouble breathing, and dizziness.	(VA, n.d.)
National Institutes of Health (NIH)	**Post-acute sequelae of SARS CoV-2 infection**	Ongoing, relapsing, or new symptoms, or other health effects occurring after the acute phase of SARS-CoV-2 infection (i.e., present four or more weeks after the acute infection). The definition will be revised in an iterative manner based on existing and new data, medical literature, and feedback from the scientific community.	(RECOVER, 2023)

continued

ANNEX TABLE 1-1 Continued

Source	Term	Definition	Reference
Food and Drug Administration (FDA)	**Post-COVID conditions (plural)**	While most people with COVID-19 have resolution of their symptoms within weeks of their illness, some people experience post-COVID conditions. Post-COVID conditions are new, returning, or ongoing health problems people can experience four or more weeks after initial infection with the SARS-CoV-2 virus. These conditions have also been termed long COVID, long-haul COVID, postacute sequelae of COVID-19, long-term effects of COVID, or chronic COVID. Post-COVID conditions have been observed in people with mild to severe COVID-19 infection, and can present with localized and systemic symptoms impacting nearly all organ systems.	(FDA, 2021)
World Health Organization (WHO)	**Post-COVID-19 condition (singular)**	Post-COVID-19 condition occurs in individuals with a history of probable or confirmed SARS-CoV-2 infection, usually 3 months from the onset of COVID-19 with symptoms that last for at least 2 months and cannot be explained by an alternative diagnosis; common symptoms include fatigue, shortness of breath, and cognitive dysfunction, and generally have an impact on everyday functioning; symptoms might be new onset after initial recovery from an acute COVID-19 episode or persist from the initial illness; symptoms might also fluctuate or relapse over time; a separate definition might be applicable for children; recognize "Long COVID"	(Soriano et al., 2022)
Broader Research Community	**Persistent symptoms or COVID-19 consequences**	Persistent signs and symptoms that continue or develop after acute COVID-19 for any period of time	(Behnood et al., 2022)

ANNEX TABLE 1-1 Continued

Source	Term	Definition	Reference
American Academy of Physical Medicine and Rehabilitation	**Post-acute sequelae of SARS CoV-2 infection (equates it with Long COVID)**	Post-Acute Sequelae of SARS-CoV-2 infection (PASC) or Long COVID is a condition that occurs in individuals who have had COVID-19 and report at least one persistent symptom after acute illness. Long COVID encompasses a constellation of varied and ongoing symptoms – even in the same patient across time – and may include neurological challenges, cognitive symptoms such as brain fog, cardiovascular and respiratory issues, fatigue, pain and mobility issues, among others.	(AAPMR, 2023)
American College of Cardiology	**Post-acute sequelae of SARS-CoV-2 infection**	PASC encompasses a constellation of symptoms that emerge or persist weeks to months after recovery from COVID-19 [referencing CDC, WHO]. Although evidence guiding the care of these patients continues to evolve, there is a need to develop common taxonomies and approaches to care that can be updated iteratively as new data become available.	(Gluckman et al., 2022)
American Thoracic Society	**Long COVID**	The term that is often used to describe these persistent symptoms. You are considered to have 'Long COVID' when you are still having symptoms at least 4 weeks after the initial infection. Long COVID may also be referred to by other names such as post-COVID conditions, PASC (post-acute sequelae of SARS-CoV-2 infection) or long-haul COVID.	(ATS, 2022)
Humana Military	**Long COVID**	While most people with COVID-19 get better within weeks, some continue to have symptoms—or develop new ones—after their initial recovery. The technical term for this is post-acute sequelae of SARS-CoV-2 infection (PASC), or simply "long COVID." People with long COVID are often called "long haulers." A person of any age who has had COVID-19 can later develop a post-virus condition.	(Humana, n.d.)

continued

ANNEX TABLE 1-1 Continued

Source	Term	Definition	Reference
Infectious Disease Society of America	**Post-COVID19 conditions (plural)**	References other definitions, Long COVID, CDC, and WHO	(IDSA, n.d.)
Wikipedia	**Long COVID**	Long COVID is a condition characterized by long-term consequences persisting or appearing after the typical convalescence period of COVID-19. It is also known as post-COVID-19 syndrome, post-COVID-19 condition, post-acute sequelae of SARS-CoV-2 infection (PASC), or chronic COVID syndrome (CCS). Long COVID can affect nearly every organ system, with sequelae including respiratory system disorders, nervous system and neurocognitive disorders, mental health disorders, metabolic disorders, cardiovascular disorders, gastrointestinal disorders, musculoskeletal pain, and anemia. A wide range of symptoms are commonly reported, including fatigue, malaise, headaches, shortness of breath, anosmia (loss of smell), parosmia (distorted smell), muscle weakness, low fever, and cognitive dysfunction.	(Wikipedia, 2023)
International Classification of Diseases (ICD)-10-CM code	**U09.9 Post-COVID condition, unspecified**	No definition is given, but the following are noted: • This code enables establishment of a link with COVID-19. • This code is not to be used in cases that are still presenting with active COVID-19. However, an exception is made in cases of reinfection with COVID-19, occurring with a condition related to prior COVID-19. • Post-acute sequelae of COVID-19	(ICD 10 Data, 2023)
National Institute for Health and Care Excellence (NICE)*	**Ongoing symptomatic COVID-19**	Signs and symptoms of COVID-19 from 4 weeks up to 12 weeks	(NICE, 2020)

ANNEX TABLE 1-1 Continued

Source	Term	Definition	Reference
National Institute for Health and Care Excellence (NICE)**	**Post-COVID19 syndrome**	Signs and symptoms that develop during or after an infection consistent with COVID-19, continue for more than 12 weeks and are not explained by an alternative diagnosis; it usually presents with clusters of symptoms, often overlapping, which can fluctuate and change over time and can affect any system in the body; post-COVID-19 syndrome might be considered before 12 weeks while the possibility of an alternative underlying disease is also being assessed	(NICE, 2020)

NOTE: Adapted from the table titled, "Commonly used terminology in the research of COVID-19 sequelae" in Munblit, D., M. O'Hara, and A. Akrami, et al. 2022. Long COVID: Aiming for a consensus. *The Lancet Respiratory Medicine* S2213-2600(22):135-137. https://www.thelancet.com/action/showPdf?pii=S2213-2600%2822%2900135-7 (accessed June 21, 2022).

*United Kingdom National Institute for Health and Care Excellence (NICE)

**NICE also states that: "In addition to the clinical case definitions, the term 'long COVID' is commonly used to describe signs and symptoms that continue or develop after acute COVID-19. It includes both ongoing symptomatic COVID-19 (from 4 to 12 weeks) and post-COVID-19 syndrome (12 weeks or more)."

SOURCE: HHS, 2022, Appendix C.

2

Diagnosis of SARS-CoV-2 Infection

When Long COVID occurs, it follows an acute infection with SARS-CoV-2, the virus responsible for the COVID-19 pandemic. This chapter addresses the request in the committee's statement of task (Box 1-1 in Chapter 1) to identify and describe the tests, findings, and signs currently clinically accepted to establish a history of COVID-19, including tests for SARS-CoV-2, findings of other diagnostic tests, and signs consistent with COVID-19. It also addresses the request to identify any methods generally accepted by the medical community for establishing a history of COVID-19 in patients who are not covered by a report of a positive viral test for SARS-CoV-2, a diagnostic test with findings consistent with COVID-19 (e.g., chest x-ray with lung abnormalities), or a diagnosis of COVID-19 based on signs consistent with COVID-19 (e.g., fever, cough). In addressing these tasks, the chapter provides context surrounding the evolution of the diagnosis of COVID-19, beginning with the gold-standard approach of viral testing specifically for SARS-CoV-2. The chapter then reviews the diagnosis of COVID-19 based on signs, symptoms, and diagnostic surrogates prior to the advent of specific testing for SARS-CoV-2 infection.

Diagnosis of acute COVID-19 differs from that of Long COVID. Given the absence of a consensus-based definition and the ongoing evidence-based research on best practices for diagnosing Long COVID, this chapter focuses primarily on the early and current diagnostic measures of acute COVID-19.

VIRAL TESTING

Over the course of the pandemic, diagnostic tests specific to SARS-CoV-2 were developed and became more readily available, although disparities in socioeconomic status and geographical location still impacted access to such testing (Dalva-Baird et al., 2021; Rentsch et al., 2020; Romero et al., 2020). As of this writing, a viral test is necessary to confirm a diagnosis of SARS-CoV-2 infection. The primary method used today is direct measurement through molecular or antigen testing. Early in the pandemic, indirect measurement was possible through serological (antibody) studies, but today, viral culture is reserved mainly for research purposes.

Nucleic Acid Amplification (Molecular) Tests

Nucleic acid amplification tests (NAATs), sometimes called molecular tests, detect nucleic acids (genetic material) from the single-stranded RNA SARS-CoV-2 virus. These tests are now considered the gold-standard for diagnosis of COVID-19 in the clinical setting because of their high sensitivity and specificity (CDC, 2023d; Hayden et al., 2023; Hellou et al., 2021; Lieberman et al., 2020; NIH, 2023). NAATs can use various methods to amplify and detect virus genes, including reverse transcriptase polymerase chain reaction (PCR) and isothermal amplification (e.g., loop-mediated isothermal amplification [LAMP], clustered regularly interspaced short palindromic repeats [CRISPR]) technologies (CDC, 2023d). Commercial tests generally detect at least two genes' targets on the virus. Many molecular diagnostic tests for COVID-19 are authorized by the U.S. Food and Drug Administration (FDA); platforms used for the testing can differ around the world (FDA, 2023b). The turnaround time for results ranges from 15 minutes (rapid or some isothermal amplification platforms) to several hours (real-time reverse transcription-PCR [RT-PCR]) (Ganguli et al., 2020; Hayden et al., 2023).

It may take up to 5 days following exposure before NAATs can detect viral particles in an infected person (NIH, 2023). A positive test confirms the diagnosis of COVID-19; however, false positives, although rare, can occur (FDA, 2021). False negatives also have been documented, and repeat testing is indicated if clinically appropriate (CDC, 2023d; FDA, 2023a; Long et al., 2021). An inconclusive or indeterminate result indicates that only one of the two or more genes that the NAAT targets was identified. If the person is early in the disease course, repeat testing can help confirm the result (Hayden et al., 2023). The FDA monitors variants resulting from new mutations that may impact the performance of the NAAT (NIH, 2023). The pooled sensitivity of the SARS-CoV-2 NAAT has been estimated at 97 percent (95% CI 93 to 99); pooled specificity was 100 percent (CI 96 to 100) (Hayden et al., 2023). Viral RNA may be detectable for up to 90 days after initial infection irrespective of active infection; thus, NAATs should not be used to test someone for active infection who has already tested positive in the past 90 days (CDC, 2024b).

Antigen Tests

Antigen tests detect certain proteins (antigens) from the virus via immunoassay. In these tests, synthetic antibodies probe a person's respiratory sample for evidence of viral proteins, which confirms an active infection (Center for Health Security, 2023). Antigen tests typically provide rapid results (in as little as 15 minutes), allow the patient to test at home and other points of care, and are therefore more accessible and convenient than NAATs (FDA, 2023a; Hayden et al., 2023); they are also less expensive (CDC, 2024).

A positive antigen test indicates active COVID infection. Sensitivity is highest in symptomatic individuals within 5 to 7 days of symptom onset (NIH, 2023; Parvu et al., 2021). Although the sensitivity of antigen testing is higher in symptomatic than in asymptomatic individuals, it remains lower than that of NAATs (Hayden et al., 2023). Sensitivity is improved with repeated antigen testing (Hayden et al., 2023). A negative antigen test in persons with signs or symptoms of COVID-19 should be confirmed by NAAT (CDC, 2024). False positive antigen tests are rare (CDC, 2023a).

Both molecular and antigen tests can be performed by trained personnel in laboratory facilities or in point-of-care settings, such as clinics and hospitals, pharmacies, schools, and nursing or rehabilitation facilities (Hayden et al., 2023). Some NAATs can be self-administered by the patient (e.g., at home) and shipped to a laboratory for testing. Antigen tests can be self-administered and performed at home; thus, results may not be officially recorded in a medical record (CDC, 2023c; NIH, 2023).

Nasopharyngeal specimens remain the recommended samples for SARS-CoV-2 diagnostic testing; other sampling sites, such as nasal mid-turbinate, anterior nasal, or oropharyngeal swabs, are acceptable alternatives (CDC, 2023c; Hayden et al., 2023; Hellou et al., 2021; NIH, 2023). Some tests can be performed on saliva or mouth gargle specimens (FDA, 2023a). With both NAATs and antigen tests, clinical performance, and thus sensitivity and specificity, depends on how well the specimen is collected, the actual site of sampling, and the duration of illness at the time of testing (Brümmer et al., 2021; Dinnes et al., 2022; Hayden et al., 2023; Hellou et al., 2021; Kucirka et al., 2020; Mallett et al., 2020; NIH, 2023; Parvu et al., 2021; Tsang et al., 2021). Because NAATs can detect molecular parts of SARS-CoV-2 for up to 3 months after an infection, even when live virus is no longer present (Rhee et al., 2021), antigen testing is particularly helpful for individuals with a recent history of COVID infection who need to test following a new exposure to document active infection (CDC, 2022b; Hayden et al., 2023).

Antibody Tests (Serology)

Antibody (immunoglobulin) tests, or serology, are an indirect method of demonstrating recent exposure to SARS-CoV-2. Early in the pandemic, prior to the availability of at-home antigen tests and the facility of molecular testing, antibody tests were used to help diagnose SARS-CoV-2 infection.

Several types of antibodies are produced after infection, including IgM, a short-term immunoglobulin that becomes undetectable weeks to months following infection, and IgG, which is usually produced after two or more weeks and may confer long-term protection and/or remain positive for a long time even if not offering protection.

Antibody tests can be used to detect prior SARS-CoV-2 infection and/ or prior vaccination. Different tests target different protein parts of the virus, such as the spike protein or the nucleocapsid protein (CDC, 2022). Because COVID-19 vaccines are engineered using the viral spike protein, vaccinated persons will test positive for the IgG antibody. Individuals with previous infection may also mount a positive serum IgM or IgG spike protein response. Antibodies to the nucleocapsid protein are generated only by infection, so a specific antibody test (IgG or IgM) against the nucleocapsid protein can be used to document prior infection in a vaccinated individual as long as the antibodies are still positive (CDC, 2022). Antibodies (IgG or IgM) against the SARS-CoV-2 virus are typically measurable two or more weeks after the onset of symptoms. Hence, negative antibody testing during the acute phase of the disease cannot rule out the disease, and convalescent titers may be helpful (CDC, 2022). An IgG response to the spike protein has been reported to remain stable over 6+ months (Dan et al., 2021).

For diagnostic or epidemiological purposes, the grade of evidence for the use of antibody tests is very low to moderate (Hayden et al., 2024). Both serum IgM and IgG tests have variable levels of sensitivity and specificity depending on the timeline of evaluation, and the predictive value of a diagnostic test depends not only on the characteristics of the test but also on the prevalence of the disease, which varies greatly depending on fluctuations of SARS-CoV-2 prevalence in different geographic locations and points in time. The method used to quantify antibodies can also impact accuracy, with a large systematic review and meta-analysis performed in 2022 showing better performance with respect to sensitivity for tests performed through ELISA (enzyme-linked immunosorbent assays) (81–82 percent) or CLIA (chemiluminescent immunoassays) (77–79 percent) than through LFIA (lateral flow immunoassays) (69–70 percent) (Zheng et al., 2022).

Seroprevalence data from November 2022 show that 96.7 percent of the U.S. population aged 16 and older had been vaccinated for or infected with SARS-CoV-2. Therefore, serological testing is not currently indicated to establish an active infection (CDC, 2024a).

One important topic with regard to the accuracy of serologic testing is recognition of patients worldwide who have primary and secondary immunodeficiencies. Those conditions may result in an inability to produce, or propensity to lose, antibodies, which may lead to false negatives on serology testing and/or require immunoglobulin replacement therapies, which may lead to false positives on serology testing. Assessment of serologic testing performed on patients with humoral defects indicates that vaccination is safe and cellular immunity is stimulated, but with an inadequate response in terms of production of antibodies and low-quality antibodies in a large number of the patients who do produce them (Arroyo-Sánchez et al., 2022; Connolly and Paik, 2022; Pham et al., 2022; Van Leeuwen et al., 2022).

Other Tests

Newer tests, such as interferon-γ (IFN-γ) release assays (IGRAs), aimed at identifying the adaptive T cell immune response ("memory T cells") to SARS-CoV-2, are in development and may have potential as a more long-term marker of active/past infection compared with antibody response. More robust data are needed to determine how long the T cell immune response remains following infection and what level of protection may be provided by the presence of that response (Binayke et al., 2024; Fernández-González et al., 2022).

BEFORE VIRAL DIAGNOSTIC TESTNG

Signs and Symptoms

SARS-CoV-2 was first identified in Wuhan City, China, in December 2019. It is unclear whether, and for how long, the virus may have been in circulation prior to that time (Pekar et al., 2021, 2022). It quickly spread worldwide, and COVID-19 was officially declared a pandemic on March 11, 2020. Viral diagnostic tests were limited at the onset of the pandemic until clinical laboratories began to offer viral testing for SARS-CoV-2 in March 2020 (Greninger and Jerome, 2020), and clinicians therefore had to rely on the presenting symptoms to make a diagnosis of COVID-19. The most frequently reported symptoms at that time, for both adults and children, included fever, cough, shortness of breath, sore throat, muscle soreness, diarrhea, headache, and fever (Irfan et al., 2021; Kadirvelu et al., 2022; Kaye et al., 2021). It is noteworthy that many infected individuals experienced a loss, or disturbance, of taste and smell. The loss of taste (ageusia) and smell (anosmia) were two of the more distinctive symptoms of SARS-CoV-2 infection (Dixon et al., 2021; Mizrahi et al., 2020), particularly with earlier variants (Von Bartheld and Wang, 2023).

Infected adults and children may be asymptomatic or have mild, moderate, or severe illness (Shang et al., 2022). The severity of COVID-19 symptoms depends on the presence of underlying premorbid conditions and chronic disease, age, vaccination status, health status, and the variant causing the infection. Signs and symptoms have changed throughout the course of the pandemic and through variant mutations. Omicron variants, for example, are less associated with anosmia compared with the Delta variant (Von Bartheld and Wang, 2023; Butowt et al., 2022), and patients infected with an Omicron variant more frequently report runny nose, headache, sneezing, and sore throat relative to those with earlier variants (Public Health Agency of Canada, 2022). By October 2022, fewer than 20 percent of cases included reports of anosmia (ZOE, 2022); symptoms experienced at that time differ from those reported early in the pandemic (Public Health Agency of Canada, 2022; Whitaker et al., 2022). Even among Omicron variants, Omicron BA.2 was found more likely to be symptomatic compared with BA.1. People infected with the Delta variant experienced a longer duration of acute symptoms relative to those infected with the Omicron variant. However, symptom duration with any variant was found to be shorter among those who had received three doses of the COVID-19 vaccine (Public Health Agency of Canada, 2022).

Individual signs and symptoms alone have poor diagnostic accuracy for SARS-CoV2 infection given their overlap with those of other viral syndromes, and the presence or absence of specific signs and symptoms is not sufficient to confirm or rule out infection (Struyf et al., 2022). For this reason, and given the lack of access to and availability of viral testing, a variety of nonviral diagnostic tests were utilized early in the pandemic to help with diagnosis.

Supporting Diagnostic Testing

Although the tests described in this section are not specific to COVID-19, the consistent prevalence of certain abnormalities seen in hospitalized COVID-19 patients fostered their use in diagnosing the disease early in the pandemic. Imaging studies, pulmonary function tests, and laboratory tests are among the ancillary tests used in the diagnosis of COVID-19 (Silva et al., 2021).

Imaging Studies

Typical chest X-ray (CXR) findings for COVID-19 include bilateral peripheral and basal multifocal airspace opacities (ground-glass opacity and consolidation); however, various patterns of CXR findings may be observed (Rousan et al., 2020). Because of the higher sensitivity of chest computed tomography (CT) compared with CXR in the detection of early lung disease, disease progression, and alternative diagnosis, high-resolution CT was also used in the clinical evaluation of suspected COVID-19 pneumonia cases (Silva et al., 2021; Wiersinga et al., 2020). CT hallmarks of COVID-19 are bilateral distribution of ground glass opacities with or without consolidation in the posterior and peripheral lung, but the predominant findings in later phases include consolidations, linear opacities, "crazy-paving" pattern, "reversed halo" sign, and vascular enlargement.

The CT findings for COVID-19 can overlap with the findings of other diseases, including other causes of viral pneumonia, but were considered additional support for the diagnosis given the epidemiological context (Carotti et al., 2020). Less common findings, termed "ancillary findings," have also been seen on radiography in patients with COVID-19, reflecting the heterogeneity of this disease. These ancillary findings include intrapulmonary vessel enlargement, subpleural curvilinear lines, centrilobular solid nodules, and pleural and pericardial effusion, among others (Silva et al., 2021). A systematic review and meta-analysis of 94 studies aimed at detecting the accuracy of chest CT, CXR, and lung ultrasound in suspected COVID-19 cases showed that both chest CT (69 studies) and lung ultrasound (15 studies) correctly diagnosed COVID-19 in 87 percent of cases, and CXR (17 studies) correctly diagnosed it in 73 percent of cases (Ebrahimzadeh et al., 2022). Compared with the COVID-specific viral tests that are now available, these imaging studies are not as sensitive or specific to COVID.

Pulmonary Function Tests

Abnormal results on pulmonary function tests, called "lung diffusion capacity of carbon monoxide" or DLCO, may also be seen as a result of destruction of the alveolar air sacs or thickening of the alveolar–capillary basement membrane, which then leads to impaired gas exchange. This phenomenon has been well described in cases of COVID-19 pneumonia (Cortes-Telles et al., 2021; Lee et al., 2022; Steinbeis et al., 2022; Torres-Castro et al., 2021).

Laboratory Tests

Common laboratory abnormalities seen in COVID-19 include abnormal complete blood count (e.g., lymphopenia), abnormal coagulation (e.g., elevated D-dimer), elevated inflammatory markers (e.g., C-reactive protein), elevated serum lactate dehydrogenase, and reduced serum albumin (Greco et al., 2021).

Again, these abnormalities are not unique to SARS-CoV-2 infection, but they gained relevance in the adequate epidemiological context.

Surveillance case definitions have changed over time based on the availability of SARS-CoV2 specific diagnostic testing (CDC, 2023b). Clinical diagnosis is one of exclusion, meaning symptoms are not explained by any other probable disease. Initially, clinical criteria included

> at least two of the following symptoms: fever (measured or subjective), chills, rigors, myalgia, headache, sore throat, new olfactory and taste disorder(s)
>
> OR
>
> at least one of the following symptoms: cough, shortness of breath, or difficulty breathing
>
> OR
>
> Severe respiratory illness with at least one of the following:
>
> - Clinical or radiographic evidence of pneumonia, OR
> - Acute respiratory distress syndrome (ARDS).
>
> AND
>
> No alternative more likely diagnosis. (CDC, 2023b, 2020 Interim Case Definition, Approved April 5, 2020)

Case definitions have incorporated other clinical data, laboratory/microbiological data, and/or epidemiological linkages or exposure history—for example, travel to areas with sustained transmission, occupation as a health care worker, or a contact with a positive test. Since August 2020, case definitions have been further classified as "suspect," "probable," or "confirmed" (CDC, 2023b). Epidemiological linkage for a SARS-CoV-2 diagnosis was defined by the U.S. Centers for Disease Control and Prevention (CDC) in 2021 as "close contact—being within 6 feet for at least 15 minutes (cumulative over 24 hours) with a confirmed or probable case of COVID-19 disease" or "member of an exposed risk cohort as defined by public health authorities during an outbreak or during high community transmission" (CDC, 2023b). The presence of epidemiological linkage and meeting clinical criteria allows a case to be classified at most as "probable," but does not require confirmatory or presumptive laboratory evidence of SARS-CoV-2 infection when that evidence is not available. Of note, given the eventual expansion of viral testing, the 2023 update of the case definition for COVID-19 no longer includes epidemiological linkage (CDC, 2023b).

ESTABLISHING A HISTORY OF PRIOR COVID-19

Prior COVID-19

During the early days of the COVID-19 pandemic, testing capacity was significantly constrained in the United States (Mercer and Salit, 2021). Consequently, many people with signs and symptoms of SARS-CoV-2 infection lacked access to testing and were not formally diagnosed. As the pandemic unfolded, testing constraints eased, at-home testing kits became widely available, and testing behavior changed. As a result, many people with signs and symptoms of SARS-CoV-2 infection either did not undergo testing or self-tested at home without formal reporting to a health care system. These realities underscore that reliance on testing to diagnose COVID-19 and subsequently its long-term health effects will necessarily miss these individuals and therefore should not be used as the sole approach to ascertaining a history of SARS-CoV-2 infection. In the absence of objective laboratory testing, signs and symptoms of COVID-19 or a self-report should be considered sufficient. Among patients without positive laboratory test results, the use of non-SARS-CoV-2 specific ICD codes (e.g., generic coronavirus infection, SARS [the prior disease] utilized prior to SARS-CoV-2 specific ICD codes), alone or in combination with signs/symptoms, may be an alternative approach to support a history of prior COVID-19, combined with all the other clinical findings described above.

Future Directions

Rapid advances in biomedical research and technology make the manufacturing of a newer generation of diagnostic tools and tests for COVID-19 likely. Host DNA methylation patterns have been studied to differentiate between COVID-19–infected and –uninfected persons, and these patterns may help predict disease progression and outcomes even before the onset of symptoms (Konigsberg et al., 2021). DNA methylation entails the addition of a methyl group to the DNA molecule in the cells, which plays a crucial role in silencing gene expression, preventing DNA synthesis (Moore et al., 2013). Although neither widely used nor generally recognized presently, specific DNA methylation patterns have been shown to aid in the diagnosis of SARS-CoV-2 infection, to predict disease severity, and to establish a history of prior infection (Konigsberg et al., 2021; Pang et al., 2022). This and many novel techniques are expected to emerge. Several studies are evaluating biomarkers of both COVID-19 and Long COVID, but results are not yet conclusive.

DIAGNOSIS OF LONG COVID

There currently are no consensus-based diagnostic criteria for Long COVID. The condition is generally diagnosed on the basis of presumed history of acute SARS-CoV-2 infection (as indicated by a positive viral test or patient self-report; as of this writing, no diagnostic test for Long COVID is available), the presence of Long COVID health effects and symptoms, and consideration of other conditions that could be causing the symptoms. Continued research on and discussion of Long COVID will help inform a case definition and standardized diagnosis (Srikanth et al., 2023). There are several definitions of Long COVID that include varying time since acute SARS-CoV-2 infection, and the definitions in the literature are subject to change as research and data progress.

SUMMARY AND CONCLUSIONS

Testing to diagnose acute SARS-CoV-2 infection, as well as testing capacity and behaviors, has changed dramatically over the course of the COVID-19 pandemic. Testing was constrained during the early phase of the pandemic, but subsequently became increasingly available. The introduction of at-home testing means that many people may not have reported their positive results to health care systems. As viral infections fluctuate, as insurance coverage for at-home tests changes, and as society returns to prepandemic activities, some individuals may not even be testing for SARS-CoV-2 with at-home tests when ill. As a result of these two drivers, the diagnosis of many individuals with SARS-CoV-2 infection was not formally documented. Reliance on a documented history of SARS-CoV-2 infection when diagnosing Long COVID will miss individuals whose infection was not documented and therefore should not be used as the sole approach to establishing a diagnosis. The presence of signs and symptoms and self-reported prior infection is generally sufficient to establish a diagnosis of SARS-CoV-2 infection.

REFERENCES

Arroyo-Sánchez, D., O. Cabrera-Marante, R. Laguna-Goya, P. Almendro-Vázquez, O. Carretero, F. J. Gil-Etayo, P. Suàrez-Fernández, P. Pérez-Romero, E. Rodríguez De Frías, A. Serrano, L. M. Allende, D. Pleguezuelo, and E. Paz-Artal. 2022. Immunogenicity of anti-SARS-CoV-2 vaccines in common variable immunodeficiency. *Journal of Clinical Immunology* 42(2): 240–252.

Binayke, A., A. Zaheer, S. Vishwakarma, S. Singh, P. Sharma, R. Chandwaskar, M. Gosain, S. Raghavan, D. R. Murugesan, P. Kshetrapal, R. Thiruvengadam, S. Bhatnagar, A. K. Pandey, P. K. Garg, and A. Awasthi. 2024. A quest for universal anti-SARS-CoV-2 T-cell assay: Systematic review, meta-analysis, and experimental validation. *npj Vaccines* 9:3.

Brümmer, L. E., S. Katzenschlager, M. Gaeddert, C. Erdmann, S. Schmitz, M. Bota, M. Grilli, J. Larmann, M. A. Weigand, N. R. Pollock, A. Macé, S. Carmona, S. Ongarello, J. A. Sacks, and C. M. Denkinger. 2021. Accuracy of novel antigen rapid diagnostics for SARS-CoV-2: A living systematic review and meta-analysis. *PLoS Medicine* 18(8):e1003735.

Butowt, R., K. Bilińska, and C. von Bartheld. 2022. Why does the Omicron variant largely spare olfactory function? Implications for the pathogenesis of anosmia in coronavirus disease 2019. *Journal of Infectious Diseases* 226(8):1304–1308.

Carotti, M., F. Salaffi, P. Sarzi-Puttini, A. Agostini, A. Borgheresi, D. Minorati, M. Galli, D. Marotto, and A. Giovagnoni. 2020. Chest CT features of coronavirus disease 2019 (COVID-19) pneumonia: Key points for radiologists. *La Radiologia Medica* 125(7):636–646.

CDC (U.S. Centers for Disease Control and Prevention). 2022. *Interim guidelines for COVID-19 antibody testing.* https://www.cdc.gov/coronavirus/2019-ncov/hcp/testing/antibody-tests-guidelines.html (accessed February 14, 2024).

CDC. 2023a. *Considerations for SARS-CoV-2 antigen testing for healthcare providers testing individuals in the community.* https://www.cdc.gov/coronavirus/2019-ncov/lab/resources/antigen-tests-guidelines.html (accessed April 23, 2024).

CDC. 2023b. *Coronavirus disease 2019 (COVID-19).* https://ndc.services.cdc.gov/conditions/coronavirus-disease-2019-covid-19/ (accessed February 14, 2024).

CDC. 2023c. *Diagnosis.* https://www.cdc.gov/coronavirus/2019-ncov/hcp/clinical-care/clinical-considerations-diagnosis.html (accessed February 14, 2024).

CDC. 2023d. *Nucleic acid amplification tests (NAATs).* https://www.cdc.gov/coronavirus/2019-ncov/lab/naats.html (accessed February 14, 2024).

CDC. 2024a. *2022 nationwide COVID-19 infection- and vaccination-induced antibody seroprevalence (blood donations).* https://covid.cdc.gov/covid-data-tracker/#nationwide-blood-donor-seroprevalence-2022 (accessed January 18, 2024).

CDC. 2024b. *Overview of testing for SARS-CoV-2, the virus that causes COVID-19.* https://www.cdc.gov/coronavirus/2019-ncov/hcp/testing-overview.html (accessed February 14, 2024).

Center for Health Security. 2023. *Testing basics: Antigen tests.* https://covid19testingtoolkit.centerforhealthsecurity.org/basics/types-of-covid-19-tests/diagnostic-tests/antigen-tests (accessed February 14, 2024).

Connolly, C. M., and J. J. Paik. 2022. SARS-CoV-2 vaccination in the immunocompromised host. *Journal of Allergy and Clinical Immunology* 150(1):56–58.

Cortes-Telles, A., S. Lopez-Romero, E. Figueroa-Hurtado, Y. N. Pou-Aguilar, A. W. Wong, K. M. Milne, C. J. Ryerson, and J. A. Guenette. 2021. Pulmonary function and functional capacity in COVID-19 survivors with persistent dyspnoea. *Respiratory Physiology & Neurobiology* 288:103644.

Dalva-Baird, N. P., W. M. Alobuia, E. Bendavid, and J. Bhattacharya. 2021. Racial and ethnic inequities in the early distribution of U.S. COVID-19 testing sites and mortality. *European Journal of Clinical Investigation* 51(11):e13669.

Dan, J. M., J. Mateus, Y. Kato, K. M. Hastie, E. D. Yu, C. E. Faliti, A. Grifoni, S. I. Ramirez, S. Haupt, A. Frazier, C. Nakao, V. Rayaprolu, S. A. Rawlings, B. Peters, F. Krammer, V. Simon, E. O. Saphire, D. M. Smith, D. Weiskopf, A. Sette, and S. Crotty. 2021. Immunological memory to SARS-CoV-2 assessed for up to 8 months after infection. *Science* 371(6529):eabf4063.

Dinnes, J., P. Sharma, S. Berhane, S. S. van Wyk, N. Nyaaba, J. Domen, M. Taylor, J. Cunningham, C. Davenport, and S. Dittrich. 2022. Rapid, point-of-care antigen tests for diagnosis of SARS-CoV-2 infection. *Cochrane Database of Systematic Reviews* 7(7):CD013705.

Dixon, B. E., K. K. Wools-Kaloustian, W. F. Fadel, T. J. Duszynski, C. Yiannoutsos, P. K. Halverson, and N. Menachemi. 2021. Symptoms and symptom clusters associated with SARS-CoV-2 infection in community-based populations: Results from a statewide epidemiological study. *PLoS ONE* 16(3):e0241875.

Ebrahimzadeh, S., N. Islam, H. Dawit, J. P. Salameh, S. Kazi, N. Fabiano, L. Treanor, M. Absi, F. Ahmad, P. Rooprai, A. Al Khalil, K. Harper, N. Kamra, M. M. Leeflang, L. Hooft, C. B. van der Pol, R. Prager, S. S. Hare, C. Dennie, R. Spijker, J. J. Deeks, J. Dinnes, K. Jenniskens, D. A. Korevaar, J. F. Cohen, A. Van den Bruel, Y. Takwoingi, J. van de Wijgert, J. Wang, E. Pena, S. Sabongui, M. D. McInnes, and Cochrane COVID-19 Diagnostic Test Accuracy Group. 2022. Thoracic imaging tests for the diagnosis of COVID-19. *Cochrane Database of Systematic Reviews* 5(5):CD013639.

FDA (Food and Drug Administration). 2021. *False positive results with BD SARS-CoV-2 reagents for the BD Max System—Letter to clinical laboratory staff and health care providers.* https://public4.pagefreezer.com/content/FDA/08-02-2022T03:01/https://www.fda.gov/medical-devices/letters-health-care-providers/false-positive-results-bd-sars-cov-2-reagents-bd-max-system-letter-clinical-laboratory-staff-and (accessed April 23, 2024).

FDA. 2023a. *COVID-19 test basics.* https://www.fda.gov/consumers/consumer-updates/covid-19-test-basics (accessed April 23, 2024).

FDA. 2023b. *In vitro diagnostics EUAs—Molecular diagnostic tests for SARS-CoV-2.* https://www.fda.gov/medical-devices/covid-19-emergency-use-authorizations-medical-devices/in-vitro-diagnostics-euas-molecular-diagnostic-tests-sars-cov-2 (accessed February 14, 2024).

Fernández-González, M., V. Agulló, S. Padilla, J. A. García, J. García-Abellán, Á. Botella, P. Mascarell, M. Ruiz-García, M. Masiá, and F. Gutiérrez. 2022. Clinical performance of a standardized severe acute respiratory syndrome coronavirus 2 (SARS-CoV-2) interferon-γ release assay for simple detection of T-cell responses after infection or vaccination. *Clinical Infectious Diseases* 75(1):e338–e346.

Ganguli, A., A. Mostafa, J. Berger, M. Y. Aydin, F. Sun, S. A. S. D. Ramirez, E. Valera, B. T. Cunningham, W. P. King, and R. Bashir. 2020. Rapid isothermal amplification and portable detection system for SARS-CoV-2. *Proceedings of the National Academy of Sciences of the United States of America* 117(37):22727–22735.

Greco, M., S. Suppressa, R. A. Lazzari, F. Sicuro, C. Catanese, and G. Lobreglio. 2021. sFlt-1 and CA 15.3 are indicators of endothelial damage and pulmonary fibrosis in SARS-CoV-2 infection. *Scientific Reports* 11(1):19979.

Greninger, A. L., and K. R. Jerome. 2020. The first quarter of SARS-CoV-2 testing: The University of Washington Medicine experience. *Journal Clinical Microbiology* 58(8):e01416-20.

Hayden, M. K., K. E. Hanson, J. A. Englund, M. J. Lee, M. Loeb, F. Lee, D. Morgan, R. Patel, I. El Mikati, S. Iqneibi, F. Alabed, J. Amarin, R. Mansour, P. Patel, Y. Falck-Ytter, V. Lavergne, R. L. Morgan, M. H. Murad, S. Sultan, A. Bhimraj, and R. A. Mustafa. 2023. *Infectious Diseases Society of America guidelines on the diagnosis of COVID-19: Molecular diagnostic testing.* https://www.idsociety.org/practice-guideline/covid-19-guideline-diagnostics/ (accessed April 23, 2024).

Hayden, M. K., I. K. El Mikati, K. E. Hanson, J. A. Englund, R. M. Humphries, F. Lee, M. Loeb, D. J. Morgan, R. Patel, O. Al Ta'ani, J. Nazzal, S. Iqneibi, J. Z. Amarin, S. Sultan, Y. Falck-Ytter, R. L. Morgan, M. H. Murad, A. Bhimraj, and R. A. Mustafa. 2024. Infectious Diseases Society of America guidelines on the diagnosis of COVID-19: Serologic testing. *Clinical Infectious Diseases*:ciae121.

Hellou, M. M., A. Górska, F. Mazzaferri, E. Cremonini, E. Gentilotti, P. De Nardo, I. Poran, M. M. Leeflang, E. Tacconelli, and M. Paul. 2021. Nucleic acid amplification tests on respiratory samples for the diagnosis of coronavirus infections: A systematic review and meta-analysis. *Clinical Microbiology and Infection* 27(3):341–351.

Irfan, O., F. Muttalib, K. Tang, L. Jiang, Z. S. Lassi, and Z. Bhutta. 2021. Clinical characteristics, treatment and outcomes of paediatric COVID-19: A systematic review and meta-analysis. *Archives of Disease in Childhood* 106(5):440–448.

Kadirvelu, B., G. Burcea, J. K. Quint, C. E. Costelloe, and A. A. Faisal. 2022. Variation in global COVID-19 symptoms by geography and by chronic disease: A global survey using the COVID-19 symptom mapper. *eClinicalMedicine* 45:101317.

Kaye, A. D., E. M. Cornett, K. C. Brondeel, Z. I. Lerner, H. E. Knight, A. Erwin, K. Charipova, K. L. Gress, I. Urits, and R. D. Urman. 2021. Biology of COVID-19 and related viruses: Epidemiology, signs, symptoms, diagnosis, and treatment. *Best Practice & Research Clinical Anaesthesiology* 35(3):269–292.

Konigsberg, I. R., B. Barnes, M. Campbell, E. Davidson, Y. Zhen, O. Pallisard, M. P. Boorgula, C. Cox, D. Nandy, S. Seal, K. Crooks, E. Sticca, G. F. Harrison, A. Hopkinson, A. Vest, C. G. Arnold, M. G. Kahn, D. P. Kao, B. R. Peterson, S. J. Wicks, D. Ghosh, S. Horvath, W. Zhou, R. A. Mathias, P. J. Norman, R. Porecha, I. V. Yang, C. R. Gignoux, A. A. Monte, A. Taye, and K. C. Barnes. 2021. Host methylation predicts SARS-CoV-2 infection and clinical outcome. *Communications Medicine* 1(1):42.

Kucirka, L. M., S. A. Lauer, O. Laeyendecker, D. Boon, and J. Lessler. 2020. Variation in false-negative rate of reverse transcriptase polymerase chain reaction–based SARS-CoV-2 tests by time since exposure. *Annals of Internal Medicine* 173(4):262–267.

Lee, J. H., J.-J. Yim, and J. Park. 2022. Pulmonary function and chest computed tomography abnormalities 6-12 months after recovery from COVID-19: A systematic review and meta-analysis. *Respiratory Research* 23(1):233.

Lieberman, J. A., G. Pepper, S. N. Naccache, M. L. Huang, K. R. Jerome, and A. L. Greninger. 2020. Comparison of commercially available and laboratory-developed assays for in vitro detection of SARS-CoV-2 in clinical laboratories. *Journal of Clinical Microbiology* 58(8):e00821–e00820.

Long, D. R., S. Gombar, C. A. Hogan, A. L. Greninger, V. O'Reilly-Shah, C. Bryson-Cahn, B. Stevens, A. Rustagi, K. R. Jerome, and C. S. Kong. 2021. Occurrence and timing of subsequent severe acute respiratory syndrome coronavirus 2 reverse-transcription polymerase chain reaction positivity among initially negative patients. *Clinical Infectious Diseases* 72(2):323–326.

Mallett, S., A. J. Allen, S. Graziadio, S. A. Taylor, N. S. Sakai, K. Green, J. Suklan, C. Hyde, B. Shinkins, Z. Zhelev, J. Peters, P. J. Turner, N. W. Roberts, L. F. Di Ruffano, R. Wolff, P. Whiting, A. Winter, G. Bhatnagar, B. D. Nicholson, and S. Halligan. 2020. At what times during infection is SARS-CoV-2 detectable and no longer detectable using RT-PCR-based tests? A systematic review of individual participant data. *BioMed Central Medicine* 18(1):346.

Mercer, T. R., and M. Salit. 2021. Testing at scale during the COVID-19 pandemic. *Nature Reviews Genetics* 22(7):415–426.

Mizrahi, B., S. Shilo, H. Rossman, N. Kalkstein, K. Marcus, Y. Barer, A. Keshet, N. A. Shamir-Stein, V. Shalev, A. E. Zohar, G. Chodick, and E. Segal. 2020. Longitudinal symptom dynamics of COVID-19 infection. *Nature Communications* 11(1):6208.

Moore, L. D., T. Le, and G. Fan. 2013. DNA methylation and its basic function. *Neuropsychopharmacology* 38(1):23–38.

NIH (National Institutes of Health). 2023. *Testing for SARS-CoV-2 infection.* https://www.covid19treatmentguidelines.nih.gov/overview/sars-cov-2-testing/ (accessed April 23, 2024).

Pang, A. P. S., A. T. Higgins-Chen, F. Comite, I. Raica, C. Arboleda, H. Went, T. Mendez, M. Schotsaert, V. Dwaraka, R. Smith, M. E. Levine, L. C. Ndhlovu, and M. J. Corley. 2022. Longitudinal study of DNA methylation and epigenetic clocks prior to and following test-confirmed COVID-19 and mRNA vaccination. *Frontiers in Genetics* 13:819749.

Parvu, V., D. S. Gary, J. Mann, Y. C. Lin, D. Mills, L. Cooper, J. C. Andrews, Y. C. Manabe, A. Pekosz, and C. K. Cooper. 2021. Factors that influence the reported sensitivity of rapid antigen testing for SARS-CoV-2. *Frontiers in Microbiology* 12:714242.

Pekar, J., M. Worobey, N. Moshiri, K. Scheffler, and J. O. Wertheim. 2021. Timing the SARS-CoV-2 index case in Hubei province. *Science* 372(6540):412–417.

Pekar, J. E., A. Magee, E. Parker, N. Moshiri, K. Izhikevich, J. L. Havens, K. Gangavarapu, L. M. Malpica Serrano, A. Crits-Christoph, N. L. Matteson, M. Zeller, J. I. Levy, J. C. Wang, S. Hughes, J. Lee, H. Park, M.-S. Park, K. Ching Zi Yan, R. T. P. Lin, M. N. Mat Isa, Y. M. Noor, T. I. Vasylyeva, R. F. Garry, E. C. Holmes, A. Rambaut, M. A. Suchard, K. G. Andersen, M. Worobey, and J. O. Wertheim. 2022. The molecular epidemiology of multiple zoonotic origins of SARS-CoV-2. *Science* 377(6609):960–966.

Pham, M. N., K. Murugesan, N. Banaei, B. A. Pinsky, M. Tang, E. Hoyte, D. B. Lewis, and Y. Gernez. 2022. Immunogenicity and tolerability of COVID-19 messenger RNA vaccines in primary immunodeficiency patients with functional B-cell defects. *Journal of Allergy and Clinical Immunology* 149(3):907–911.e3.

Public Health Agency of Canada. 2022. *COVID-19 signs, symptoms and severity of disease: A clinician guide.* https://www.canada.ca/en/public-health/services/diseases/2019-novel-coronavirus-infection/guidance-documents/signs-symptoms-severity.html (accessed February 14, 2024).

Rentsch, C. T., F. Kidwai-Khan, J. P. Tate, L. S. Park, J. T. King, M. Skanderson, R. G. Hauser, A. Schultze, C. I. Jarvis, M. Holodniy, V. Lo Re, K. M. Akgün, K. Crothers, T. H. Taddei, M. S. Freiberg, and A. C. Justice. 2020. Patterns of COVID-19 testing and mortality by race and ethnicity among United States veterans: A nationwide cohort study. *PLoS Medicine* 17(9):e1003379.

Rhee, C., S. Kanjilal, M. Baker, and M. Klompas. 2021. Duration of severe acute respiratory syndrome coronavirus 2 (SARS-CoV-2) infectivity: When is it safe to discontinue isolation? *Clinical Infectious Diseases* 72(8):1467–1474.

Romero, L., L. Z. Pao, H. Clark, C. Riley, S. Merali, M. Park, C. Eggers, S. Campbell, C. Bui, J. Bolton, X. Le, R. N. Fanfair, M. Rose, A. Hinckley, and C. Siza. 2020. Health center testing for SARS-CoV-2 during the COVID-19 pandemic—United States, June 5–October 2, 2020. *Morbidity and Mortality Weekly Report* 69(50):1895-1901.

Rousan, L. A., E. Elobeid, M. Karrar, and Y. Khader. 2020. Chest x-ray findings and temporal lung changes in patients with COVID-19 pneumonia. *BioMed Central Pulmonary Medicine* 20(1):245.

Shang, W., L. Kang, G. Cao, Y. Wang, P. Gao, J. Liu, and M. Liu. 2022. Percentage of asymptomatic infections among SARS-CoV-2 Omicron variant-positive individuals: A systematic review and meta-analysis. *Vaccines (Basel)* 10(7):1049.

Silva, M., R. E. Ledda, M. Schiebler, M. Balbi, S. Sironi, F. Milone, P. Affanni, G. Milanese, and N. Sverzellati. 2021. Frequency and characterization of ancillary chest CT findings in COVID-19 pneumonia. *British Journal of Radiology* 94(1118):20200716.

Srikanth, S., J. R. Boulos, T. Dover, L. Boccuto, and D. Dean. 2023. Identification and diagnosis of Long COVID-19: A scoping review. *Progress in Biophysics and Molecular Biology* 182:1–7.

Steinbeis, F., C. Thibeault, F. Doellinger, R. M. Ring, M. Mittermaier, C. Ruwwe-Glösenkamp, F. Alius, P. Knape, H.-J. Meyer, L. J. Lippert, E. T. Helbig, D. Grund, B. Temmesfeld-Wollbrück, N. Suttorp, L. E. Sander, F. Kurth, T. Penzkofer, M. Witzenrath, and T. Zoller. 2022. Severity of respiratory failure and computed chest tomography in acute COVID-19 correlates with pulmonary function and respiratory symptoms after infection with SARS-CoV-2: An observational longitudinal study over 12 months. *Respiratory Medicine* 191:106709.

Struyf, T., J. J. Deeks, J. Dinnes, Y. Takwoingi, C. Davenport, M. M. Leeflang, R. Spijker, L. Hooft, D. Emperador, J. Domen, A. Tans, S. Janssens, D. Wickramasinghe, V. Lannoy, S. R. A. Horn, and A. Van Den Bruel. 2022. Signs and symptoms to determine if a patient presenting in primary care or hospital outpatient settings has COVID-19. *Cochrane Database of Systematic Reviews* 5(5):CD013665.

Torres-Castro, R., L. Vasconcello-Castillo, X. Alsina-Restoy, L. Solis-Navarro, F. Burgos, H. Puppo, and J. Vilaro. 2021. Respiratory function in patients post-infection by COVID-19: A systematic review and meta-analysis. *Pulmonology* 27(4):328-337.

Tsang, N. N. Y., H. C. So, K. Y. Ng, B. J. Cowling, G. M. Leung, and D. K. M. Ip. 2021. Diagnostic performance of different sampling approaches for SARS-CoV-2 RT-PCR testing: A systematic review and meta-analysis. *The Lancet Infectious Diseases* 21(9):1233–1245.

Van Leeuwen, L. P. M., C. H. Geurtsvankessel, P. M. Ellerbroek, G. J. De Bree, J. Potjewijd, A. Rutgers, H. Jolink, F. Van De Veerdonk, E. C. M. Van Gorp, F. De Wilt, S. Bogers, L. Gommers, D. Geers, A. H. W. Bruns, H. L. Leavis, J. W. Van Haga, B. A. Lemkes, A. Van Der Veen, S. F. J. De Kruijf-Bazen, P. Van Paassen, K. De Leeuw, A. A. J. M. Van De Ven, P. H. Verbeek-Menken, A. Van Wengen, S. M. Arend, A. J. Ruten-Budde, M. W. Van Der Ent, P. M. Van Hagen, R. W. Sanders, M. Grobben, K. Van Der Straten, J. A. Burger, M. Poniman, S. Nierkens, M. J. Van Gils, R. D. De Vries, and V. A. S. H. Dalm. 2022. Immunogenicity of the mRNA-1273 COVID-19 vaccine in adult patients with inborn errors of immunity. *Journal of Allergy and Clinical Immunology* 149(6):1949–1957.

Von Bartheld, C. S., and L. Wang. 2023. Prevalence of olfactory dysfunction with the Omicron variant of SARS-CoV-2: A systematic review and meta-analysis. *Cells* 12(3):430.

Whitaker, M., J. Elliott, B. Bodinier, W. Barclay, H. Ward, G. Cooke, C. A. Donnelly, M. Chadeau-Hyam, and P. Elliott. 2022. Variant-specific symptoms of COVID-19 in a study of 1,542,510 adults in England. *Nature Communications* 13(1):6856.

Wiersinga, W. J., A. Rhodes, A. C. Cheng, S. J. Peacock, and H. C. Prescott. 2020. Pathophysiology, transmission, diagnosis, and treatment of coronavirus disease 2019 (COVID-19). *JAMA* 324(8):782-793.

Zheng, X., R. H. Duan, F. Gong, X. Wei, Y. Dong, R. Chen, M. Yue Liang, C. Tang, and L. Lu. 2022. Accuracy of serological tests for COVID-19: A systematic review and meta-analysis. *Frontiers in Public Health* 10:923525.

ZOE. 2022. *Is the Omicron COVID variant less severe than Delta?* https://health-study.joinzoe.com/blog/covid-omicron-less-severe (accessed April 4, 2024).

3

Selected Long-Term Health Effects Stemming from COVID-19 and Functional Implications

Long COVID is associated with a wide range of new or worsening health conditions and encompasses more than 200 symptoms involving many different organ systems (Davis et al., 2021; Lubell, 2022). Given the extensive range of symptoms, there have been attempts to cluster these health effects, but to date no consensus in this regard has been reached.

This chapter begins with an overview of the full range of symptoms and health effects associated with Long COVID and a summary of the condition's epidemiology. The chapter then focuses on three health effects of Long COVID that may not be captured in SSA's Listing of Impairments but can significantly affect one's ability to participate in work or school: chronic fatigue and post-exertional malaise (PEM), post–COVID-19 cognitive impairment (PCCI), and autonomic dysfunction. Although a great number of Long COVID health effects could impact function, the committee thinks it will be useful for SSA to become familiar with these three, as they are particularly challenging to treat because of their multisystem nature. (See Chapter 5 for an overview of similar multisystem chronic conditions.) These are the novel conditions for which people seek out Long COVID clinics. For each of these three health effects, the chapter provides an overview of

- the frequency and distribution of their severity and duration in the general population, as well as any differences along racial, ethnic, sex, gender, geographic, or socioeconomic dimensions, or differences specific to populations with particular preexisting or comorbid conditions;
- clinical standards for diagnosis and measurement of each of these health effects;

55

- any special considerations regarding identification and management of these health effects in special populations, including pregnant people and those with underlying health conditions;
- best practices for quantifying the functional impacts of these health effects; and
- identified challenges for clinicians in evaluating persons with these health effects.

The symptoms and health effects discussed in detail in this chapter do not represent the full range of effects experienced by patients with Long COVID. In an effort to be inclusive, the committee includes at the end of this chapter annex tables organized by body system of selected health effects associated with Long COVID, along with their potential functional impacts and selected management guidelines.

OVERVIEW OF HEALTH EFFECTS
ASSOCIATED WITH LONG COVID

Epidemiology of the Long-Term Health Effects of SARS-CoV-2 Infection

Data from the U.S. Centers for Disease Control and Prevention's (CDC's) National Health Interview Survey show that in 2022, 6.9 percent of U.S. adults and 1.3 percent of children had Long COVID at some point, while 3.4 percent of adults and 0.5 percent of children had Long COVID at the time of interview (Adjaye-Gbewonyo et al., 2023; Vahratian et al., 2023). Based on these surveys, it is estimated that approximately 8.9 million adults and 362,000 children reported Long COVID symptoms in the United States in 2022 (Adjaye-Gbewonyo et al., 2023; Vahratian et al., 2023). Among adults in the United States, data from the CDC's Household Pulse Survey show that the prevalence of Long COVID declined from 7.5 percent in June 2022 to 5.9 percent reported in January 2023, then increased to 6.8 percent in January 2024 (NCHS, 2024). Despite an overall decline in prevalence since June 2022, Long COVID's disease burden remains substantial. In January of 2024, approximately 22 percent of adults with Long COVID reported significant activity limitations (NCHS, 2024).

The body of epidemiological research shows great variation in the incidence and prevalence of the long-term effects of SARS-CoV-2 infection. These variations reflect the dynamic changes in the pandemic itself, as the virus has evolved and spawned many variants and subvariants throughout the pandemic's course; the effect of vaccines, which were introduced in December 2020 and later shown to reduce the risk of long-term health effects; and the effect of treatments for acute infection (e.g., steroids, antivirals), which may reduce the risk of long-term health effects. In addition, since awareness about Long COVID in the medical community and the public is still lacking, reported prevalence may be an underestimate.

Adding to this complexity is the broad multisystem nature of the long-term health effects of SARS-CoV-2 and the fact that these effects are expressed differently in different age groups and sexes and by baseline health (Maglietta et al., 2022; Rayner et al., 2023; Tsampasian et al., 2023; Wong et al., 2023). Variation in incidence and prevalence estimates also stems from heterogeneities in study designs, including choice of control groups (e.g., whether studies included people with negative SARS-CoV-2 tests or no known SARS-CoV-2 as controls); methods used to account for the effect of baseline health in ascertaining whether the emergence of specific health effects following infection represents new disease; specification of outcomes; and other methodological differences.

Because of the considerable variation in estimates of the long-term health effects seen in Long COVID, the committee presents average estimates for different body systems based on the published literature. Among people who had COVID-19, most estimates of long-term cardiovascular health effects, which comprise a broad array of sequelae, regress around 4 percent (Xie et al., 2022b). Neurological and psychiatric conditions are also common among people who had COVID-19, with estimates of around 6 percent (Harrison and Taquet, 2023; Ley et al., 2023; Taquet et al., 2021, 2022; Wulf Hanson et al., 2022; Xie et al., 2022a; Xu et al., 2022). The reported incidence of gastrointestinal disorders post–COVID-19 is highly variable, but estimates suggest 6 percent (Xu et al., 2023). Respiratory problems persist in some people following SARS-CoV-2 infection, and prevalence studies at 6 months to 2 years suggest estimates of 2–4 percent (Wulf Hanson et al., 2022). Endocrine conditions are estimated to affect 1–2 percent of people previously infected with SARS-CoV-2 (Ssentongo et al., 2022). Similarly, estimates of the prevalence of genitourinary disorders is around 1 percent (Kayaaslan et al., 2021).

Terminology

The committee considers a *health condition* to be a state, including injury, illness, or physical or mental diagnosis, that adversely affects a person's physical and/or mental health and well-being. A *symptom* is a subjective manifestation of disease experienced and reported by a patient, while a *sign* is an objective manifestation of disease that an examining practitioner can observe or measure (King, 1968; NIH, n.d.). In the context of this study, the committee uses *health effects* as an umbrella term that includes symptoms, health conditions, and other sequelae caused by or associated with prior infection with SARS-CoV-2.

Full Range of Health Effects

SARS-CoV-2 infection can lead to post-acute and long-term health effects in nearly every organ system (see Figure 3-1). As described in Chapter 1, the *International Classification of Functioning, Disability and Health* model of disability identifies three domains of functioning: body functions and structures (i.e., physiological functions of the body, including psychological functions, and functioning of body structures), activity (i.e., actions or tasks), and participation (i.e., performance of tasks in a social context, such as school or work), all of which are mediated by personal and environmental factors that can either enhance or diminish an individual's activity and participation (WHO, 2023b). Health effects associated with Long COVID may manifest as impairments in body structures and

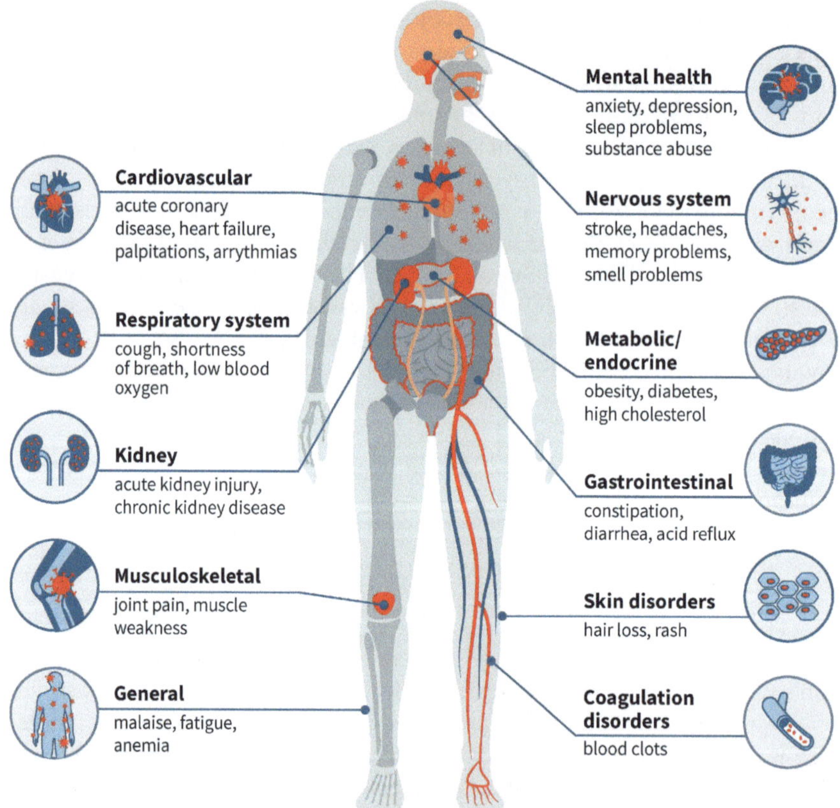

FIGURE 3-1 Lasting impact of COVID-19.
SOURCE: Washington University School of Medicine in St. Louis.

physiological functions, with resulting activity limitations and restrictions on participation. The impairments associated with Long COVID may affect mental (e.g., cognitive, psychosocial, emotional) functioning as well as physical functioning. In addition, individuals with Long COVID may experience multiple and potentially overlapping symptoms and conditions, including PEM, PCCI, and autonomic dysfunction. A number of preexisting conditions (e.g., diabetes, heart failure, chronic obstructive pulmonary disease, dementia) can increase the risk of adverse outcomes from SARS-CoV-2 infection, both during and following acute infection (Awatade et al., 2023; Dubey et al., 2023; Núñez-Gil et al., 2023; Steenblock et al., 2022; Treskova-Schwarzbach et al., 2021). Although persistent health effects associated with SARS-CoV-2 infection may include worsening of preexisting conditions, this chapter focuses primarily on newly acquired conditions. Health care providers and patients need to be aware of potential worsening of preexisting conditions and continue to monitor and treat them as needed. Additionally, the variable health effects of Long COVID may have different impacts on different patients depending on the burden of the preexisting condition, further emphasizing the need for a patient-specific approach for monitoring and treatment of health conditions.

Annex Tables 3-1 through 3-11 at the end of this chapter list selected health conditions associated with Long COVID in adults, organized by body system. Annex Table 3-12 lists selected health effects that are not organ system–specific, including chronic fatigue and PEM, ME/CFS, and fever. These tables include a summary of the potential functional implications of the conditions, selected clinical guidelines for their diagnosis and management, and potentially relevant SSA Listings for adults, where applicable. For the functional implications, the committee chose to focus on the kind of information that SSA collects about functioning in adults, which comes from a variety of sources, including the applicant, medical providers, employers, and other third parties with knowledge of the applicant. Information collected about physical functioning encompasses such activities as sitting, standing, walking, lifting, carrying, reaching, gross manipulation (e.g., handling large objects), fine manipulation (e.g., handling small objects, writing, typing), climbing, and low work (e.g., stooping, crouching, kneeling, crawling) (SSA, 2020). Annex Table 3-13 lists the physical; vison, hearing, and speaking; and mental activities the committee considered in populating the tables, along with their definitions. The committee populated the column on potential functional limitations based on the members' collective expertise. SSA also collects information about the applicant's ability to perform various daily activities, such as dressing, bathing, self-feeding, and using the toilet, as well as preparing meals, doing house- and yardwork, getting around, and shopping.

The long-term health effects associated with Long COVID can affect people across race, ethnicity, sex, gender, and age groups. Generally, the risk—on the relative scale—of these long-term health effects increases according to the severity of acute infection: the risk is 2–3 times greater in people who were versus were not hospitalized, and greatest in people who required intensive care (Núñez-Seisdedos et al., 2022; Xie et al., 2022b). However, because most people infected with SARS-CoV-2 experience mild or moderate disease that does not require hospitalization, those with mild or moderate cases constitute the majority of individuals with long-term adverse health effects of SARS-CoV-2 (Lai et al., 2023; Spagnuolo et al., 2020). Rates of Long COVID among pregnant women who had COVID-19 during pregnancy are similar to those of the general population (Kandemir et al., 2024). In addition, among pregnant women with COVID-19 at delivery, rates of caesarean delivery and frequency of maternal complications increased (Knight et al., 2020; Prabhu et al., 2020). The risk of Long COVID among adult females is about twice that among adult males (Munblit et al., 2021; Perlis et al., 2022; Sudre et al., 2021). Some pediatric studies also report a higher prevalence of Long COVID in female compared to male children and adolescents, although the exact risk is still undefined (Vahratian et al., 2023; Zheng et al., 2023).

Some of the long-term health effects of acute SARS-CoV-2 infection are chronic and can negatively impact individuals' quality of life; ability to participate in the labor market or school; and, in some cases, life expectancy. The extent to which the long-term health effects of infection will have a functional impact on a person's life and ability to work or participate in school can depend on health and functional status prior to COVID-19 and the severity of the medical condition(s). In addition, symptoms and related functional limitations may fluctuate, waxing and waning over time.

Clustering of Health Effects

Given the vast number of symptoms and health effects associated with Long COVID, several research groups have attempted to cluster patients with similar effects to better understand the disease (see Table 3-1).

The committee found that the evidence on clustering of the post-acute and long-term health effects of SARS-CoV-2 remains inconsistent across studies as a result of differences in study designs, populations studied, enrollment criteria, the era in which the study was undertaken (reflecting the possible differential effect of variants, changes in clinical care, and vaccination on phenotypic clusters), specification of post-acute and long-term health effects of SARS-CoV-2 infection, methodological approaches to clustering, and other factors. These differences yielded inconsistent results

TABLE 3-1 Research on Clusters of Long COVID Health Effects

Reference	Population and Study Type	Time after Initial COVID-19 Infection	Clustering Methodology	Proposed Long COVID Symptom Clusters	Notes
Canas et al. (2023)	Prospective cohort study, 9,804 UK-based adults	84 days	Unsupervised clustering analysis of time-series data, additional testing using data from Covid Symptom Study Biobank	(1) cardiorespiratory, (2) central neurological, and (3) multi-organ systemic inflammatory	Subclusters determined for wild-type variant in unvaccinated people, alpha variant in unvaccinated people, and delta variant in vaccinated people.
Evans et al. (2021)	PHOSP-COVID cohort, 1,077 UK adults	2 and 7 months	Clustering large applications k-medoids approach	(1) very severe, (2) severe, (3) moderate with cognitive impairment, (4) mild	46% in the mild cluster. Full recovery reached in 3% of the very severe cluster, 7% of the severe cluster, 36% of the moderate cluster, and 43% of the mild cluster. Elevated serum C-reactive protein was positively associated with cluster severity.
Fischer et al. (2022)	Predi-COVID cohort in Luxembourg, 288 participants	12 months	Hierarchical ascendant classification	(1) mild (less severe initial infection, fewer comorbidities, fewer persisting symptoms), (2) moderate (mean of 11 persisting symptoms, poor sleep, poor respiratory quality of life), (3) severe (higher number of symptoms especially vascular, urinary, skin)	48% in the mild cluster. Severe cluster had a higher proportion of women and smokers.

continued

TABLE 3-1 Continued

Reference	Population and Study Type	Time after Initial COVID-19 Infection	Clustering Methodology	Proposed Long COVID Symptom Clusters	Notes
Frontera et al. (2022)	242 patients hospitalized with COVID-19	12 months	Unsupervised hierarchical cluster analysis	(1) few symptoms, mostly headache, (2) many symptoms including high levels of depression and anxiety, (3) shortness of breath, headache, and cognitive symptoms	The study administered psychological therapy and medications to cluster 2 and PT or OT to cluster 3. They found 100% of those who received psychiatric therapy, 97% who received PT/OT, and 83% who received few interventions improved over time
Goldhaber et al. (2022)	UC San Diego health system, 999 respondents	Unspecified	Exploratory factor analysis	(1) gastrointestinal, (2) musculoskeletal, (3) neurocognitive, (4) airway, (5) cardiopulmonary	Neurocognitive burden associated with depression and anxiety. Musculoskeletal burden associated with older age
Kenny et al. (2022)	Multicenter prospective cohort, 233 individuals, 77% mild initial illness	4 weeks or more	Multiple correspondence analysis on the most common self-reported symptoms and hierarchical clustering	(1) pain symptoms including joint pain, myalgia, headache, (2) cardiovascular symptoms with chest pain, shortness of breath, palpitations, (3) significantly fewer symptoms than clusters 1 and 2	Clusters 1 and 2 had greater functional impairment, longer work absence
Kisiel et al. (2023)	506 patients from 3 Swedish cohorts, mostly hospitalized	12 weeks or more	K-means cluster analysis and ordinal logistic regression were used to create PCS scores	(1) mild, (2) moderate, (3) severe (predominating symptoms were fatigue, cognitive impairment, and depression)	59% in the mild cluster. Cluster 3 had the most reduced work ability. Smoking, high BMI, diabetes, and COVID-19 onset severity were predictors of cluster 3.

Study	Population	Time since infection	Method	Symptoms/clusters	Findings
Thaweethai et al. (2023)	Prospective cohort study of 9,764 adults at 85 enrolling sites in 33 states plus Washington, DC, and Puerto Rico	6 months or more	Unsupervised machine learning	(1) post-exertional malaise (PEM) and fatigue, (2) brain fog and PEM, (3) brain fog, PEM, and fatigue, (4) fatigue, PEM, dizziness, brain fog, GI symptoms, and palpitations	Using least absolute shrinkage and selection operator (LASSO), found most representative Long COVID symptoms to be smell/taste, PEM, chronic cough, brain fog, and thirst.
Tsuchida et al. (2023)	Adolescents and adults in an outpatient clinic in Japan	2 months or more	Cluster analysis was performed using CLUSTER (SAS Ver 9.4, SAS Institute Inc., Cary, NC, USA), and cluster classification was performed.	(1) fatigue only, (2) fatigue, dyspnea, chest pain, palpitations, forgetfulness, (3) fatigue, headache, insomnia, anxiety, motivation loss, low mood, forgetfulness, (4) hair loss, (5) taste and smell disorders	Clusters 2 and 3 had higher proportions of autonomic nervous system disorders and leave of absence from work and school
Wulf Hanson et al. (2022)	Pooled 54 studies and 2 medical record databases with data for 1.2 million individuals from 22 countries	3 months	Selected based on reporting frequency in published studies and availability of health state in Global Burden of Disease study	(1) fatigue, bodily pain, and depression and anxiety, (2) cognitive problems (inability to concentrate and remember), and (3) ongoing respiratory problems such as shortness of breath, cough, and chest pain	Among individuals with COVID-19, 6.2% had long COVID at 3 months: 10.6% for female adults, 5.4% for male adults, 2.8% for children and young people.
Yong and Liu (2022)	Review of 43 studies on Long COVID	3 months or more	"narrative review" of the literature (not systematic)	(1) non-severe COVID-19 multi-organ sequelae (NSC-MOS), (2) pulmonary fibrosis sequelae (PFS), (3) myalgic encephalomyelitis or chronic fatigue syndrome (ME/CFS), (4) POTS, (5) post-intensive care syndrome (PICS) and (6) medical or clinical sequelae (MCS)	Among individuals with Long COVID symptoms 3 months after symptomatic SARS-CoV-2 infection, an estimated 15% continued to experience symptoms at 12 months.

across studies, making it challenging to weave the evidence into a coherent narrative to inform policy discussions and clinical care. The heterogeneity of results reflects both the nascency of the field (less than 3.5 years old) and the complexity of Long COVID itself. The generation of better-quality and more consistent evidence will require consensus on terms, definitions, and methodological approaches.

SELECTED MULTISYSTEM HEALTH EFFECTS ASSOCIATED WITH LONG COVID

Three health effects associated with Long COVID that have a significant effect on functioning and are particularly challenging to manage—chronic fatigue and PEM, PCCI, and autonomic dysfunction—are reviewed in this section. There is significant overlap among the symptoms associated with these conditions.

Chronic Fatigue and Post-Exertional Malaise

PEM, also called post-exertional symptom exacerbation, is characterized by a severe worsening of fatigue and other symptoms following physical, mental, social, or emotional exertion that would not typically cause such a reaction in healthy individuals. This exacerbation of symptoms can occur immediately after the stressor or can be somewhat delayed (hours to days). In addition, an episode of PEM can last for days or even weeks. The specific symptoms that worsen vary among individuals, but often can go beyond fatigue to include muscle or joint pain, cognitive difficulties, sleep disturbances, headaches, flu-like symptoms, and/or gastrointestinal disturbances (Vernon et al., 2023).

Fatigue, broadly defined as a distressing or persistent tiredness that is neither proportional to recent activity nor alleviated by rest (Sandler et al., 2021; Twomey et al., 2022), is the most dominant symptom of Long COVID in several studies, ranging from 19 percent to 76.3 percent of patients (Cheung et al., 2023; Hartung et al., 2022; Ho et al., 2023; Kayaaslan et al., 2021; Líška et al., 2022; Sánchez-García et al., 2023; Štěpánek et al., 2023). Of the many descriptive studies that have captured fatigue and other symptoms seen in Long COVID, only a small proportion make a point of measuring PEM. In a large cross-sectional sample of adults who were selected from post–COVID-19 online groups, PEM was reported by 89.1 percent (95% confidence interval [CI] 88–90%); for most participants, PEM lasted a few days (Davis et al., 2021). A recent analysis of the National Institutes of Health Researching COVID to Enhance Recovery (RECOVER) longitudinal study was aimed at developing and validating a quantitative definition of Long COVID using multiple symptoms. In that study, PEM was reported in 87 percent of patients identified as having Long COVID (Thaweethai et al., 2023).

Diagnosis

Both post-COVID fatigue and PEM are generally diagnosed based on patient-reported symptoms and a detailed medical history. Typically, a thorough medical evaluation—which may include blood tests, imaging studies, and other diagnostic tests—is conducted to rule out other possible causes or contributing factors.

In clinical settings, health care providers typically evaluate chronic fatigue and PEM by asking patients to describe their symptoms in detail, including by inquiring about the type of exertion (physical, emotional, or mental) that leads to worsening of symptoms; the duration and severity of the symptom worsening that follows those stressors; how long it takes for the symptoms to return to baseline; what symptoms are experienced; and whether there is a prodrome related to the worsening of the symptoms. Multiple validated questionnaires can be used to measure a person's perception and severity of fatigue and PEM (Davenport et al., 2023; FACIT, 2021), such as the DePaul Symptom Questionnaire–Post-Exertional Malaise (DSQ-PEM), which captures the frequency and severity of PEM symptoms (Bedree et al., 2019; Cotler et al., 2018; Davenport et al., 2023; FACIT, 2021).

One approach to diagnosing PEM, investigated in myalgic encephalitis/chronic fatigue syndrome (ME/CFS) but not yet in Long COVID, involves two consecutive days of cardiopulmonary exercise testing (CPET) (Stevens et al., 2018). Deconditioned adults and those with other chronic conditions show minimal variation between the first and second day of CPET measurement. In ME/CFS patients with PEM, multiple studies reveal a significant decline in oxygen consumption ($\dot{V}O_2$) at peak performance and the ventilatory anaerobic threshold on the second day of CPET testing (Davenport et al., 2019; Stevens et al., 2018). The ventilatory anaerobic threshold reflects a person's ability to sustain continuous work and is more related to everyday exertion. This drop in $\dot{V}O_2$ between the first- and second-day CPET measurements suggests that patients with PEM risk entering anaerobic metabolism during activities they could have completed without it just the day before (Stevens et al., 2018). In ME/CFS, symptoms most associated with PEM after exercise include cognitive dysfunction, reduced self-reported daily functioning, and mood disturbances (Chu et al., 2018). Although 2-day CPET helps with understanding the physiologic response to exercise in patients with PEM generally, there are health system and patient-level barriers that potentially limit the broad implementation of 2-day CPET in diagnosing PEM in Long COVID and ME/CFS. The health system barriers include limited or inequitable access to CPET, with even fewer trained clinicians who can apply and interpret 2-day CPET to diagnose PEM. Patient-level barriers include prolonged recovery from testing and the prohibitive cost of testing without adequate insurance coverage. Several studies have explored the role of CPET in Long COVID, but not all have used PEM as an inclusion criterion (Baratto et al., 2021; Durstenfeld et al., 2022; Evers et al., 2022; Wernhart et al., 2023). Although much of the existing research on 2-day CPET in PEM has been in patients with ME/CFS, the findings should be expected to generalize, regardless of suspected onset. Nevertheless, additional research is needed to compare 2-day CPET results in Long COVID versus ME/CFS.

Functional Impacts

Chronic fatigue symptoms in Long COVID impact a person's ability to work and perform activities of daily living, which makes clinical care and rehabilitation a priority for these patients (Walker et al., 2023). They can also impact productivity by preventing a return to pre-COVID functional levels, thereby affecting the social and economic health of the impacted individual. A cross-sectional observational study on the impact of fatigue on function in 3,754 Long COVID patients, conducted at 31 post-COVID clinics in the United Kingdom, found that 94 percent (3,541) were of working age (18–65 years). Half (n = 1,321/2,600, 50.8 percent) of those who completed the "working days lost" questionnaire reported the loss of at least 1 day of work in the last month. Approximately 20 percent (20.3 percent) reported losing 20–28 days of work, and 20 percent also reported the inability to work completely. These results were associated mainly with fatigue (Walker et al., 2023). Symptoms of chronic fatigue in Long COVID may also influence a person's attitudes toward leisure time, thereby impacting mental health functioning and perceived stress.

Since PEM is considered a hallmark symptom for diagnosing ME/CFS (CDC, 2021b; IOM, 2015; NICE, 2021d), Long COVID patients with PEM may also fit criteria for ME/CFS. Understanding the functional impact of PEM is made more challenging by the fluctuating nature of the symptom complex and the fact that often people can compensate for limitations in function by first making compensatory changes in the time, effort, and resources they ascribe to certain tasks or by making compensatory changes in their social or leisure activity patterns (NICE, 2021d).

One recent study comparing PEM symptoms in Long COVID with those in ME/CFS found that the PEM symptoms were more likely to improve over 1 year in individuals with Long COVID, while there was no improvement in those with ME/CFS. However, 51 percent of the individuals with ME/CFS in this study had already had symptoms for >4 years, while 82 percent of those with Long COVID had had symptoms for <1 year (Oliveira et al., 2023). In a large cross-sectional sample of adults selected from post–COVID-19 online groups, those participants who had versus those who did not have PEM at 6 months or more after their COVID-19 illness had a significantly higher average number of Long COVID symptoms that persisted beyond 6 months (Davis et al., 2021). In a smaller cross-sectional analysis of more than 200 adults with at least 4 weeks of persistent symptoms after acute COVID-19 illness, PEM was associated with more severe fatigue and a higher risk of work status limitations, no or low physical activity, lower general health, and lower social functioning (Twomey et al., 2022). In a population-based longitudinal cohort study, PEM was associated with increased risk of other symptoms, such as insomnia, cognitive impairment, headache, and generalized pain, compared with those with fatigue without PEM. The presence of PEM was also associated with increased risk of functional impairment, reduced work capacity, and reduced physical activity (Nehme et al., 2023). Similarly, another population-based longitudinal study conducted in Switzerland describing the long-term trajectory of post-COVID symptoms in adults at 1, 2, 6, 9, 12, 18, and 24 months after SARS-CoV-2 infection found that PEM was more likely in those who had worsening of or no change in their perceived health status compared with those who reported improvement or showed continued recovery (Ballouz et al., 2023).

Treatment

When PEM is identified, the focus of treatment turns to comprehensively assessing and managing the functional impact of these symptoms, along with other Long COVID–related symptoms. When PEM is present, rehabilitation interventions and other treatment approaches may need to be personalized to enhance patient safety (Herrera et al., 2021; WHO, 2023a). For physical activity, the anerobic threshold can be used as the physical activity ceiling for safe activity to avoid PEM, recognizing that the nature of PEM is that the anerobic threshold may vary based on the patient's previous activities and other recent stressors (Davenport et al., 2010).

In addition to using self-report questionnaires to capture the severity of patients' fatigue and functional limitations, clinicians may ask patients to track their activities in detailed diaries to better capture the types of activities that are most likely to trigger PEM for each individual. Preventing PEM or lessening its severity may require identifying those triggering factors, such as physical, mental, and emotional stressors; orthostatic intolerance; hormonal factors in women; environmental factors (humidity and extreme temperatures); sensory stimuli (light, noise, and smells); certain foods; and infections, including reinfections with SARS-CoV-2. Teaching patients to respect their physiological limits is an important aspect of managing PEM. An important aspect of rehabilitation for people living with PEM is the provision and use of assistive products and environmental modifications to prevent PEM and its functional impact (WHO, 2023a). Therefore, another important aspect of management is facilitating work or school accommodations that may be necessary to prevent PEM (e.g., flexible hours, telecommuting options, specialized equipment to reduce physical or cognitive exertion).

Selected Populations

To date, few research studies have explored differences in PEM's prevalence, severity, and functional impact by race/ethnicity, rurality, or other social factors. A study using the TriNetX database to look at the use of outpatient rehabilitation for a post-COVID condition did find that Hispanic individuals had a significantly higher incidence of fatigue (Hentschel et al., 2022). There also is a scarcity of information on Long COVID fatigue and PEM and the impact of the condition in pregnant and lactating women, even though women appear to be at higher risk for the condition (Pagen et al., 2023).

Post-COVID-19 Cognitive Impairment

Cognitive impairment has emerged as one of the most commonly reported health effects associated with Long COVID, potentially portending significant consequences for patient functioning and quality of life. Cognitive impairment is defined as difficulties with thinking processes that can impact various cognitive domains, including memory, attention, processing speed, language, visuospatial, and executive functions (e.g., multitasking, judgment, problem solving). In patients with Long COVID, cognitive impairment has been characterized primarily by deficits in executive functioning (Becker et al., 2023). Cognitive impairment associated with Long COVID can vary in severity, from mild to severe, and often has an impact on instrumental activities of daily living.

Studies have reported varied rates of PCCI ranging from 8 to 80 percent (Becker et al., 2021), likely the result of varying measurement of cognition, including self-reported versus objective neuropsychological measures; use of cognitive screeners (which are insensitive to milder forms of impairment) (Lynch et al., 2022); and telephonic or online administration of measures versus validated, in-person assessments. However, the most robust studies have found PCCI to occur in approximately 24 percent of patients post COVID-19, across the spectrum of acute COVID severity (Becker et al., 2021). These cognitive deficits have been found to persist several months following SARS-CoV-2 infection (Becker et al., 2021, 2023), with some studies reporting long-term persistence beyond 1 year (Cavaco et al., 2023). While the severity of PCCI is relatively mild in comparison to the deficits seen in neurodegenerative diseases and severe traumatic brain injuries, it can still contribute to significant functional disability in those impacted (Delgado-Alonso et al., 2022).

PCCI can occur regardless of age, preexisting comorbidities, vaccination status, and COVID-19 variant. However, vulnerability to the condition appears to be greater in Black, Hispanic, female, and older-aged populations (Jacobs et al., 2023; Valdes et al., 2022), a finding that has substantial implications for occupational and social functioning. Female sex has also been associated with a greater probability of PCCI (Jacobs et al., 2023; Valdes et al., 2022). Differences have been found among racial and ethnic groups, such that Black and Hispanic individuals may be more likely to experience Long COVID and PCCI compared with non-Hispanic White individuals (Jacobs et al., 2023). Fewer years of education, Black race, and unemployment with baseline disability have likewise been found to confer a greater risk of PCCI (Valdes et al., 2022). Finally, preexisting conditions, including headaches (Jacobs et al., 2023), cognitive impairment (Valdes et al., 2022), neurological disease (Hartung et al., 2022), and renal disease (Bucholc et al., 2022), all appear to confer greater risk of PCCI. Conversely, some data suggest that the COVID-19 vaccine may reduce the risk of PCCI (Gao et al., 2022).

While the term "brain fog" has been deemed synonymous with cognitive impairment in the Long COVID literature, the two may be distinct clinical entities (McWhirter et al., 2023; Orfei et al., 2022). Brain fog is not a recognized medical diagnosis in itself, but rather a debilitating symptom that is usually seen in association with other factors, such as fatigue, psychosocial stress, and both physical and mental conditions (Jennings et al., 2022). Brain fog seen in patients following SARS-CoV-2 infection has anecdotally been described as inattention, forgetfulness, difficulty concentrating, and difficulty finding words (McWhirter et al., 2023). While these difficulties are often observed in formal neuropsychological assessments, it is well known that patients' subjective cognitive reports may sometimes be discrepant with objective neuropsychological findings (Schild et al., 2023). Nevertheless, it is important to note that individuals with cognitive impairment may report brain fog as a symptom, and that brain fog and PCCI may be equally functionally disabling in patients with Long COVID.

Diagnosis

The prevalence of cognitive impairment, including mild cognitive impairment (MCI) and more severe forms of cognitive impairment (e.g., dementia), increases with age. It is generally uncommon (i.e., less than 3 percent of the population) before age 65 and increases dramatically after age 75 (Casagrande et al., 2022; U.S. Preventive Services Task Force, 2020). The prevalence of MCI can be difficult to estimate due to several factors. There are varying diagnostic criteria for MCI. Additionally, as the population ages, some cases of MCI return to normal cognition with ongoing follow-up while others progress to dementia (Casagrande et al., 2022; U.S. Preventive Services Task Force, 2020). In addition to a comprehensive medical history, the clinical standard for diagnosis of cognitive impairment includes a comprehensive neuropsychological evaluation consisting of standardized tests that have well-established normative data (Becker et al., 2023; Casaletto and Heaton, 2017). These tests allow a clinician to compare an individual's scores with those of a normative population, adjusted for age; education; and sometimes other factors, such as sex. An individual's performance on these tests is often categorized according to standard deviations (SDs) below the mean of the normative sample. Scores within 1 SD below the mean are considered "average," whereas scores between 1 and 1.5 SDs below the mean are considered "mildly impaired" or "below average," and those more than 2 SDs below the mean are considered "moderately to severely impaired." A neuropsychological evaluation often tests all cognitive domains, including attention, working memory, processing speed, executive functions, language, visuospatial abilities, and learning and memory (Becker et al., 2023).

Many clinical challenges are involved in the evaluation and diagnosis of individuals with PCCI. As noted above, some individuals with Long COVID may report brain fog or other cognitive concerns and experience functional impairment, while not necessarily meeting the clinical diagnostic threshold for cognitive impairment (Davis et al., 2023). This may occur for several reasons.

First, most neuropsychological measures were developed to assess individuals with neurodegenerative disorders or traumatic brain injury (Casaletto and Heaton, 2017; Harvey, 2012) and may not adequately capture the often subtle impairment that can result from COVID-19. Similarly, many caveats apply to the normative data with respect to the populations that are considered "normal," as norms may not always account adequately for such factors as education, cultural background, language proficiency, and other individual differences.

Second, the theory of cognitive reserve posits that individual differences in the ability to cope with brain pathology or damage are influenced by the brain's resilience and adaptability, which is often related to such factors as educational attainment, occupational complexity, lifelong learning and stimulation, and social engagement (Stern et al., 2019). Individuals with a high cognitive reserve may not immediately show impairment on neuropsychological tests for several reasons: (1) they may be adept at using alternative cognitive strategies or recruiting additional brain resources to compensate for those areas that are impaired; (2) they may have started with a higher baseline of cognitive abilities, and thus will still score within the "normal" range on tests even if they have experienced some decline; and (3) their brain may be better able to cope with or resist damage because of its adaptability (Stern et al., 2019). At the same time, however, by the time these individuals' cognitive symptoms become apparent or manifest on neuropsychological tests, the underlying brain pathology may be quite advanced. In some cases, individuals with high cognitive reserve may report subjective cognitive decline; they feel that their cognitive abilities have diminished even if they still score well on formal testing. This subjective feeling may be attributable to patients' awareness of subtle changes or difficulties that are not yet detectable with standardized tests, a phenomenon that may be consistent with the concept of brain fog. This phenomenon underscores the importance of considering a comprehensive clinical picture, including subjective reports, daily functioning, and other factors, in conjunction with neuropsychological test scores. Without prior neuropsychological testing, it can be challenging to determine the degree of decline or change from an individual's baseline cognitive abilities, especially if those baseline abilities were above-average.

Third, performance validity can sometimes be an issue in the clinical evaluation of PCCI. That is, an individual's performance on neuropsychological tests can be influenced by various factors unrelated to PCCI, such as anxiety, depression, fatigue, or even the specific circumstances of the testing day. Such conditions as sleep disorders or chronic pain, medications, or other medical issues can influence cognitive performance and may lead to inconsistent test results, complicating their interpretation. In some cases, an individual's effort on a test may be called into question; that is, some individuals may have difficulty fully engaging with the evaluation, usually because of psychological or situational factors. It is also possible that individuals may purposely underperform (e.g., for secondary gain, such as disability claims). Fortunately, neuropsychologists have performance validity measures that can detect suboptimal effort.

Finally, it is important to note that other conditions can mimic the symptoms of PCCI. For example, depression may increase one's perception of brain fog and contribute to poor attention and concentration (Cristillo et al., 2022). Identifying whether cognitive deficits are due to PCCI or other factors can therefore be challenging. For this reason, a thorough medical history can be extremely useful in ruling in or out other potentially contributing factors.

Functional Impacts

Quantifying the functional impacts of PCCI involves integrating a comprehensive medical history, results of objective neuropsychological tests, subjective symptom reports, and real-world observations. A neuropsychological evaluation can help in identifying specific areas of cognitive strength and weakness and in predicting where an individual may have the most difficulty from day to day.

Several instruments (e.g., Instrumental Activities of Daily Living scale) can be used to gauge how PCCI may be impacting daily tasks, such as managing finances, following instructions, or planning activities. Other self-report tools can help capture individuals' perceptions of their cognitive and functional challenges. For example, numerous self-report instruments have been shown to adequately capture the severity and functional impact of symptoms associated with self-reported brain fog, such as the Neuro-QOL Scale (Shirley Ryan AbilityLab, 2019), the Cogstate (Maruff et al., 2009), or the Everyday Cognition scale (ECog) (Farias et al., 2008). Feedback from family members, coworkers, or educators can also provide a comprehensive view of an individual's functioning by offering insight into observed challenges in task completion, time management, or problem solving in real-world settings. Similarly, review of work performance evaluations or school assessments can be helpful in delineating where an individual may be struggling. Especially in complex cases, a neuropsychologist may work closely with other professionals (e.g., occupational therapists, speech therapists, educators, vocational counselors) to provide a holistic understanding of the individual's functional challenges.

Selected Populations

Research on PCCI in selected populations is limited. As described above, several studies have found racial and ethnic differences in the incidence of PCCI, whereby minoritized populations may be disproportionately impacted (Jacobs et al., 2023). While a neuropsychological evaluation can be extremely valuable in quantifying PCCI and its functional impact, it may not always be accessible to all individuals, and there are many barriers to care. First, because of high demand and a limited number of trained neuropsychologists, there can be extended wait times for an evaluation. Second, many neuropsychologists practice in urban areas or academic medical centers. Therefore, people living in rural or remote areas may not have easy access to a neuropsychologist and may have to travel significant distances for an evaluation. Third, neuropsychological assessments can be costly, and not all insurance plans cover them adequately; individuals without insurance may not be able to afford the evaluation. Finally, in certain cultures or communities, stigma may be associated with seeking psychological or neuropsychological services, preventing some individuals from pursuing an evaluation.

In addition, certain populations may not derive the same benefit from an evaluation. Several cultural nuances come into play here. First, individuals who speak languages other than English and those whose cultural background differs from that of the majority U.S. population may not have access to appropriate and culturally sensitive evaluations or even to neuropsychologists or interpreters with whom they can communicate, which can lead to misinterpretation of results. Second, most neuropsychological tests were developed and standardized on English-speaking populations, and appropriate normative data may not be available for the individual in question. In this case, an individual's performance can be over- or underestimated. Finally, in some cultures, cognitive challenges may be expressed more in somatic or physical terms, which can affect self-report measures, clinical interviews, and even effort on the neuropsychological tests. Thus, data derived from neuropsychological evaluations in such populations must often be interpreted with some caution.

Autonomic Dysfunction

Orthostatic intolerance and autonomic dysfunction have emerged as a distinct symptom cluster in Long COVID (El-Rhermoul et al., 2023). Autonomic dysfunction is any disturbance of the autonomic nervous system, inclusive of postural orthostatic tachycardia syndrome (POTS). POTS has increasingly been observed in patients following SARS-CoV-2 infection (Amekran et al., 2022). Other, less frequent types of autonomic dysfunction observed in patients with Long COVID include neurocardiogenic syncope (NCS) and orthostatic hypotension (OH) (Blitshteyn and Whitelaw, 2021). When objective tests do not confirm an established autonomic disorder (i.e., POTS, NCS, or OH), but autonomic symptoms arise upon assuming an upright posture and are relieved by being supine, then the diagnosis of orthostatic intolerance can be given. Some symptoms of autonomic dysfunction, such as lightheadedness, improve quickly upon lying down, but other symptoms, such as fatigue and brain fog, can persist for hours or days at a time and can impact activities of daily living (Fedorowski, 2019; Vernino et al., 2021).

Although POTS is itself a diagnosable multisystem disorder, it also has emerged as a distinct phenotype of Long COVID (El-Rhermoul et al., 2023). POTS is characterized by a sustained heart rate of 30 beats per minute or more in the absence of orthostatic hypotension (Amekran et al., 2022). Like Long COVID, POTS is a multisystem disorder; common symptoms include fatigue, nausea, dizziness, palpitations, chest pain, and exercise intolerance. POTS, and autonomic dysfunction generally, often present secondary to viral infections. Some studies have suggested that POTS could contribute to the pathophysiology of Long COVID, explaining the persistence of symptoms such as fatigue and cognitive issues in Long COVID patients, although the evidence for this hypothesis is limited (Amekran et al., 2022; Barizien et al., 2021; El-Rhermoul et al., 2023; Isaac et al., 2023). Mechanisms of action may include direct tissue damage, immune dysregulation, hormonal disturbances, elevated cytokine levels, and persistent low-grade infection (Carmona-Torre et al., 2022). Autonomic dysfunction appears to play a significant role in Long COVID and its potential neurological complications (Buoite Stella et al., 2022; Diekman and Chung, 2023).

The prevalence of POTS in the general U.S. population varies, with estimates ranging from 0.1 to 1 percent and a higher incidence among females, although in the general population is likely significantly under-diagnosed (Arnold et al., 2018; Bhatia et al., 2016; Shaw et al., 2019). POTS occurs most frequently in females aged 12–50 and is less common in young children (Amekran et al., 2022). Among people with Long COVID, one study reports 4.1 percent of respondents had received a diagnosis of POTS by the time of the survey, and 33.9 percent of those who reported tachycardia had symptoms suggestive of POTS (Davis et al., 2021). Another study reported 12 percent of individuals with Long COVID who underwent standard autonomic testing had results consistent with POTS (Bryarly et al., 2022). Studies indicate that 25–66 percent of Long COVID patients report autonomic dysfunction (Ladlow et al., 2022; Larsen et al., 2022). One study found orthostatic hypotension in 14 percent of subjects with Long COVID symptoms (Buoite Stella et al., 2022). Kavi (2022) cites unpublished data indicating that Long COVID clinics report 15–50 percent of patients having postural symptoms. These numbers should be taken as preliminary estimates given that most of the data to date came from small retrospective studies that vary in timing after initial SARS-COV-2 infection, definitions of POTS and autonomic dysfunction, and testing protocols.

Diagnosis

The diagnostic criteria for POTS are

- a sustained increase in heart rate upon assuming an upright position of ≥30 beats per minute in adults or ≥40 beats per minute in adolescents aged 12–19,
- the presence of chronic symptoms of orthostatic intolerance for at least 3 months, and
- the absence of orthostatic hypotension (Kavi, 2022; Raj et al., 2021, 2022).

In addition to a detailed medical history and physical examination, evaluating for orthostatic intolerance includes autonomic function tests and questionnaires. Autoantibody testing can provide supporting evidence.

Two forms of standing tests are used to diagnose POTS in Long COVID patients. These tests assess heart rate and blood pressure changes upon assuming an upright position, providing insight into autonomic dysfunction and orthostatic intolerance. In the active stand test, patients rest supine for 5 minutes, then immediately stand up, and their blood pressure and heart rate are measured at 2, 5, and 10 minutes. This test captures the immediate response to standing and helps identify orthostatic tachycardia and associated symptoms (Espinosa-Gonzalez et al., 2023). Another potentially useful test is the National Aeronautics and Space Administration's (NASA's) lean test, which involves the patient leaning against a wall after resting supine, with blood pressure and heart rate measured every minute for 10 minutes. This posture minimizes the impact of skeletal muscle pump effects on the cardiovascular system (Espinosa-Gonzalez et al., 2023; Kavi, 2022). These standing tests can be conducted in the primary care setting and may provide valuable information for diagnosing POTS without the need for specialist consultation or specialized equipment (Kavi, 2022).

The head-up tilt test is a specialized assessment used in secondary or tertiary health care settings to investigate autonomic dysfunction (Espinosa-Gonzalez et al., 2023). Head-up tilt table testing is usually performed with a motorized table with a foot board for weight bearing (Benditt et al., 1996). The patient lies supine, loosely restrained by safety straps to prevent injury if loss of consciousness occurs. After a variable period of supine rest, usually 15 minutes but in some studies up to 60 minutes, the tilt table is brought upright, usually to 60–70 degrees. This test, designed to explore the underlying causes of loss of consciousness, is the accepted method for investigating fainting in controlled laboratory conditions. During the test, the patient is positioned on a table equipped with motorized tilting capability. Blood pressure and heart rate measurements are taken while the patient is in a supine position and then gradually tilted upward to approximately 60 degrees for a duration of up to 45 minutes (Espinosa-Gonzalez et al., 2023). If syncope or presyncope occurs, the patient is promptly returned to the supine position. While this specialized test is not essential for a straightforward diagnosis of orthostatic tachycardia, it is useful in investigating specific symptoms, such as unexplained syncope. Not all individuals with orthostatic symptoms require head-up tilt testing.

COMPASS-31 is a standardized, easy-to-complete autonomic questionnaire used to screen for autonomic dysfunction and track symptom changes over time (Larsen et al., 2022). Questions fall into one of six domains: orthostatic intolerance, vasomotor, secretomotor, gastrointestinal, bladder, and pupillomotor function. The questionnaire generates a weighted score from 0 to 100, with a score of ≥20 suggesting moderate to severe autonomic dysfunction (Larsen et al., 2022). COMPASS-31 is frequently used to assess symptoms of autonomic dysfunction in Long COVID research (Bryarly et al., 2022; Buoite Stella et al., 2022; Seeley et al., 2023). Individuals with Long COVID could benefit from screening for symptoms of autonomic dysfunction (e.g., through use of the COMPASS-31 questionnaire), and those experiencing symptoms of orthostatic intolerance would benefit from further evaluation for disorders such as POTS or orthostatic hypotension (Larsen, Stiles, and Miglis, 2021).

Autoantibody testing can provide supporting evidence for diagnosis, although it is currently not particularly sensitive or specific (Carmona-Torre et al., 2022). A feature of POTS following SARS-CoV-2 infection is a high prevalence of specific circulating autoantibodies, including G-protein-coupled receptor (GPCR) antibodies (such as adrenergic, muscarinic, and angiotensin II type-1 receptors) and the ganglionic neuronal nicotinic acetylcholine receptor (g-AChR). Other recognized autoantibodies in POTS include circulating antinuclear, antithyroid, anti-NMDA-type glutamate receptor, anticardiac protein, anti-phospholipid, and Sjögren's antibodies (Carmona-Torre et al., 2022).

Functional Impacts

Symptoms resulting from autonomic dysfunction following SARS-CoV-2 infection have a substantial impact on individuals' functioning and quality of life in the short, medium, and long terms (Carmona-Torre et al., 2022). Symptoms are associated with loss of school and work participation, especially in young women (Bourne et al., 2021). In a study involving 20 adult Long COVID patients (70 percent female), residual autonomic symptoms persisted in 85 percent of participants 6–8 months after SARS-CoV-2 infection, with 60 percent being unable to return to work (Blitshteyn and Whitelaw, 2021). Haloot and colleagues (2022) investigated a sample of 40 Long COVID patients who were diagnosed with POTS and found that disabling symptoms persisted in 100 percent of previously high-functioning participants even after 6 months, indicating the enduring impact of the condition. McDonald and colleagues (2014) assert that young adults with POTS experience a degree of functional impairment comparable to that reported in congestive heart failure and chronic obstructive pulmonary disease, leading to a notably low quality of life. A prospective study of 99 participants—including those with post-acute sequelae of COVID-19 (PASC) (another term used for Long COVID), those with POTS, and healthy controls—revealed a high burden of autonomic dysfunction in those with PASC, leading to poor health-related quality of life and high health disutility (Seeley et al., 2023).

Approximately 50 percent of patients with POTS recover within 1–3 years, with lifestyle measures aiding recovery (Fedorowski, 2019). Exercise therapy, including rowing or cycling, has been shown to be effective in improving functioning in individuals with POTS following COVID-19. A minimum of 3 months of exercise therapy has been recommended, and symptoms often worsen before improving (Fu and Levine, 2018; Shibata et al., 2012). The course of recovery for symptoms associated with autonomic dysfunction in Long COVID entails remitting and relapsing as a result of various factors, such as comorbid conditions, stress, and overexertion (Barizien et al., 2021; Seeley et al., 2023); therefore exercise therapy must be individualized and closely monitored.

Assessing the ability to work in individuals experiencing orthostatic intolerance is challenging because of the unpredictable postexertional increase in symptoms for several days after prolonged periods of upright posture. This intolerance can significantly contribute to disability, and the ability to quantify the extent of functional impairments is limited. Self-reported symptom severity is critical in evaluating disability in individuals dealing with both orthostatic intolerance and Long COVID.

Overall functioning in chronic illnesses is often assessed in adults through self-report health-related quality of life questionnaires, such as the 36-Item Short Form Survey (SF-36), the EuroQOL, or the Patient-Reported Outcomes Measurement Information System (PROMIS) questionnaires (Cook et al., 2012; EuroQol Group, 1990; Ware and Sherbourne, 1992). A newly developed self-report questionnaire, the Malmö POTS symptom score, has shown promise for assessing symptom burden and measuring disease progression in adults with POTS (Spahic et al., 2023). For pediatric patients, age-specific instruments, such as the Functional Disability Inventory or Pediatric Quality of Life (PedsQL), are used into young adulthood, effectively distinguishing between healthy and chronically ill individuals (Claar and Walker, 2006; Varni et al., 2001; Walker and Greene, 1991). Self-reported measures of general or cognitive fatigue include the PedsQL, the Multidimensional Fatigue Inventory (MFI), the Wood Mental Fatigue Inventory, the Fatigue Severity Scale, and others (Bentall et al., 1993; Krupp et al., 1989; Varni and Limbers, 2008; Wood et al., 1991).

Selected Populations

Research on Long COVID-associated POTS in selected populations is limited. In a recent study of pregnant women with POTS not specific to Long COVID (8,941 female patients, 40 percent pregnant), the authors found that the severity of pregnancy symptoms in the first trimester could predict the severity of symptoms in the second and third trimesters

(Bourne et al., 2023). If symptoms improved in the first trimester, they were more likely to continue to improve in the later trimesters, while if symptoms worsened in the first trimester, they were likely to continue to worsen in the second and third trimesters. Other selected populations that may experience autonomic dysfunction from Long COVID and thus require health equity considerations include people with certain conditions and/or disabilities, racial and ethnic minorities, people diagnosed as overweight or obese, and uninsured or underinsured individuals. One example of clinical considerations regarding health equity is those with impaired mobility or severe orthostatic intolerance. Some of these patients may be unable to perform standard testing for autonomic dysfunction, such as a 10-minute stand test, requiring testing modifications (Blitshteyn et al., 2022).

HEALTH EFFECTS OF LONG COVID IN
CHILDREN AND ADOLESCENTS

While there are various definitions of children, adolescents, and young people, for the purposes of this report "children" or "pediatrics" will refer to the entire pediatric age range and "adolescents" to children in the older end of the spectrum (i.e., ages ~11 to 18 years). Although rates vary by age, children infected with SARS-CoV-2 usually have mild disease (COVID-19) with low rates of hospitalization (<2 percent) or death (<0.01 percent) (Bhopal et al., 2020, 2021). Nonetheless, persistent health effects following SARS-CoV-2 infection have been reported in children, with multisystem inflammatory syndrome in children (MIS-C) and Long COVID being commonly reported (Lopez-Leon et al., 2022). Additionally, Kompaniyets and colleagues (2022) found selected health effects for which children with SARS-CoV-2 infection are at increased risk: pulmonary embolism (adjusted hazard ratio [aHR] 2.01), myocarditis and cardiomyopathy (aHR 1.99), venous thromboembolic events (aHR 1.87), acute and unspecified renal failure (aHR 1.32), type 1 diabetes mellitus (aHR 1.23), coagulation and hemorrhagic disorders (aHR 1.18), smell and taste disturbances (aHR 1.17), type 2 diabetes (aHR 1.17), and cardiac dysrhythmias (aHR 1.16). Vaccination has been shown to reduce the risk of infection and protect against COVID-19–associated illness, including MIS-C, in children (Fowlkes et al., 2022; Tannis et al., 2023; Yousaf et al., 2023; Zambrano et al., 2022), although the majority of children in the United States remain unvaccinated against COVID-19 (AAP, 2023; CDC, 2021a; Zambrano et al., 2024).

Among the long-term health effects of COVID-19, type 1 diabetes has garnered specific attention, showing a higher incidence rate among children in the first year of the pandemic compared with a prepandemic period (incidence rate ratio [IRR], 1.14; 95% CI, 1.08–1.21) (D'Souza et al., 2023). This finding was mirrored in the months 13–24 of the pandemic, as shown in a meta-analysis (IRR, 1.27; 95% CI, 1.18–1.37) (D'Souza et al., 2023). The increased risk of type 1 diabetes in children after SARS-CoV-2 infection was found even when compared with diagnosis of acute respiratory infection unrelated to COVID-19 (Barrett et al., 2022; Rahmati et al., 2023; D'Souza et al., 2023). Additional studies are needed to further delineate this phenomenon.

MIS-C presents within 2–6 weeks of acute SARSs-CoV-2 infection as a systemic inflammatory illness. Criteria for case definition include severity necessitating hospitalization, fever above 100.4 degrees Fahrenheit, laboratory evidence of systemic inflammation, and multisystemic organ involvement that cannot be explained by another diagnosis (CDC, 2023a). Organ systems affected by MIS-C include gastrointestinal (80–90 percent), mucocutaneous (74–83 percent), cardiovascular (66.7–86.5 percent), hematologic (47.5 percent), respiratory (36.5 percent), and neurologic (12.2 percent) (Blatz and Randolph, 2022). Reassuringly, with MIS-C–directed treatment, the mortality rate has been 1–2 percent (Blatz and Randolph, 2022; Feldstein et al., 2021).

Although children with MIS-C present as critically ill, most inflammatory and cardiac manifestations resolve rapidly (Rao et al., 2022; Penner et al., 2021). However, some children do experience more long-lasting effects (Penner et al., 2021). One study tested children 6 months after hospitalization on the 6-minute-walk test and found that 45 percent of the patients scored below the 3rd percentile for age, demonstrating functional impairment (Penner et al., 2021). In this same study, 98 percent of the children were able to return to full-time education, but formal neuropsychological testing was not conducted to assess school performance (Penner et al., 2021). More research is needed to characterize the potential long-term effects of MIS-C.

Pediatric Long COVID is a separate entity from MIS-C. The true prevalence of Long COVID symptoms and health effects remains unclear for multiple reasons and varies widely in the literature, including limited studies and heterogeneous samples (Pellegrino et al., 2022). However, rates of pediatric Long COVID are lower than the rates of adult Long COVID (Behnood et al., 2022; CDC, 2023b; Jiang et al., 2023; Rao et al., 2022; Zheng et al., 2023). The risk of Long COVID may be associated with severe symptoms during initial infection, hospitalization, the number of organ systems involved, the number of symptoms at presentation, lack of vaccination against COVID-19, medical complexity, and body mass index ≥85th percentile for age and sex (Bygdell et al., 2023; Funk et al., 2022; Rao et al., 2022). Children with MIS-C may also develop Long COVID (Maddux et al., 2022).

Children with Long COVID may have health effects across body systems (Table 3-2). Commonly reported symptoms include fatigue (sometimes with PEM), weakness, headache, sleep disturbance, muscle and joint pain, respiratory problems, palpitations, altered sense of smell or taste, dizziness, and autonomic dysfunction (Morrow et al., 2022; Rao et al., 2022). Guidelines specific to pediatric Long COVID can aid in the diagnosis and management of the condition in children (Malone et al., 2022).

A systematic review of 22 studies (n = 23,141) from 12 countries identified fatigue (47 percent) as the most dominant Long COVID symptom in children and young people (age ≤ 19 years old), followed by headache (35 percent) (Behnood et al., 2022); these findings are consistent with those of several adult studies (Cheung et al., 2023; Líška et al., 2022; Sánchez-García et al., 2023; Štěpánek et al., 2023). In another systematic review and meta-analysis of 21 pediatric studies (n = 80,071), the prevalence of Long COVID was reported as 25.24 percent, with fatigue (9.66 percent) being the second most dominant clinical manifestation, behind mood symptoms (16.50 percent). Sleep disorders (8.42 percent), headache (7.84 percent), and respiratory symptoms (7.62 percent) were among the top-ranked Long COVID manifestations (Lopez-Leon et al., 2022). It is important to note that for this systematic review and meta-analysis, Long COVID criteria included symptoms lasting for at least 4 weeks, which likely contributed to the higher reported prevalence compared with findings of other studies. Studies have shown that isolation, increased stress, and loss of parents and caregivers significantly impacted children's development during the pandemic and may lead to a future rise in mental illnesses (Lopez-Leon et al., 2022) and other Long COVID sequelae.

Fatigue and PEM present similarly in pediatric populations compared to adults and are common in children with Long COVID; however, data from pediatric populations with ME/CFS indicate better long-term recovery compared with adults (Carruthers et al., 2011). In a cohort observational study of nearly 800 children, ME/CFS had a mean duration of 5 years, with 54 percent of patients reporting recovery between 5–10 years, and 68 percent of patients reporting recovery after more than 10 years (Rowe, 2019); this issue has not been explicitly studied in children with Long COVID.

POTS and other forms of autonomic dysfunction have also been reported in children with Long COVID (Morrow et al., 2022). Presentations and symptomatology, including orthostatic dizziness, palpitations, chest pain, diaphoresis, and nausea, are similar to those in adults. However, the diagnostic criteria for POTS are different in children and in adults: for individuals aged 12–19, the required heart rate increment is an increase of at least 40 beats/minute on a standing tolerance test, compared with 30 beats/minute in adults (Morrow et al., 2022; Vernino et al., 2021). One study compared 29 adolescents with Long COVID who developed

TABLE 3-2 Common Long COVID Symptoms in Children and Adolescents by Body System

Respiratory	Shortness of breath or dyspnea Chest (thoracic) pain or tightness Cough Difficulty with activity/exercise intolerance
Cardiovascular	Palpitations or tachycardia Dizziness/lightheadedness Syncope Chest pain Difficulty with activity/exercise intolerance
Neurological	Headache Dizziness/lightheadedness or vertigo Orthostatic intolerance Syncope or presyncope Tremulousness Paresthesia or numbness Difficulty with attention/concentration Difficulty with memory Cognitive impairment or brain fog
Special Senses	Abnormal or loss of smell or taste
Musculoskeletal	Weakness Muscle, bone, or joint pain
Gastrointestinal	Nausea Vomiting/reflux Abdominal pain Bowel irregularities (constipation/diarrhea) Weight loss Lack of appetite
Mental Health	Anxiety Depression/low mood Increased somatic symptoms School avoidance Regression of academic or social milestones
No specific organ system	Fatigue (general); Post-exertional malaise Exercise intolerance Sleep disturbances Fever

SOURCES: Behnood et al., 2022; Borch et al., 2022; Drogalis-Kim et al., 2022; Funk et al., 2022; Jiang et al., 2023; Kompaniyets et al., 2022; Kostev et al., 2022; Leftin Dobkin et al., 2021; Lopez-Leon et al., 2022; Malone et al., 2022; Mariani et al., 2023; Morrow et al., 2022; Pellegrino et al., 2022; Radtke et al., 2021; Riera Canales and Llanos-Chca, 2023; Roessler et al., 2022; Sansone et al., 2023.

an inappropriate sinus tachycardia or POTS with 64 adolescents who developed autonomic dysfunction prior to the COVID-19 pandemic. The authors concluded that, at least with regard to heart-rate variability, adolescents with POTS diagnosed following SARS-CoV-2 infection were not significantly different from the prepandemic controls (Buchhorn, 2023). Management of POTS is similar for children and for adults, with lifestyle interventions and physical therapy protocols being first line, augmented by medications when indicated.

Post–COVID-19 cognitive impairment (PCCI) or brain fog is reported in children with Long COVID and may manifest in behavioral changes and declining school performance. Limited research has focused on the chronic cognitive effects of COVID-19 in children. Objective neuropsychological data in pediatric patients have shown increased attention deficits in these patients and elevated mood/anxiety concerns (Luedke et al., 2024; Morrow et al., 2021; Ng et al., 2022; Tarantino et al., 2022), although these data came from small, single-center studies. In a survey of 510 children with ages ranging from 1–18 years, 61 percent had poor concentration, 46 percent had difficulty remembering information, 40 percent struggled with completing everyday tasks, and 33 percent had difficulties with information processing (Buonsenso et al., 2022). Importantly, other factors, such as fatigue and mental health problems, should be evaluated when cognitive problems are suspected, as these and other factors can contribute to poor attention and other cognitive difficulties.

With respect to management, a cognitive rehabilitation approach should be considered to improve attention regulation and help the child develop compensatory strategies. Whenever possible, support and accommodations should be offered in school settings to prevent the child from falling further behind academically. Periodic reassessment of cognitive functions is also prudent to monitor progress over time. Finally, screening for mental health problems is critical in children with post-COVID cognitive impairment, as PCCI can greatly impact quality of life.

Children with Long COVID may experience new or worsening mental health conditions, such as anxiety and depression. One study with 236 pediatric Long COVID patients found that irritability, mood changes, and anxiety or depression were found in 24.3 percent, 23.3 percent, and 13.1 percent of the cohort, respectively, suggesting a high prevalence of persistent psychiatric symptoms (Roge et al., 2021). Children may experience anxiety and depression differently from adults. Signs of depression can include behavioral problems at school, changes in eating or sleeping habits, and lack of interest in fun activities, while signs of anxiety in children can include fear of being away from a parent, physical symptoms of panic, and refusal to go to school. Diagnosis involves ruling out other conditions that may affect mood, and often includes interviews with the child and their caregivers (Cleveland Clinic, 2023). Management of mood disorders for pediatric patients with Long COVID is the same as management for those without Long COVID (e.g., psychotherapy, medications); however, special consideration is warranted for the other comorbid Long COVID symptoms and how they may interact with mood disorders or their treatment. The most common antidepressants for children are selective serotonin reuptake inhibitors (SSRIs), which increase the level of serotonin in the brain.

Although there may be overlap between pediatric and adult presentations and intervention options, particularly among adolescents, pediatric management of Long COVID entails specific considerations: developmentally, some young children and those with developmental disabilities may have difficulty describing their symptoms, and patient histories may come from parents and others outside the home, such as caregivers, coaches, or teachers. Compared with adults, children are healthier, with fewer preexisting chronic health conditions. Conditions that may increase the risk of Long COVID in adults, such as type 2 diabetes, are rarely seen in pediatrics, and Long COVID may therefore represent a large change from baseline for previously healthy children (Malone et al., 2022).

In addition to adverse effects of pediatric Long COVID on participation and performance in school, sports, and other activities (Morello et al., 2023; Pellegrino et al., 2022), it also has been shown to negatively affect family functioning as a whole (Chen et al. 2023). Management of pediatric Long COVID is focused on symptomatic support and from a functional perspective, on activities of daily living, such as participation in school and in activities and hobbies. Additionally, the American Heart Association and American Academy of Pediatrics recommend that those treating pediatric patients with moderate or severe acute SARS-CoV-2 infection or with any prolonged cardiac symptoms (e.g., fatigue, syncope, palpitations) use a screen to assess for the possibility of cardiac complications before recommending a return to physical activity (AAP, 2022a).

While the trajectory for children affected by Long COVID is more favorable than that for adults, additional studies are needed to better understand and characterize the diversity of presentations in children and long-term implications related to quality of life and function. The National Institutes of Health's (NIH's) RECOVER initiative currently has ongoing clinical trials and studies under way aimed at further understanding how to treat and prevent Long COVID in children in addition to adults (NIH, 2023). However, more research is still needed (Long COVID and kids: More research is urgently needed, 2022).

As detailed in Chapter 1, SSA's definition and determination of disability in children and adolescents (<18 years) differs from those in adults. "Disability" for adults in the SSA context centers on work disability or an inability to perform work-related activities (see, e.g., Annex Table 3-13 at the end of this chapter) and to participate in work "in an ordinary work setting, on a regular and continuing basis, and for 8 hours per day, 5 days per week, or an equivalent work schedule" (SSA, 2021). In contrast, the definition and determination of disability in children incorporates the concept of functioning more broadly (i.e., a child's qualifying impairment(s) must cause "marked and severe functional limitations"[1]). When evaluating the effects of an impairment or combination of impairments on a child's functioning, SSA considers "how appropriately, effectively, and independently" the child performs their activities (everything they do at home, at school, and in the community) "compared to the performance of other children [their] age who do not have impairments."[2] In particular, SSA considers functioning in six domains: "(i) acquiring and using information, (ii) attending and completing tasks, (iii) interacting and relating with others, (iv) moving about and manipulating objects, (v) caring for [oneself], and (vi) health and physical well-being."[3]

SELECTED GUIDANCE STATEMENTS SPECIFIC TO LONG COVID

In addition to the diagnosis and management guidelines included in Annex Tables 3-1 through 3-12, selected guidance statements specific to Long COVID are listed in Table 3-3. The CDC (2024) maintains a webpage with information on Long COVID (which the CDC refers to as Post-COVID conditions) for health care providers and the general public, covering the topics of assessment and testing, management, documentation, research, and tools and resources. The latter includes a list of "medical professional organization expert opinion and consensus statements." The World Health Organization (WHO) (2023a) also maintains a webpage on "clinical management of COVID-19," which includes a link to the most recent version of its *COVID-19 Clinical Management: Living Guidance* document. This publication contains "the most up-to-date recommendations for the clinical management of people with COVID-19" and includes a section on the "care of COVID-19 patients after acute illness" (WHO, 2023a).

In the United Kingdom, the National Institute for Health and Care Excellence, the Scottish Intercollegiate Guidelines Network, and the Royal College of General Practitioners jointly developed a guideline addressing identification, assessment, and management of the long-term effects of COVID-19 and offering "recommendations about care in all healthcare settings for adults, children and young people who have new or ongoing

---

[1] 20 CFR 416.906.
[2] 20 CFR 416.926a.
[3] 20 CFR 416.926a.

TABLE 3-3 Selected Guidance Statements on Long COVID

Author	Title	Last revised	Source
U.S. Centers for Disease Control and Prevention	*Post-COVID conditions: Information for healthcare providers*	February 6, 2024	CDC (2024)
World Health Organization	*Clinical management of COVID-19: Living guideline, 18 August 2023*	August 18, 2023	WHO (2023a)
National Institute for Health and Care Excellence, Scottish Intercollegiate Guidelines Network, and Royal College of General Practitioners	*COVID-19 rapid guideline: Managing the long-term effects of COVID-19*	November 11, 2021	NICE (2021a)
Catalan Society of Family and Community Medicine Long COVID-19 Study Group	*Long Covid-19: Proposed primary care clinical guidelines for diagnosis and disease management*	April 20, 2021	Sisó-Almirall et al. (2021)
American Academy of Pediatrics	*Post-COVID-19 conditions in children and adolescents*	September 2, 2022	AAP (2022b)
American Academy of Physical Medicine and Rehabilitation (AAPMR) PASC Multi-Disciplinary Collaborative Pediatric Work Group	*Multi-disciplinary collaborative consensus guidance statement on the assessment and treatment of postacute sequelae of SARS CoV-2 infection (PASC) in children and adolescents*	August 11, 2022	Malone et al. (2022)
AAPMR PASC Multi-Disciplinary Collaborative Writing Group	*Multidisciplinary collaborative consensus guidance statement on the assessment and treatment of fatigue in postacute sequelae of SARS-CoV-2 infection (PASC) patients*	July 26, 2021	Herrera et al. (2021)
AAPMR PASC Multi-Disciplinary Collaborative Writing Group	*Multi-disciplinary collaborative consensus guidance statement on the assessment and treatment of breathing discomfort and respiratory sequelae in patients with post-acute sequelae of SARS-CoV-2 infection (PASC)*	November 29, 2021	Maley et al. (2022)
AAPMR PASC Multi-Disciplinary Collaborative Writing Group	*Multi-disciplinary collaborative consensus guidance statement on the assessment and treatment of cognitive symptoms in patients with post-acute sequelae of SARS-CoV-2 infection (PASC)*	December 1, 2021	Fine et al. (2022)

continued

TABLE 3-3 Continued

Author	Title	Last revised	Source
AAPMR PASC Multi-Disciplinary Collaborative Writing Group	*Multi-disciplinary collaborative consensus guidance statement on the assessment and treatment of cardiovascular complications in patients with post-acute sequelae of SARS-CoV-2 infection (PASC)*	May 27, 2022	Whiteson et al. (2022)
AAPMR PASC Multi-Disciplinary Collaborative Writing Group	*Multi-disciplinary collaborative consensus guidance statement on the assessment and treatment of autonomic dysfunction in patients with post-acute sequelae of SARS-CoV-2 infection (PASC)*	June 3, 2022	Blitshteyn et al. (2022)
AAPMR PASC Multi-Disciplinary Collaborative Writing Group	*Multidisciplinary collaborative consensus guidance statement on the assessment and treatment of neurologic sequelae in patients with post-acute sequelae of SARS-CoV-2 infection (PASC)*	March 29, 2023	Melamed et al. (2023)
AAPMR PASC Multi-Disciplinary Collaborative Writing Group	*Multidisciplinary collaborative consensus guidance statement on the assessment and treatment of mental health symptoms in patients with post-acute sequelae of SARS-CoV-2 infection (PASC)*	November 8, 2023	Cheng et al. (2023)

symptoms 4 weeks or more after the start of acute COVID-19" (NICE, 2021a). Likewise, a Long COVID study group of the Catalan Society of Family and Community Medicine (Spain) issued proposed primary care clinical guidelines for the diagnosis and management of the condition in 2021 (Sisó-Almirall et al., 2021). The stated primary objective of the guidelines is the identification of individuals "with signs and symptoms of long COVID-19 . . . through a protocolized diagnostic process that studies possible etiologies and establishes an accurate differential diagnosis" (Sisó-Almirall et al., 2021, p. 4350).

Pediatric guidance on Long COVID in the United States includes statements from the American Academy of Pediatrics (AAP, 2022b) and a pediatric work group in alliance with the American Academy of Physical Medicine and Rehabilitation (AAPMR) PASC Multi-Disciplinary Collaborative (Malone et al., 2022). The AAP guidance provides information on

Long COVID in children and adolescents and evaluation and management of some of the potential ongoing symptoms. To assist primary care physicians and assist in initial specialty evaluations for children and adolescents with Long COVID, the AAPMR pediatric guidance statement addresses the initial evaluation of children and adolescents with Long COVID and potential health effects in different body systems, as well as return to play or activity and accommodations for school and activities (Malone et al., 2022). Work groups of the AAPMR PASC Multi-Disciplinary Collaborative have also issued guidance statements on the diagnosis and management of health effects of Long COVID in specific areas: fatigue, breathing discomfort and respiratory sequelae, cognitive symptoms, cardiovascular complications, autonomic dysfunction, neurologic sequelae, and mental health (Blitshteyn et al., 2022; Cheng et al., 2023; Fine et al., 2022; Herrera et al., 2021; Maley et al., 2022; Melamed et al., 2023; Whiteson et al., 2022).

OVERVIEW OF BODY SYSTEMS POTENTIALLY AFFECTED IN LONG COVID

In addition to the information in Annex Tables 3-1 through 3-12 on selected health effects associated with Long COVID, the following narratives, organized by body system, provide a high-level overview of diagnostic, management, and other information potentially relevant to adults with Long COVID. It is important to note that symptoms and health conditions may cross two or more body systems.

Respiratory System

Persistent respiratory symptoms and conditions are common in patients with Long COVID (Evans et al., 2023). The underlying pathophysiology for these symptoms and conditions is complex and multifactorial, encompassing persistent cardiac, pulmonary, or vascular dysfunction. The diagnostic approach to patients with these symptoms and conditions in Long COVID involves a clinical history and physical examination, and may include blood, radiologic, and other diagnostic tests, such as the 1-minute sit-to-stand test, chest X-ray, and pulmonary function testing (Daines et al., 2022). Computed tomography pulmonary angiography (CTPA) or ventilation perfusion (VQ) scintigraphy and VQ single-photon emission computed tomography (Daines et al., 2022; Kim et al., 2022) may be used to identify pulmonary vascular manifestations after acute SARS-CoV-2 infection. In general, the management approaches for all these respiratory symptoms and conditions in Long COVID are not specific to Long COVID, although some studies indicate the use of steroids to improve radiological, subjective, and functional outcomes in selected patients with post-COVID-19 pulmonary involvement (Dhooria et al., 2022; Goel et al., 2021; Mizera et al., 2024; Myall et al., 2021). Management of respiratory symptoms and conditions associated with Long COVID varies based on the severity of the symptoms, the level of functional impairment, comorbid illnesses, and other clinical factors.

Cardiovascular System

Cardiovascular symptoms and conditions are common following acute SARS-CoV-2 infection, and can include cardiopulmonary symptoms (e.g., chest pain, dyspnea, or palpitations), cardio-neuro symptoms, cardiac inflammatory diseases (e.g., myocarditis and pericarditis), and collateral damage from acute coronary syndromes (DePace and Colombo, 2022; Satterfield et al., 2022). Diagnostic approaches for cardiovascular symptoms and conditions related to Long COVID include electrocardiogram (ECG); transthoracic echocardiography; echocardiography; stress testing; event monitoring; and laboratory assessments such as cardiac biomarkers, cell counts, inflammatory markers, and coagulation markers. Functional tests, such as the 3-minute active stand test, 10-minute POTS assessment, and 6-minute walking test, may be administered. Cardiac magnetic resonance (CMR) can be used to determine abnormalities in ventricular and systolic function; pericardial effusion; and such abnormalities as myocarditis, epicarditis, pericarditis, and endocarditis (Satterfield et al., 2022; Von Knobelsdorff-Brenkenhoff and Schulz-Menger, 2023). Cardiopulmonary exercise testing can be used to better understand the relevant factors contributing to post-COVID diminished exercise capacity. As mentioned in the earlier discussion of PEM, two consecutive days of CPET can help diagnose PEM in individuals with ME/CS (Davenport et al., 2019; Stevens et al., 2018). Long COVID patients may exhibit various ECG abnormalities, including sinus tachycardia, ST changes, T-wave abnormalities, prolonged QT interval, low voltage, and bundle branch block.

Management of cardiovascular issues related to Long COVID currently involves symptom management and rehabilitation. Although there are no specific guidelines for cardiac inflammatory diseases such as myocarditis, ongoing research is exploring the use of antivirals, steroids, and nonsteroidal anti-inflammatory drugs in this condition (Raman et al., 2022). In general, the management approaches for all the cardiovascular symptoms and conditions in Long COVID, are not specific to Long COVID and treatment approaches generally follow the routine guidelines for the underlying condition.

Neurological System

A growing body of evidence indicates that Long COVID can manifest as neurological sequelae, affecting the central and/or peripheral nervous system. Some manifestations occur during the acute phase in hospitalized patients or as sequelae of a major neurological event, such as a stroke, while other relevant symptoms and conditions either continue or emerge weeks after infection. The neurological abnormalities observed in Long COVID likely arise from a multifaceted interplay of direct viral effects, autoimmunity, inflammation, mitochondrial dysfunction, vascular changes and thrombosis, hormonal imbalances, and persistent viral presence. A comprehensive understanding of these pathophysiological mechanisms is essential for the development of targeted therapeutic strategies for managing and alleviating the neurological sequelae of Long COVID. Management can include pharmacological interventions; physical therapy; pacing; occupational therapy, including lifestyle modifications; and psychological therapy (Tana et al., 2022).

Special Senses

Research on the specific abnormalities of the special senses such as vision, hearing, balance, taste, and smell in Long COVID is still emerging, and understanding of these abnormalities is evolving. Some individuals with Long COVID have reported persistent alterations in taste and smell, conditions known as anosmia (loss of smell) and ageusia (loss of taste). Additionally, studies have found visual and auditory disturbances, such as blurry vision, tinnitus, or hearing loss, in some Long COVID patients. These sensory changes can impact quality of life and may persist after acute SARS-CoV-2 infection even after other COVID-19 symptoms have resolved. In addition to diminishing quality of life, impaired or loss of smell and taste may lead to changes in eating habits (Ferrulli et al., 2022), potentially resulting in weight loss and worsening of other symptoms, including fatigue. Abnormalities of the special senses should be assessed in patients suspected of having Long COVID; however, a thorough medical history and physical examination are always advisable.

There are no well-established treatments for dysfunctions of the special senses due to Long COVID. The authors of a systematic review (Khani et al., 2021) propose several potential medications for treating Long COVID anosmia and ageusia, including pentoxifylline, zinc, omega-3, intranasal fluticasone, intranasal insulin, statins, and melatonin.

Musculoskeletal System

Individuals with Long COVID frequently report musculoskeletal and pain conditions alongside a range of other symptoms, complicating their pain experience and impacting their function and quality of life. Skeletal muscle abnormalities have been associated with lower exercise capacity, and exercise-induced myopathy has been noted with PEM (Appelman et al., 2024).

Diagnosis of musculoskeletal manifestations of Long COVID requires a thorough workup that ranges from noninvasive techniques (e.g., radiology/imaging) to invasive maneuvers (e.g., biopsy). A detailed medical history and physical examination is the first step, before any diagnostic test. Evidence is currently insufficient to recommend or advise against tests including creatine kinase, lactate dehydrogenase, c-reactive protein (CRP), rheumatologic factor, and antinuclear antibody in patients with arthralgia and myalgia lasting more than 12 weeks after COVID-19 (Kim et al., 2022).

There currently is no specific treatment for the musculoskeletal manifestations of Long COVID; patient-centered symptomatic management aimed at improving the quality of life is the goal by default (Calabrese et al., 2022). In a systematic review, Balcom and colleagues (2021) report that Long COVID myositis showed a favorable response to steroids, intravenous immunoglobulin, and tocilizumab. Baricitinib, an anti-inflammatory drug used to treat rheumatoid arthritis, has shown promising results; however, its association with increased risk for the development of malignancy has warranted further investigation (Assadiasl et al., 2021). Physical therapy (low-intensity aerobic training exercises) and psychological measures have proven to be effective in improving muscle strength (Nambi et al., 2022). Of note, people with Long COVID can exhibit changes in skeletal muscle mitochondrial function and metabolism that can further deteriorate with PEM; therefore, engaging in intense exercise is not advisable for some individuals with Long COVID (Appelman et al., 2024).

Endocrine System

Several conditions consistent with endocrine dysfunction, including diabetes mellitus (DM), dyslipidemia, thyroid dysfunction, adrenal dysfunction, and reproductive hormone dysfunction, have been noted in patients with Long COVID. The interplay between the endocrine system and Long COVID can be bidirectional: studies have shown a higher risk of developing Long COVID in patients with DM or those who are overweight, but have also shown that treatments, such as corticosteroids, potentially used both for acute SARS-CoV-2 infection and Long COVID may increase the risk of developing endocrine and metabolic disease (Bornstein et al., 2022).

Thyroid dysfunction has also been reported in Long COVID. Findings are mixed, however, as to the true role played by thyroid dysfunction and even the presence of antithyroid antibodies in Long COVID patients (Lui et al., 2023; Sunada et al., 2022).

Adrenal dysfunction has also been postulated as a relevant feature in patients with Long COVID. Of note, lower levels of serum cortisol have been described in patients with Long COVID compared with non–Long COVID healthy controls (Klein et al., 2023).

Finally, the presence of reproductive hormonal dysfunction in patients with Long COVID has been hypothesized, due mainly to epidemiological factors and to a high incidence (74 percent of females) of patient-reported changes in menstrual cycle as part of the Long COVID complex of symptoms. However, no clear entity has been identified to define a clear diagnostic pathway (Lott et al., 2023).

The diagnosis and treatment of endocrine dysfunction is similar for individuals with and without Long COVID.

Immune System

The immune system is an integral part of the response to SARS-CoV-2 infection itself, as its proper function is critical for the ability to contain and eliminate the infection prior to any additional therapeutic support. Given its role in the control and containment of the primary infection, it is not surprising that dysregulation of the immune system has been reported by patients with Long COVID.

Different levels of immune dysregulation have been identified in patients with Long COVID, including differences in the levels of circulating myeloid and lymphocyte populations compared with control patients without Long COVID; increased levels of antibody response to SARS-CoV-2; and increased levels of antibody response to other pathogens, especially Epstein-Barr virus (Klein et al., 2023). Notably, these abnormalities are not diagnostic of Long COVID, but are observations that support immune dysregulation among Long COVID patients.

Immune dysregulation is a broad theme. The immune system overlaps with all the other body systems and functions, and so the dysregulation noted in patients with Long COVID is hypothesized to potentially affect viral persistence and replication and gut microbiota dysbiosis, and to lead to autoimmunity and immune priming, blood clotting and endothelial abnormalities, and dysfunctional neurological signaling (Bellanti et al., 2023).

Patients with Long COVID frequently report symptoms compatible with mast cell activation syndrome (MCAS). Several of the symptoms frequently seen in Long COVID overlap with those seen in MCAS, which can lead to diagnostic confusion. The diagnostic criteria for MCAS are well established by international societies and are applied similarly in Long COVID patients (Valent et al., 2021).

Treatment of MCAS depends on the individual's symptoms. It involves, first, guaranteeing anaphylaxis management ability through education and permanent availability of an epinephrine auto-injector and additionally controlling the different mast cell mediators. Treatment is standardized by society guidelines and applies to all patients with MCAS, regardless of the presence of Long COVID (Valent et al., 2020).

Gastrointestinal System

Individuals with Long COVID frequently report gastrointestinal symptoms, in isolation or combined with other symptoms. These symptoms may be compatible with such diagnoses as gastroesophageal reflux disease and irritable bowel syndrome, with similar presentations and management.

Genitourinary System

The relationship between chronic kidney disease and COVID-19 is bidirectional: chronic kidney disease increases susceptibility to COVID-19 infection and risk for severe disease, and Long COVID increases the risk of chronic kidney disease, even independently of acute kidney injury (Schiffl and Lang, 2023). The risk of renal dysfunction increases proportional to the severity of the acute COVID-19 infection (nonhospitalized, hospitalized, or ICU), although the risk extends to all patients, including those with milder cases of COVID-19 (Bowe et al., 2021). Kidney dysfunction is often a silent problem that can progress without being discovered. It is therefore important to monitor kidney function in Long COVID patients who are at higher risk of kidney disease. Diagnosis involves a combination of medical history, physical examination, laboratory tests, and imaging studies, as used in the general population.

Kidney care is an integral part of post-acute care for COVID-19. Treatment and management depend on the disease (i.e., chronic kidney disease or acute kidney injury) and stage, and those protocols are also applied to patients with and without Long COVID according to standardized guidelines.

Integumentary System

Cutaneous manifestations of Long COVID are relatively mild and last an average of 7 to 15 days (Freeman et al., 2023; Martora et al., 2023 Mass General, 2022; Polly and Fernandez, 2022). These conditions would most likely not rise to the level of a disabling impairment.

Mental Health

Because SARS-CoV-2 infection can affect the brain, some of its post-acute sequelae may manifest in the form of neuropsychiatric disorders, including depression, anxiety, and adjustment and stress disorders. These disorders are likely driven by structural and/or functional brain alterations following infection and should not be misconstrued as evidence of a psychological basis for Long COVID. That said, mental health problems can also arise as a secondary or tertiary effect of Long COVID, as well as of the global pandemic more broadly. That is, with the rapid spread of SARS-CoV-2 arose the strict implementation of widespread social restrictions (e.g., quarantine, social distancing measures), often coupled with occupational loss and economic hardships. These factors should also be considered, as they could certainly play a role in initiating and/or exacerbating mental health problems in a subset of individuals. Along those lines, having Long COVID may predispose individuals to mental health problems by virtue of their new onset limitations. Finally, preexisting mental health problems may also be exacerbated following SARS-CoV-2 infection. Overall, determining whether mental health problems in those infected by SARS-CoV-2 differ from those not infected but merely affected by the global pandemic remains an ongoing challenge.

Regardless of their precise etiology, it is advisable for all clinicians to screen for new-onset anxiety and depression in Long COVID patients as they can have profound functional implications. Diagnosis of mental health problems may range from brief screening assessments in medical settings to more thorough clinical assessments by mental health professionals. Thorough assessments involve a review of symptoms, medical history, and psychosocial context. Criteria for diagnosis of mental health disorders are outlined in the *Diagnostic and Statistical Manual of Mental Disorders*, Fifth Edition, Text Revision (DSM-5-TR) (APA, 2022) or the *International Classification of Diseases*, Eleventh Revision (ICD-11) (WHO, 2023b). These criteria are used to diagnose anxiety, depression, posttraumatic stress disorder (PTSD), and other metal health disorders that may be pertinent in Long COVID.

The treatment of mental health disorders in patients with Long COVID can vary widely depending on the specific disorder, its severity, and the individual's unique needs and comorbid symptoms. The most common, evidence-based approaches include psychotherapy (e.g., cognitive-behavioral therapy), medications (e.g., antidepressants, antipsychotics), or a combination of the two (Cleveland Clinic, 2023). Importantly, given the multimorbidity of Long COVID, it is critical for clinicians to consider the potential interaction effects of certain medications, as well as their impact on other Long COVID symptoms.

SUMMARY AND CONCLUSIONS

Long COVID comprises hundreds of health effects caused by or associated with acute SARS-CoV-2 infection that manifest in many different body systems. Evidence on clustering of the post-acute and long-term health effects of SARS-CoV-2 remains inconsistent across studies, and consensus is needed on terms, definitions, and methodological approaches for generating better-quality and more consistent evidence. Health effects associated with Long COVID may manifest as impairments in body structures and physiological functions, potentially affecting mental (e.g., cognitive, psychosocial, emotional) functioning as well as physical functioning. In addition, individuals with Long COVID may experience multiple and potentially overlapping symptoms and conditions, including chronic fatigue and PEM, PCCI, and autonomic dysfunction. Some health effects can be sufficiently severe to interfere with an individual's day-to-day functioning, including participation and performance in work and school activities. There is some overlap between SSA's current Listing of Impairments (Listings) and health effects associated with Long COVID, such as impaired lung and heart function. However, it is likely that most individuals with Long COVID applying for Social Security disability benefits will do so on the basis of health effects not covered in the Listings. Three frequently reported health effects that can significantly interfere with the ability to perform work or school activities and may not be captured in SSA's Listings are chronic fatigue and PEM, PCCI, and autonomic dysfunction, all of which can be difficult to assess clinically in terms of their severity and effects on a person's functioning.

Children with Long COVID also may experience health effects across many body systems. Commonly reported symptoms include fatigue, weakness, headache, sleep disturbance, muscle and joint pain, respiratory problems, palpitations, altered sense of smell or taste, dizziness, and autonomic dysfunction. Although pediatric presentations and intervention options may overlap with those in adults, particularly among adolescents, who may be more likely to mimic adult presentation and trajectories, pediatric management of Long COVID entails specific considerations related to developmental age and/or disabilities and history gathering. In general, children have fewer preexisting chronic health conditions than adults; thus, Long COVID may represent a substantial change from their baseline, particularly for those who were previously healthy. Management of pediatric Long COVID, as with adults, is focused on symptomatic support and, from a functional perspective, on activities of daily living, such as participation in school and in activities and hobbies.

REFERENCES

AAP (American Academy of Pediatrics). 2022a. *COVID-19 interim guidance: Return to sports and physcial activity.* https://www.aap.org/en/pages/2019-novel-coronavirus-covid-19-infections/clinical-guidance/covid-19-interim-guidance-return-to-sports/#:~:text=The%20 AAP%20recommends%20not%20returning,physician%20evaluation%20has%20 been%20completed (accessed January 12, 2024).

AAP. 2022b. *Post-COVID-19 conditions in children and adolescents* https://www.aap.org/ en/pages/2019-novel-coronavirus-covid-19-infections/clinical-guidance/post-covid-19-conditions-in-children-and-adolescents/ (accessed January 17, 2024).

AAP. 2023. *Children and COVID-19 vaccination trends.* https://www.aap.org/en/pages/2019-novel-coronavirus-covid-19-infections/children-and-covid-19-vaccination-trends/ (accessed January 16, 2024).

AAPM (American Academy of Pain Medicine). 2023. *Clinical guidelines.* https://painmed.org/clinical-guidelines/ (accessed July 5, 2024).

ACOG (American College of Obstetricians and Gynecologists). 2018. *Dysmenorrhea and endometriosis in the adolescent–Committee opinion number 760.* https://www.acog.org/clinical/clinical-guidance/committee-opinion/articles/2018/12/dysmenorrhea-and-endometriosis-in-the-adolescent (accessed March 26, 2024).

ACR (American College of Rheumatology). 2021. *Vasculitis clinical practice guidelines* https://rheumatology.org/vasculitis-guideline (accessed November 9, 2023).

Adjaye-Gbewonyo, D., A. Vahratian, C. G. Perrine, and J. Bertolli. 2023. Long COVID in adults: United States, 2022. *NCHS Data Brief* (480):1–8.

Amekran, Y., N. Damoun, and A. J. El Hangouche. 2022. Postural orthostatic tachycardia syndrome and post-acute COVID-19. *Global Cardiology Science and Practice* 2022(1-2): e202213.

American College of Gastroenterology. 2023. *ACG's gastroenterology guidelines.* https://gi.org/guidelines/ (accessed November 14, 2023).

American Epilepsy Society. 2019. *AES clinical practice guideline development manual.* https://aesnet.org/clinical-care/clinical-guidance/guidelines (accessed April 4, 2024).

Ammirati, E., M. Frigerio, E. D. Adler, C. Basso, D. H. Birnie, M. Brambatti, M. G. Friedrich, K. Klingel, J. Lehtonen, J. J. Moslehi, P. Pedrotti, O. E. Rimoldi, H.-P. Schultheiss, C. Tschöpe, L. T. Cooper, and P. G. Camici. 2020. Management of acute myocarditis and chronic inflammatory cardiomyopathy: An expert consensus document. *Circulation: Heart Failure* 13(11):e007405.

Angeli, P., M. Bernardi, C. Villanueva, C. Francoz, R. P. Mookerjee, J. Trebicka, A. Krag, W. Laleman, and P. Gines. 2018. EASL clinical practice guidelines for the management of patients with decompensated cirrhosis. *Journal of Hepatology* 69(2):406–460.

APA (American Psychiatric Association). 2022. *Diagnostic and statistical manual of mental disorders, Fifth Edition, Text Revision (DSM-5-TR).* Washington, DC: APA.

Appelman, B., B. T. Charlton, R. P. Goulding, T. J. Kerkhoff, E. A. Breedveld, W. Noort, C. Offringa, F. W. Bloemers, M. Van Weeghel, B. V. Schomakers, P. Coelho, J. J. Posthuma, E. Aronica, W. Joost Wiersinga, M. Van Vugt, and R. C. I. Wüst. 2024. Muscle abnormalities worsen after post-exertional malaise in long COVID. *Nature Communications* 15(1):17.

Arnold, A. C., J. Ng, and S. R. Raj. 2018. Postural tachycardia syndrome–Diagnosis, physiology, and prognosis. *Autonomic Neuroscience* 215(December):3–11.

ASHA (American Speech-Language-Hearing Association). 2016. *Diagnosis and management of balance vestibular disorder* https://www.asha.org/articles/diagnosis-and-management-of-balance-vestibular-disorder/ (accessed November 10, 2023).

Assadiasl, S., Y. Fatahi, B. Mosharmovahed, B. Mohebbi, and M. H. Nicknam. 2021. Baricitinib: From rheumatoid arthritis to COVID-19. *Journal of Clinical Pharmacology* 61(10):1274–1285.

Avasthi, A., S. Grover, and T. S. Sathyanarayana Rao. 2017. Clinical practice guidelines for management of sexual dysfunction. *Indian Journal of Psychiatry* 59(Suppl 1):S91–S115.

Awatade, N. T., P. A. B. Wark, A. S. L. Chan, S. Mamun, N. Y. Mohd Esa, K. Matsunaga, C. K. Rhee, P. M. Hansbro, and S. S. Sohal,. 2023. The complex association between COPD and COVID-19. *Journal of Clinical Medicine* 12(11):3791.

Balcom, E. F., A. Nath, and C. Power. 2021. Acute and chronic neurological disorders in COVID-19: Potential mechanisms of disease. *Brain* 144(12):3576–3588.

Ballouz, T., D. Menges, A. Anagnostopoulos, A. Domenghino, H. E. Aschmann, A. Frei, J. S. Fehr, and M. A. Puhan. 2023. Recovery and symptom trajectories up to two years after SARS-CoV-2 infection: Population based, longitudinal cohort study. *BMJ* 381:e074425.

Baratto, C., S. Caravita, A. Faini, G. B. Perego, M. Senni, L. P. Badano, and G. Parati. 2021. Impact of COVID-19 on exercise pathophysiology: A combined cardiopulmonary and echocardiographic exercise study. *Journal of Applied Physiology* (1985) 130(5):1470–1478.

Barizien, N., M. Le Guen, S. Russel, P. Touche, F. Huang, and A. Vallée. 2021. Clinical characterization of dysautonomia in long COVID-19 patients. *Scientific Reports* 11(1):14042.

Barrett, C. E., A. K. Koyama, P. Alvarez, W. Chow, E. A. Lundeen, C. G. Perrine, M. E. Pavkov, D. B. Rolka, J. L. Wiltz, L. Bull-Otterson, S. Gray, T. K. Boehmer, A. V. Gundlapalli, D. A. Siegel, L. Kompaniyets, A. B. Goodman, B. E. Mahon, R. V. Tauxe, K. Remley, and S. Saydah. 2022. Risk for newly diagnosed diabetes >30 days after SARS-CoV-2 infection among persons aged <18 years–United States, March 1, 2020–June 28, 2021. *MMWR Morbidity and Mortality Weekly Report* 71(2):59–65.

Bateman, L., A. C. Bested, H. F. Bonilla, B. V. Chheda, L. Chu, J. M. Curtin, T. T. Dempsey, M. E. Dimmock, T. G. Dowell, D. Felsenstein, D. L. Kaufman, N. G. Klimas, A. L. Komaroff, C. W. Lapp, S. M. Levine, J. G. Montoya, B. H. Natelson, D. L. Peterson, R. N. Podell, I. R. Rey, I. S. Ruhoy, M. A. Vera-Nunez, and B. P. Yellman. 2021. Myalgic encephalomyelitis/chronic fatigue syndrome: Essentials of diagnosis and management. *Mayo Clinic Proceedings* 96(11):2861–2878.

Bates, D., B. C. Schultheis, M. C. Hanes, S. M. Jolly, K. V. Chakravarthy, T. R. Deer, R. M. Levy, and C. W. Hunter. 2019. A comprehensive algorithm for management of neuropathic pain. *Pain Medicine* 20(Supplement_1):S2–S12.

Baugh, R. F., G. J. Basura, L. E. Ishii, S. R. Schwartz, C. M. Drumheller, R. Burkholder, N. A. Deckard, C. Dawson, C. Driscoll, M. B. Gillespie, R. K. Gurgel, J. Halperin, A. N. Khalid, K. A. Kumar, A. Micco, D. Munsell, S. Rosenbaum, and W. Vaughan. 2013. Clinical practice guideline: Bell's palsy. *Otolaryngology–Head and Neck Surgery* 149(S3):S1–S27.

Becker, J. H., J. J. Lin, M. Doernberg, K. Stone, A. Navis, J. R. Festa, and J. P. Wisnivesky. 2021. Assessment of cognitive function in patients after COVID-19 infection. *JAMA Network Open* 4(10):e2130645–e2130645.

Becker, J. H., J. J. Lin, A. Twumasi, R. Goswami, F. Carnavali, K. Stone, M. Rivera-Mindt, M. S. Kale, G. Naasan, J. R. Festa, and J. P. Wisnivesky. 2023. Greater executive dysfunction in patients post-COVID-19 compared to those not infected. *Brain, Behavior, and Immunity* 114:111–117.

Bedree, H., M. Sunnquist, and L. A. Jason. 2019. The Depaul Symptom Questionnaire-2: A validation study. *Fatigue: Biomedicine, Health & Behavior* 7(3):166–179.

Behnood, S. A., R. Shafran, S. D. Bennett, A. X. D. Zhang, L. L. O'Mahoney, T. J. Stephenson, S. N. Ladhani, B. L. De Stavola, R. M. Viner, and O. V. Swann. 2022. Persistent symptoms following SARS-CoV-2 infection amongst children and young people: A meta-analysis of controlled and uncontrolled studies. *Journal of Infection* 84(2):158–170.

Bellanti, J. A., P. Novak, Y. Faitelson, J. A. Bernstein, and M. C. Castells. 2023. The long road of long COVID: Specific considerations for the allergist/immunologist. *Journal of Allergy and Clinical Immunology Practice* 11(11):3335–3345.

Benditt, D. G., D. W. Ferguson, B. P. Grubb, W. N. Kapoor, J. Kugler, B. B. Lerman, J. D. Maloney, A. Raviele, B. Ross, R. Sutton, M. J. Wolk, and D. L. Wood. 1996. Tilt table testing for assessing syncope. *Journal of the American College of Cardiology* 28(1):263–275.

Bentall, R. P., G. C. Wood, T. Marrinan, C. Deans, and R. H. Edwards. 1993. A brief mental fatigue questionnaire. *British Journal of Clinical Psychology* 32(3):375–379.

Bernstein, J. A., D. M. Lang, D. A. Khan, T. Craig, D. Dreyfus, F. Hsieh, J. Sheikh, D. Weldon, B. Zuraw, D. I. Bernstein, J. Blessing-Moore, L. Cox, R. A. Nicklas, J. Oppenheimer, J. M. Portnoy, C. R. Randolph, D. E. Schuller, S. L. Spector, S. A. Tilles, and D. Wallace. 2014. The diagnosis and management of acute and chronic urticaria: 2014 update. *Journal of Allergy and Clinical Immunology* 133(5):1270–1277.

Bhatia, R., S. J. Kizilbash, S. P. Ahrens, J. M. Killian, S. A. Kimmes, E. E. Knoebel, P. Muppa, A. L. Weaver, and P. R. Fischer. 2016. Outcomes of adolescent-onset postural orthostatic tachycardia syndrome. *The Journal of Pediatrics* 173:149–153.

Bhopal, S., J. Bagaria, and R. Bhopal. 2020. Children's mortality from COVID-19 compared with all-deaths and other relevant causes of death: Epidemiological information for decision-making by parents, teachers, clinicians and policymakers. *Public Health* 185:19–20.

Bhopal, S. S., J. Bagaria, B. Olabi, and R. Bhopal. 2021. Children and young people remain at low risk of COVID-19 mortality. *The Lancet Child & Adolescent Health* 5(5):e12–e13.

Blatz, A. M., and A. G. Randolph. 2022. Severe COVID-19 and multisystem inflammatory syndrome in children in children and adolescents. *Critical Care Clinics* 38(3):571–586.

Blitshteyn, S., and S. Whitelaw. 2021. Postural orthostatic tachycardia syndrome (POTS) and other autonomic disorders after COVID-19 infection: A case series of 20 patients. *Journal of Immunologic Research* 69(2):205–211.

Blitshteyn, S., J. H. Whiteson, B. Abramoff, A. Azola, M. N. Bartels, R. Bhavaraju-Sanka, T. Chung, T. K. Fleming, E. Henning, and M. G. Miglis. 2022. Multi-disciplinary collaborative consensus guidance statement on the assessment and treatment of autonomic dysfunction in patients with post-acute sequelae of SARS-CoV-2 infection (PASC). *PM&R* 14(10):1270–1291.

BLS (Bureau of Labor Statistics). 2020. *ORS collection manual.* https://www.bls.gov/ors/information-for-survey-participants/pdf/occupational-requirements-survey-collection-manual-082020.pdf (accessed March 26, 2024).

Borch, L., M. Holm, M. Knudsen, S. Ellermann-Eriksen, and S. Hagstroem. 2022. Long COVID symptoms and duration in SARS-CoV-2 positive children—A nationwide cohort study. *European Journal of Pediatrics* 181(4):1597–1607.

Bornstein, S. R., B. Allolio, W. Arlt, A. Barthel, A. Don-Wauchope, G. D. Hammer, E. S. Husebye, D. P. Merke, M. H. Murad, C. A. Stratakis, and D. J. Torpy. 2016. Diagnosis and treatment of primary adrenal insufficiency: An Endocrine Society clinical practice guideline. *Journal of Clinical Endocrinology and Metabolism* 101(2):364–389.

Bornstein, S. R., D. Cozma, M. Kamel, M. Hamad, M. G. Mohammad, N. A. Khan, M. M. Saber, M. H. Semreen, and C. Steenblock. 2022. Long-COVID, metabolic and endocrine disease. *Hormone and Metabolic Research* 54(8):562–566.

Bourne, K. M., D. S. Chew, L. E. Stiles, B. H. Shaw, C. A. Shibao, L. E. Okamoto, E. M. Garland, A. Gamboa, A. Peltier, A. Diedrich, I. Biaggioni, R. S. Sheldon, D. Robertson, and S. R. Raj. 2021. Postural orthostatic tachycardia syndrome is associated with significant employment and economic loss. *Journal of Internal Medicine* 290(1):203–212.

Bourne, K. M., K. A. Nerenberg, L. E. Stiles, C. A. Shibao, L. E. Okamoto, E. M. Garland, A. Gamboa, A. Peltier, A. Diedrich, I. Biaggioni, R. S. Sheldon, P. S. Gibson, A. J. Kealey, and S. R. Raj. 2023. Symptoms of postural orthostatic tachycardia syndrome in pregnancy: A cross-sectional, community-based survey. *BJOG* 130(9):1120–1127.

Bowe, B., Y. Xie, E. Xu, and Z. Al-Aly. 2021. Kidney outcomes in long COVID. *Journal of the American Society of Nephrology* 32(11):2851–2862.

Brandt, L. J., P. Feuerstadt, G. F. Longstreth, and S. J. Boley. 2015. ACG clinical guideline: Epidemiology, risk factors, patterns of presentation, diagnosis, and management of colon ischemia (CI). *American Journal of Gastroenterology* 110(1):18–44.

Bryarly, M., J. Cabrera, K. Tarpara, S. Barshikar, and S. Vernino. 2022. Minimal objective autonomic dysfunction in long-COVID. *Clinical Autonomic Research* 32(5):362.

Buchhorn, R. 2023. Therapeutic approaches to dysautonomia in childhood, with a special focus on long COVID. *Children (Basel)* 10(2):316.

Bucholc, M., D. Bradley, D. Bennett, L. Patterson, R. Spiers, D. Gibson, H. Van Woerden, and A. J. Bjourson. 2022. Identifying pre-existing conditions and multimorbidity patterns associated with in-hospital mortality in patients with COVID-19. *Scientific Reports* 12(1):17313.

Budhwar, N., and Z. Syed. 2020. Chronic dyspnea: Diagnosis and evaluation. *American Family Physician* 101(9):542–548.

Buoite Stella, A., G. Furlanis, N. A. Frezza, R. Valentinotti, M. Ajcevic, and P. Manganotti. 2022. Autonomic dysfunction in post-COVID patients with and without neurological symptoms: A prospective multidomain observational study. *Journal of Neurology* 269(2):587–596.

Buonsenso, D., F. E. Pujol, D. Munblit, D. Pata, S. McFarland, and F. K. Simpson. 2022. Clinical characteristics, activity levels and mental health problems in children with long coronavirus disease: A survey of 510 children. *Future Microbiology* 17(8):577–588.

Bygdell, M., J. M. Kindblom, J. Martikainen, H. Li, and F. Nyberg. 2023. Incidence and characteristics in children with post–COVID-19 condition in Sweden. *JAMA Network Open* 6(7):e2324246–e2324246.

Calabrese, C., E. Kirchner, and L. H. Calabrese. 2022. Long COVID and rheumatology: Clinical, diagnostic, and therapeutic implications. *Best Practice & Research Clinical Rheumatology* 36(4):101794.

Canas, L. S., E. Molteni, J. Deng, C. H. Sudre, B. Murray, E. Kerfoot, M. Antonelli, K. Rjoob, J. Capdevila Pujol, L. Polidori, A. May, M. F. Österdahl, R. Whiston, N. J. Cheetham, V. Bowyer, T. D. Spector, A. Hammers, E. L. Duncan, S. Ourselin, C. J. Steves, and M. Modat. 2023. Profiling post-COVID-19 condition across different variants of SARS-CoV-2: A prospective longitudinal study in unvaccinated wild-type, unvaccinated Alpha-variant, and vaccinated Delta-variant populations. *The Lancet Digital Health* 5(7):e421–e434.

Cappel, J. A., and D. A. Wetter. 2014. Clinical characteristics, etiologic associations, laboratory findings, treatment, and proposal of diagnostic criteria of pernio (chilblains) in a series of 104 patients at Mayo Clinic, 2000 to 2011. *Mayo Clinic Proceedings* 89(2):207–215.

Carmona-Torre, F., A. Mínguez-Olaondo, A. López-Bravo, B. Tijero, V. Grozeva, M. Walcker, H. Azkune-Galparsoro, A. López de Munain, A. B. Alcaide, J. Quiroga, J. L. Del Pozo, and J. C. Gómez-Esteban. 2022. Dysautonomia in COVID-19 patients: A narrative review on clinical course, diagnostic and therapeutic strategies. *Frontiers in Neurology* 13:886609.

Carruthers, B. M., M. I. Van De Sande, K. L. De Meirleir, N. G. Klimas, G. Broderick, T. Mitchell, D. Staines, A. C. P. Powles, N. Speight, R. Vallings, L. Bateman, B. Baumgarten-Austrheim, D. S. Bell, N. Carlo-Stella, J. Chia, A. Darragh, D. Jo, D. Lewis, A. R. Light, S. Marshall-Gradisbik, I. Mena, J. A. Mikovits, K. Miwa, M. Murovska, M. L. Pall, and S. Stevens. 2011. Myalgic encephalomyelitis: International consensus criteria. *Journal of Internal Medicine* 270(4):327–338.

Cartwright, S. L., and M. P. Knudson. 2008. Evaluation of acute abdominal pain in adults. *American Family Physician* 77(7):971–978.

Casagrande, M., G. Marselli, F. Agostini, G. Forte, F. Favieri, and A. Guarino. 2022. The complex burden of determining prevalence rates of mild cognitive impairment: A systematic review. *Frontiers in Psychiatry* 13:960648.

Casaletto, K. B., and R. K. Heaton. 2017. Neuropsychological assessment: Past and future. *Journal of the International Neuropsychological Society* 23(9-10):778–790.

Castro, C., and M. Gourley. 2010. Diagnostic testing and interpretation of tests for autoimmunity. *Journal of Allergy and Clinical Immunology* 125(2 Suppl 2):S238–S247.

Cavaco, S., G. Sousa, A. Gonçalves, A. Dias, C. Andrade, D. Pereira, E. A. Aires, J. Moura, L. Silva, R. Varela, S. Malheiro, V. Oliveira, A. Teixeira-Pinto, L. F. Maia, and M. Correia. 2023. Predictors of cognitive dysfunction one-year post COVID-19. *Neuropsychology* 37(5):557–567.

CDC (U.S. Centers for Disease Control and Prevention). 2021a. *COVID-19 vaccination coverage and vaccine confidence among children.* https://www.cdc.gov/vaccines/imz-managers/coverage/covidvaxview/interactive/children.html (accessed January 12, 2024).

CDC. 2021b. *IOM 2015 diagnostic criteria.* https://www.cdc.gov/me-cfs/healthcareproviders/diagnosis/iom-2015-diagnostic-criteria.html (accessed March 7, 2024).

CDC. 2021c. *Sexually transmitted infections treatment guidelines, 2021.* https://www.cdc.gov/std/treatment-guidelines/epididymitis.htm (accessed November 14, 2023).

CDC. 2023a. *Information for healthcare providers about multisystem inflammatory syndrome in children (MIS-C).* https://www.cdc.gov/mis/mis-c/hcp_cstecdc/index.html (accessed January 12, 2024).

CDC. 2023b. *Information for pediatric healthcare providers.* https://www.cdc.gov/coronavirus/2019-ncov/hcp/pediatric-hcp.html2021#PCCs (accessed January 12, 2024).

CDC. 2024. *Post-COVID conditions: Information for healthcare providers.* https://www.cdc.gov/coronavirus/2019-ncov/hcp/clinical-care/post-covid-conditions.html (accessed January 16, 2024).

Chang, R., T. Yen-Ting Chen, S. I. Wang, Y. M. Hung, H. Y. Chen, and C. J. Wei. 2023. Risk of autoimmune diseases in patients with COVID-19: A retrospective cohort study. *EClinicalMedicine* 56:101783.

Chen, E. Y., A. K. Morrow, and L. A. Malone. 2023. Exploring the influence of pre-existing conditions and infection factors on pediatric long COVID symptoms and quality of life. *American Journal of Physical Medicine and Rehabilitation* 103(7):567–574.

Cheng, A. L., J. Anderson, N. Didehbani, J. S. Fine, T. K. Fleming, R. Karnik, M. Longo, R. Ng, Y. Re'em, S. Sampsel, J. Shulman, J. K. Silver, J. Twaite, M. Verduzco-Gutierrez, and M. Kurylo. 2023. Multi-disciplinary collaborative consensus guidance statement on the assessment and treatment of mental health symptoms in patients with post-acute sequelae of SARS-CoV-2 infection (PASC). *PM&R* 15(12):1588–1604.

Cheung, J., K. Nordmeier, S. Kelland, M. Harrington, J. Williman, M. Storer, B. Beaglehole, L. Beckert, S. T. Chambers, M. J. Epton, J. Freeman, D. R. Murdoch, A. M. Werno, and M. J. Maze. 2023. Symptom persistence and recovery among COVID-19 survivors during a limited outbreak in Canterbury, New Zealand: A prospective cohort study. *Internal Medicine Journal* 53(1):37–45.

Chiabrando, J. G., A. Bonaventura, A. Vecchié, G. F. Wohlford, A. G. Mauro, J. H. Jordan, J. D. Grizzard, F. Montecucco, D. H. Berrocal, A. Brucato, M. Imazio, and A. Abbate. 2020. Management of acute and recurrent pericarditis. *Journal of the American College of Cardiology* 75(1):76–92.

Chu, L., I. J. Valencia, D. W. Garvert, and J. G. Montoya. 2018. Deconstructing post-exertional malaise in myalgic encephalomyelitis/chronic fatigue syndrome: A patient-centered, cross-sectional survey. *PLoS ONE* 13(6):e0197811.

Claar, R. L., and L. S. Walker. 2006. Functional assessment of pediatric pain patients: Psychometric properties of the functional disability inventory. *Pain* 121(1-2):77–84.

Cleveland Clinic. 2023. *Depression in children.* https://my.clevelandclinic.org/health/diseases/14938-depression-in-children (accessed October 10, 2023).

Cook, K. F., A. M. Bamer, D. Amtmann, I. R. Molton, and M. P. Jensen. 2012. Six Patient-Reported Outcome Measurement Information System short form measures have negligible age- or diagnosis-related differential item functioning in individuals with disabilities. *Archives of Physical Medicine and Rehabilitation* 93(7):1289–1291.

Cotler, J., C. Holtzman, C. Dudun, and L. A. Jason. 2018. A brief questionnaire to assess post-exertional malaise. *Diagnostics* 8(3):66.

Crawford, P., and E. E. Zimmerman. 2011. Differentiation and diagnosis of tremor. *American Family Physician* 83(6):697–702.

Cristillo, V., A. Pilotto, S. C. Piccinelli, S. Gipponi, M. Leonardi, M. Bezzi, and A. Padovani. 2022. Predictors of "brain fog" 1 year after COVID-19 disease. *Neurological Sciences* 43(10):5795–5797.

Crockett, S. D., S. Wani, T. B. Gardner, Y. Falck-Ytter, A. N. Barkun, S. Crockett, Y. Falck-Ytter, J. Feuerstein, S. Flamm, Z. Gellad, L. Gerson, S. Gupta, I. Hirano, J. Inadomi, G. C. Nguyen, J. H. Rubenstein, S. Singh, W. E. Smalley, N. Stollman, S. Street, S. Sultan, S. S. Vege, S. B. Wani, and D. Weinberg. 2018. American Gastroenterological Association institute guideline on initial management of acute pancreatitis. *Gastroenterology* 154(4):1096–1101.

D'Souza, D., J. Empringham, P. Pechlivanoglou, E. M. Uleryk, E. Cohen, and R. Shulman. 2023. Incidence of diabetes in children and adolescents during the COVID-19 pandemic: A systematic review and meta-analysis. *JAMA Network Open* 6(6): e2321281–e2321281.

Daines, L., B. Zheng, P. Pfeffer, J. R. Hurst, and A. Sheikh. 2022. A clinical review of long-COVID with a focus on the respiratory system. *Current Opinion in Pulmonary Medicine* 28(3):174–179.

Dalrymple, S. N., J. H. Row, and J. Gazewood. 2023. Bell palsy: Rapid evidence review. *American Family Physician* 107(4):415–420.

Davenport, T. E., S. R. Stevens, M. J. VanNess, C. R. Snell, and T. Little. 2010. Conceptual model for physical therapist management of chronic fatigue syndrome/myalgic encephalomyelitis. *Physical Therapy* 90(4):602–614.

Davenport, T. E., M. Lehnen, S. R. Stevens, J. M. VanNess, J. Stevens, and C. R. Snell. 2019. Chronotropic intolerance: An overlooked determinant of symptoms and activity limitation in myalgic encephalomyelitis/chronic fatigue syndrome? *Frontiers in Pediatrics* 7:82.

Davenport, T. E., S. R. Stevens, J. Stevens, C. R. Snell, and J. M. Van Ness. 2023. Development and measurement properties of the PEM/PESE Activity Questionnaire (PAQ). *Work* 74(4):1187–1197.

Davis, H. E., G. S. Assaf, L. McCorkell, H. Wei, R. J. Low, Y. Re'em, S. Redfield, J. P. Austin, and A. Akrami. 2021. Characterizing long COVID in an international cohort: 7 months of symptoms and their impact. *EClinicalMedicine* 38:101019.

Davis, H. E., L. McCorkell, J. M. Vogel, and E. J. Topol. 2023. Long COVID: Major findings, mechanisms and recommendations. *Nature Reviews Microbiology* 21(3):133–146.

Day, G. S., N. Scarmeas, R. Dubinsky, K. Coerver, A. Mostacero, B. West, S. R. Wessels, and M. J. Armstrong. 2022. Aducanumab use in symptomatic Alzheimer disease evidence in focus: A report of the AAN Guidelines Subcommittee. *Neurology* 98(15):619–631.

Degen, C. V., M. Mikuteit, J. Niewolik, D. Schröder, K. Vahldiek, U. Mücke, S. Heinemann, F. Müller, G. M. N. Behrens, and F. Klawonn. 2022. Self-reported tinnitus and vertigo or dizziness in a cohort of adult long COVID patients. *Frontiers in Neurology* 13:884002.

Delgado-Alonso, C., C. Cuevas, S. Oliver-Mas, M. Díez-Cirarda, A. Delgado-Álvarez, M. J. Gil-Moreno, J. Matías-Guiu, and J. A. Matias-Guiu. 2022. Fatigue and cognitive dysfunction are associated with occupational status in post-COVID syndrome. *International Journal of Environmental Research and Public Health* 19(20):13368.

Dent, E., J. E. Morley, A. J. Cruz-Jentoft, H. Arai, S. B. Kritchevsky, J. Guralnik, J. M. Bauer, M. Pahor, B. C. Clark, M. Cesari, J. Ruiz, C. C. Sieber, M. Aubertin-Leheudre, D. L. Waters, R. Visvanathan, F. Landi, D. T. Villareal, R. Fielding, C. W. Won, O. Theou, F. C. Martin, B. Dong, J. Woo, L. Flicker, L. Ferrucci, R. A. Merchant, L. Cao, T. Cederholm, S. M. L. Ribeiro, L. Rodríguez-Mañas, S. D. Anker, J. Lundy, L. M. Gutiérrez Robledo, I. Bautmans, I. Aprahamian, J. Schols, M. Izquierdo, and B. Vellas. 2018. International clinical practice guidelines for sarcopenia (ICFSR): Screening, diagnosis and management. *Journal of Health and Aging* 22(10):1148–1161.

DePace, N. L., and J. Colombo. 2022. Long-COVID syndrome and the cardiovascular system: A review of neurocardiologic effects on multiple systems. *Current Cardiology Reports* 24(11):1711–1726.

Dhooria, S., S. Chaudhary, I. S. Sehgal, R. Agarwal, S. Arora, M. Garg, N. Prabhakar, G. D. Puri, A. Bhalla, V. Suri, L. N. Yaddanapudi, V. Muthu, K. T. Prasad, and A. N. Aggarwal. 2022. High-dose *versus* low-dose prednisolone in symptomatic patients with post-COVID-19 diffuse parenchymal lung abnormalities: An open-label, randomised trial (the COLDSTER trial). *European Respiratory Journal* 59(2):2102930.

Diekman, S., and T. Chung. 2023. Post-acute sequelae of SARS-CoV-2 syndrome presenting as postural orthostatic tachycardia syndrome. *Clinical and Experimental Emergency Medicine* 10(1):18–25.

Drogalis-Kim, D., C. Kramer, and S. Duran. 2022. Ongoing dizziness following acute COVID-19 infection: A single center pediatric case series. *Pediatrics* 150(2):e2022056860.

Dubey, S., S. Das, R. Ghosh, M. J. Dubey, A. P. Chakraborty, D. Roy, G. Das, A. Dutta, A. Santra, S. Sengupta, and J. Benito-León. 2023. The effects of SARS-CoV-2 infection on the cognitive functioning of patients with pre-existing dementia. *Journal of Alzheimers Disease Reports* 7(1):119–128.

Durstenfeld, M. S., K. Sun, P. Tahir, M. J. Peluso, S. G. Deeks, M. A. Aras, D. J. Grandis, C. S. Long, A. Beatty, and P. Y. Hsue. 2022. Use of cardiopulmonary exercise testing to evaluate long COVID-19 symptoms in adults: A systematic review and meta-analysis. *JAMA Network Open* 5(10):e2236057.

EASL (European Association for the Study of the Liver). 2009. EASL clinical practice guidelines: Management of cholestatic liver diseases. *Journal of Hepatology* 51(2):237–267.

Elmunzer, B. J., J. L. Maranki, V. Gómez, A. Tavakkoli, B. G. Sauer, B. N. Limketkai, E. A. Brennan, E. M. Attridge, T. J. Brigham, and A. Y. Wang. 2023. ACG clinical guideline: Diagnosis and management of biliary strictures. *American Journal of Gastroenterology* 118(3):405–426.

El-Rhermoul, F. Z., A. Fedorowski, P. Eardley, P. Taraborrelli, D. Panagopoulos, R. Sutton, P. B. Lim, and M. Dani. 2023. Autoimmunity in long COVID and POTS. *Oxford Open Immunology* 4(1):iqad002.

ElSayed, N. A., G. Aleppo, V. R. Aroda, R. R. Bannuru, F. M. Brown, D. Bruemmer, B. S. Collins, J. L. Gaglia, M. E. Hilliard, D. Isaacs, E. L. Johnson, S. Kahan, K. Khunti, J. Leon, S. K. Lyons, M. L. Perry, P. Prahalad, R. E. Pratley, J. J. Seley, R. C. Stanton, and R. A. Gabbay, on behalf of the American Diabetes Association. 2023. 2. Classification and diagnosis of diabetes: *Standards of care in diabetes—2023*. *Diabetes Care* 46(Supplement 1):S19–S40.

ENTHealth. 2020. *Dysgeusia.* https://www.enthealth.org/conditions/dysgeusia/ (accessed December 5, 2023).

Espinosa-Gonzalez, A. B., H. Master, N. Gall, S. Halpin, N. Rogers, and T. Greenhalgh. 2023. Orthostatic tachycardia after COVID-19. *BMJ* 380:e073488.

EuroQol Group. 1990. EuroQol—A new facility for the measurement of health-related quality of life. *Health Policy* 16(3):199–208.

Evans, R. A., H. McAuley, E. M. Harrison, A. Shikotra, A. Singapuri, M. Sereno, O. Elneima, A. B. Docherty, N. I. Lone, O. C. Leavy, L. Daines, J. K. Baillie, J. S. Brown, T. Chalder, A. De Soyza, N. Diar Bakerly, N. Easom, J. R. Geddes, N. J. Greening, N. Hart, L. G. Heaney, S. Heller, L. Howard, J. R. Hurst, J. Jacob, R. G. Jenkins, C. Jolley, S. Kerr, O. M. Kon, K. Lewis, J. M. Lord, G. P. McCann, S. Neubauer, P. J. M. Openshaw, D. Parekh, P. Pfeffer, N. M. Rahman, B. Raman, M. Richardson, M. Rowland, M. G. Semple, A. M. Shah, S. J. Singh, A. Sheikh, D. Thomas, M. Toshner, J. D. Chalmers, L.-P. Ho, A. Horsley, M. Marks, K. Poinasamy, L. V. Wain, C. E. Brightling, on behalf of the PHOSP-COVID Collaborative Group. 2021. Physical, cognitive, and mental health impacts of COVID-19 after hospitalisation (PHOSP-COVID): A UK multicentre, prospective cohort study. *The Lancet Respiratory Medicine* 9(11):1275–1287.

Evans, R., A. Pick, R. Lardner, V. Masey, N. Smith, and T. Greenhalgh. 2023. Breathing difficulties after COVID-19: A guide for primary care. *BMJ* 381:e074937.

Evers, G., A. B. Schulze, I. Osiaevi, K. Harmening, R. Vollenberg, R. Wiewrodt, R. Pistulli, M. Boentert, P.-R. Tepasse, and J. R. Sindermann. 2022. Sustained impairment in cardiopulmonary exercise capacity testing in patients after COVID-19: A single center experience. *Canadian Respiratory Journal* 2022:2466789.

Expert Panel Working Group of the National Heart, Lung, and Blood Institute (NHLBI) administered and coordinated National Asthma Education and Prevention Program Coordinating Committee (NAEPPCC), M. M. Cloutier, A. P. Baptist, K. V. Blake, E. G. Brooks, T. Bryant-Stephens, E. DiMango, A. E. Dixon, K. S. Elward, T. Hartert, and J. A. Krishnan. 2020. 2020 focused updates to the asthma management guidelines: A report from the National Asthma Education and Prevention Program Coordinating Committee Expert Panel Working Group. *Journal of Allergy and Clinical Immunology* 146(6):1217–1270.

FACIT Group. 2021. *Functional assessment of chronic illness therapy—Fatigue*. https://www.facit.org/measures/facit-f (accessed March 22, 2024).

Farias, S. T., D. Mungas, B. R. Reed, D. Cahn-Weiner, W. Jagust, K. Baynes, and C. Decarli. 2008. The measurement of everyday cognition (ECog): Scale development and psychometric properties. *Neuropsychology* 22(4):531–544.

Fedorowski, A. 2019. Postural orthostatic tachycardia syndrome: Clinical presentation, aetiology and management. *Journal of Internal Medicine* 285(4):352–366.

Feldstein, L. R., M. W. Tenforde, K. G. Friedman, M. Newhams, E. B. Rose, H. Dapul, V. L. Soma, A. B. Maddux, P. M. Mourani, and C. Bowens. 2021. Characteristics and outcomes of U.S. children and adolescents with multisystem inflammatory syndrome in children (MIS-C) compared with severe acute COVID-19. *JAMA* 325(11):1074–1087.

Ferreira, J. J., T. A. Mestre, K. E. Lyons, J. Benito-León, E. K. Tan, G. Abbruzzese, M. Hallett, D. Haubenberger, R. Elble, and G. Deuschl. 2019. MDS evidence-based review of treatments for essential tremor. *Movement Disorders* 34(7):950–958.

Ferrulli, A., P. Senesi, I. Terruzzi, and L. Luzi. 2022. Eating habits and body weight changes induced by variation in smell and taste in patients with previous SARS-CoV-2 infection. *Nutrients* 14(23):5068.

Fine, J. S., A. F. Ambrose, N. Didehbani, T. K. Fleming, L. Glashan, M. Longo, A. Merlino, R. Ng, G. J. Nora, and S. Rolin. 2022. Multi-disciplinary collaborative consensus guidance statement on the assessment and treatment of cognitive symptoms in patients with post-acute sequelae of SARS-CoV-2 infection (PASC). *PM&R* 14(1):96–111.

Fischer, A., N. Badier, L. Zhang, A. Elbéji, P. Wilmes, P. Oustric, C. Benoy, M. Ollert, and G. Fagherazzi. 2022. Long COVID classification: Findings from a clustering analysis in the Predi-COVID cohort study. *International Journal of Environmental Research Public Health* 19(23):16018.

Ford, B., M. Dore, and E. Harris. 2021. Outpatient Primary Care Management of Headaches: Guidelines from the VA/DoD. *American Family Physician* 104(3):316–320.

Fowlkes, A. L., S. K. Yoon, K. Lutrick, L. Gwynn, J. Burns, L. Grant, A. L. Phillips, K. Ellingson, M. V. Ferraris, and L. B. LeClair. 2022. Effectiveness of 2-dose BNT162b2 (Pfizer BioN-Tech) mRNA vaccine in preventing SARS-CoV-2 infection among children aged 5–11 years and adolescents aged 12–15 years—Protect cohort, July 2021–February 2022. *MMWR Morbidity and Mortality Weekly Report* 71(11):422.

Fraenkel, L., J. M. Bathon, B. R. England, E. W. St Clair, T. Arayssi, K. Carandang, K. D. Deane, M. Genovese, K. K. Huston, G. Kerr, J. Kremer, M. C. Nakamura, L. A. Russell, J. A. Singh, B. J. Smith, J. A. Sparks, S. Venkatachalam, M. E. Weinblatt, M. Al-Gibbawi, J. F. Baker, K. E. Barbour, J. L. Barton, L. Cappelli, F. Chamseddine, M. George, S. R. Johnson, L. Kahale, B. S. Karam, A. M. Khamis, I. Navarro-Millán, R. Mirza, P. Schwab, N. Singh, M. Turgunbaev, A. S. Turner, S. Yaacoub, and E. A. Akl. 2021. 2021 American College of Rheumatology guideline for the treatment of rheumatoid arthritis. *Arthritis Care and Research* 73(7):924–939.

Freeman, E. E., I. Garcia-Doval, L. Naldi, and R. J. Hay. 2023. Three years on, COVID-19 and the skin: Long-term impacts, emerging trends and clinical practice. *British Journal of Dermatology* 189(1):1–3.

Frontera, J. A., L. E. Thorpe, N. M. Simon, A. de Havenon, S. Yaghi, S. B. Sabadia, D. Yang, A. Lewis, K. Melmed, L. J. Balcer, T. Wisniewski, and S. L. Galetta. 2022. Post-acute sequelae of COVID-19 symptom phenotypes and therapeutic strategies: A prospective, observational study. *PLoS ONE* 17(9):e0275274.

Funk, A. L., N. Kuppermann, T. A. Florin, D. J. Tancredi, J. Xie, K. Kim, Y. Finkelstein, M. I. Neuman, M. I. Salvadori, A. Yock-Corrales, K. A. Breslin, L. Ambroggio, P. P. Chaudhari, K. R. Bergmann, M. A. Gardiner, J. R. Nebhrajani, C. Campos, F. A. Ahmad, L. F. Sartori, N. Navanandan, N. Kannikeswaran, K. Caperell, C. R. Morris, S. Mintegi, I. Gangoiti,

V. J. Sabhaney, A. C. Plint, T. P. Klassen, U. R. Avva, N. P. Shah, A. C. Dixon, M. M. Lunoe, S. M. Becker, A. J. Rogers, V. Pavlicich, S. R. Dalziel, D. C. Payne, R. Malley, M. L. Borland, A. K. Morrison, M. Bhatt, P. B. Rino, I. Beneyto Ferre, M. Eckerle, A. J. Kam, S. L. Chong, L. Palumbo, M. Y. Kwok, J. C. Cherry, N. Poonai, M. Waseem, N. J. Simon, and S. B. Freedman, for the Pediatric Emergency Research Network–COVID-19 Study Team. 2022. Post-COVID-19 conditions among children 90 days after SARS-CoV-2 infection. *JAMA Network Open* 5(7):e2223253.

Fu, Q., and Levine, B. D. Exercise and non-pharmacological treatment of POTS. *Autonomic Neuroscience* 215:20–27.

Gao, P., J. Liu, and M. Liu. 2022. Effect of COVID-19 vaccines on reducing the risk of long COVID in the real world: A systematic review and meta-analysis. *International Journal of Environmental Research and Public Health* 19(19):12422.

Geerts, M., J. G. J. Hoeijmakers, C. M. L. Gorissen-Brouwers, C. G. Faber, and I. S. J. Merkies. 2023. Small fiber neuropathy: A clinical and practical approach. *Journal for Nurse Practitioners* 19(4):104547.

Georgesen, C., L. P. Fox, and J. Harp. 2020. Retiform purpura: A diagnostic approach. *Journal of the American Academy of Dermatology* 82(4):783–796.

Gibbs, M. B., J. C. English, and M. J. Zirwas. 2005. Livedo reticularis: An update. *Journal of the American Academy of Dermatology* 52(6):1009–1019.

Goel, N., N. Goyal, R. Nagaraja, and R. Kumar. 2021. Systemic corticosteroids for management of "long-COVID": An evaluation after 3 months of treatment. *Monaldi Archives for Chest Disease* 92(2). https://doi.org/10.4081/monaldi.2021.1981 (accessed April 29, 2024).

Goldhaber, N. H., J. N. Kohn, W. S. Ogan, A. Sitapati, C. A. Longhurst, A. Wang, S. Lee, S. Hong, and L. E. Horton. 2022. Deep dive into the long haul: Analysis of symptom clusters and risk factors for post-acute sequelae of COVID-19 to inform clinical care. *International Journal of Environmental Research and Public Health* 19(24):16841.

Gole, S., and A. Anand. 2023. Autoimmune encephalitis. In *StatPearls*. Treasure Island, FL: StatPearls Publishing.

Grover, A., F. Choi, and S. Pei-Wang. 2022. 33624 Long-term cutaneous manifestations in COVID-19 patients: A systematic review. *Journal of the American Academy of Dermatology* 87(3):AB76.

Grach, S. L., J. Seltzer, T. Y. Chon, and R. Ganesh. 2023. Diagnosis and management of myalgic encephalomyelitis/chronic fatigue syndrome. *Mayo Clinic Proceedings* 98(10): 1544–1551.

Grundy, S. M., N. J. Stone, A. L. Bailey, C. Beam, K. K. Birtcher, R. S. Blumenthal, L. T. Braun, S. De Ferranti, J. Faiella-Tommasino, D. E. Forman, R. Goldberg, P. A. Heidenreich, M. A. Hlatky, D. W. Jones, D. Lloyd-Jones, N. Lopez-Pajares, C. E. Ndumele, C. E. Orringer, C. A. Peralta, J. J. Saseen, S. C. Smith, L. Sperling, S. S. Virani, and J. Yeboah. 2019. 2018 AHA/ACC/AACVPR/AAPA/ABC/ACPM/ADA/AGS/APHA/ASPC/NLA/PCNA guideline on the management of blood cholesterol: A report of the American College of Cardiology/American Heart Association Task Force on Clinical Practice Guidelines. *Circulation* 139:e1082–e1143.

Gülen, T., C. Akin, P. Bonadonna, F. Siebenhaar, S. Broesby-Olsen, K. Brockow, M. Niedoszytko, B. Nedoszytko, H. N. G. Oude Elberink, J. H. Butterfield, W. R. Sperr, I. Alvarez-Twose, H.-P. Horny, K. Sotlar, J. Schwaab, M. Jawhar, R. Zanotti, G. Nilsson, J. J. Lyons, M. C. Carter, T. I. George, O. Hermine, J. Gotlib, A. Orfao, M. Triggiani, A. Reiter, K. Hartmann, M. Castells, M. Arock, L. B. Schwartz, D. D. Metcalfe, and P. Valent. 2021. Selecting the right criteria and proper classification to diagnose mast cell activation syndromes: A critical review. *Journal of Allergy and Clinical Immunology: In Practice* 9(11):3918–3928.

Haloot, J., M. Kabbani, M. Verduzco-Gutierrez, R. Bhavaraju-Sanka, and J. Pillarisetti. 2022. CE-541-02 post-COVID and postural orthostatic tachycardia syndrome. *Heart Rhythm* 19(5):S54.

Harrison, P. J., and M. Taquet. 2023. Neuropsychiatric disorders following SARS-CoV-2 infection. *Brain* 146(6):2241–2247.

Hartung, T. J., C. Neumann, T. Bahmer, I. Chaplinskaya-Sobol, M. Endres, J. Geritz, K. G. Haeusler, P. U. Heuschmann, H. Hildesheim, A. Hinz, S. Hopff, A. Horn, M. Krawczak, L. Krist, J. Kudelka, W. Lieb, C. Maetzler, A. Mehnert-Theuerkauf, F. A. Montellano, C. Morbach, S. Schmidt, S. Schreiber, F. Steigerwald, S. Störk, W. Maetzler, and C. Finke. 2022. Fatigue and cognitive impairment after COVID-19: A prospective multicentre study. *EClinicalMedicine* 53:101651.

Harvey, P. D. 2012. Clinical applications of neuropsychological assessment. *Dialogues in Clinical Neuroscience* 14(1):91–99.

Heidenreich, P. A., B. Bozkurt, D. Aguilar, L. A. Allen, J. J. Byun, M. M. Colvin, A. Deswal, M. H. Drazner, S. M. Dunlay, L. R. Evers, J. C. Fang, S. E. Fedson, G. C. Fonarow, S. S. Hayek, A. F. Hernandez, P. Khazanie, M. M. Kittleson, C. S. Lee, M. S. Link, C. A. Milano, L. C. Nnacheta, A. T. Sandhu, L. W. Stevenson, O. Vardeny, A. R. Vest, and C. W. Yancy. 2022. 2022 AHA/ACC/HFSA guideline for the management of heart failure: A report of the American College of Cardiology/American Heart Association Joint Committee on Clinical Practice Guidelines. *Circulation* 145:e876–e894.

Hentschel, C. B., B. A. Abramoff, T. R. Dillingham, and L. E. Pezzin. 2022. Race, ethnicity, and utilization of outpatient rehabilitation for treatment of post COVID-19 condition. *PM&R* 14(11):1315–1324.

Herrera, J. E., W. N. Niehaus, J. Whiteson, A. Azola, J. M. Baratta, T. K. Fleming, S. Y. Kim, H. Naqvi, S. Sampsel, J. K. Silver, M. Verduzco-Gutierrez, J. Maley, E. Herman, and B. Abramoff. 2021. Multidisciplinary collaborative consensus guidance statement on the assessment and treatment of fatigue in postacute sequelae of SARS-CoV-2 infection (PASC) patients. *PM&R* 13(9):1027–1043.

Ho, F. F., S. Xu, T. M. H. Kwong, A. S. Li, E. H. Ha, H. Hua, C. Liong, K. C. Leung, T. H. Leung, Z. Lin, S. Y. Wong, F. Pan, and V. C. H. Chung. 2023. Prevalence, patterns, and clinical severity of long COVID among Chinese medicine telemedicine service users: Preliminary results from a cross-sectional study. *International Journal of Environmental Research and Public Health* 20(3):1827.

Holguin, F., J. C. Cardet, K. F. Chung, S. Diver, D. S. Ferreira, A. Fitzpatrick, M. Gaga, L. Kellermeyer, S. Khurana, S. Knight, V. M. McDonald, R. L. Morgan, V. E. Ortega, D. Rigau, P. Subbarao, T. Tonia, I. M. Adcock, E. R. Bleecker, C. Brightling, L.-P. Boulet, M. Cabana, M. Castro, P. Chanez, A. Custovic, R. Djukanovic, U. Frey, B. Frankemölle, P. Gibson, D. Hamerlijnck, N. Jarjour, S. Konno, H. Shen, C. Vitary, and A. Bush. 2020. Management of severe asthma: A European Respiratory Society/American Thoracic Society guideline. *European Respiratory Journal* 55(1):1900588.

Hopkins, C., M. Alanin, C. Philpott, P. Harries, K. Whitcroft, A. Qureishi, S. Anari, Y. Ramakrishnan, A. Sama, E. Davies, B. Stew, S. Gane, S. Carrie, I. Hathorn, R. Bhalla, C. Kelly, N. Hill, D. Boak, and B. Nirmal Kumar. 2021. Management of new onset loss of sense of smell during the COVID-19 pandemic—BRS consensus guidelines. *Clinical Otolaryngology* 46(1):16–22.

Hughes, R., E. Wijdicks, R. Barohn, E. Benson, D. Cornblath, A. F. Hahn, J. Meythaler, R. Miller, J. Sladky, and J. Stevens. 2003. Practice parameter: Immunotherapy for Guillain-Barré syndrome: Report of the Quality Standards Subcommittee of the American Academy of Neurology. *Neurology* 61(6):736–740.

Humbert, M., G. Kovacs, M. M. Hoeper, R. Badagliacca, R. M. F. Berger, M. Brida, J. Carlsen, A. J. S. Coats, P. Escribano-Subias, P. Ferrari, D. S. Ferreira, H. A. Ghofrani, G. Giannakoulas, D. G. Kiely, E. Mayer, G. Meszaros, B. Nagavci, K. M. Olsson, J. Pepke-Zaba, J. K.

Quint, G. Rådegran, G. Simonneau, O. Sitbon, T. Tonia, M. Toshner, J. L. Vachiery, A. Vonk Noordegraaf, M. Delcroix, S. Rosenkranz, on behalf of ESC/ERS Scientific Document Group. 2022. 2022 ESC/ERS guidelines for the diagnosis and treatment of pulmonary hypertension. *European Heart Journal* 43(38):3618–3731.

IOM (Institute of Medicine). 2015. *Beyond myalgic encephalomyelitis/chronic fatigue syndrome: Redefining an illness*. Washington, DC: The National Academies Press.

Isaac, R. O., J. Corrado, and M. Sivan. 2023. Detecting orthostatic intolerance in long COVID in a clinic setting. *International Journal of Environmental Research and Public Health* 20(10):5804.

Jacobs, M. M., E. Evans, and C. Ellis. 2023. Racial, ethnic, and sex disparities in the incidence and cognitive symptomology of long COVID-19. *Journal of the National Medical Association* 115(2):233–243.

Jafari, Z., B. E. Kolb, and M. H. Mohajerani. 2022. Hearing loss, tinnitus, and dizziness in COVID-19: A systematic review and meta-analysis. *Canadian Journal of Neurological Sciences* 49(2):184–195.

Jennings, G., A. Monaghan, F. Xue, E. Duggan, and R. Romero-Ortuño. 2022. Comprehensive clinical characterisation of brain fog in adults reporting long COVID symptoms. *Journal of Clinical Medicine* 11(12):3440.

Jiang, L., X. Li, J. Nie, K. Tang, and Z. A. Bhutta. 2023. A systematic review of persistent clinical features after SARS-CoV-2 in the pediatric population. *Pediatrics* 152(2):e2022060351.

Kandemir, H., G. A. Bülbül, E. Kirtiş, S. Güney, C. Y. Sanhal, and İ. Mendilcioğlu. 2024. Evaluation of long-COVID symptoms in women infected with SARS-CoV-2 during pregnancy. *International Journal of Gynaecology and Obstetrics* 164(1):148–156.

Kavi, L. 2022. Postural tachycardia syndrome and long COVID: An update. *British Journal of General Practice* 72(714):8–9.

Kayaaslan, B., F. Eser, A. K. Kalem, G. Kaya, B. Kaplan, D. Kacar, I. Hasanoglu, B. Coskun, and R. Guner. 2021. Post-COVID syndrome: A single-center questionnaire study on 1007 participants recovered from COVID-19. *Journal of Medical Virology* 93(12):6566–6574.

KDIGO (Kidney Disease Improving Global Outcomes). 2012. KDIGO clinical practice guideline for acute kidney injury. *Official Journal of the International Society of Nephrology* 2(1).

KDIGO. 2013. KDIGO clinical practice guideline for the evaluation and management of chronic kidney disease. *Kidney International Supplements* 3:1–150.

Kenny, G., K. McCann, C. O'Brien, S. Savinelli, W. Tinago, O. Yousif, J. S. Lambert, C. O'Broin, E. R. Feeney, E. De Barra, P. Doran, and P. W. G. Mallon. 2022. Identification of distinct long COVID clinical phenotypes through cluster analysis of self-reported symptoms. *Open Forum of Infectious Diseases* 9(4):ofac060.

Khani, E., S. Khiali, S. Beheshtirouy, and T. Entezari-Maleki. 2021. Potential pharmacologic treatments for COVID-19 smell and taste loss: A comprehensive review. *European Journal of Pharmacology* 912:174582.

Kim, Y., S. E. Kim, T. Kim, K. W. Yun, S. H. Lee, E. Lee, J.-W. Seo, Y. H. Jung, and Y. P. Chong. 2022. Preliminary guidelines for the clinical evaluation and management of long COVID. *Infection & Chemotherapy* 54(3):566.

King, L. S. 1968. Signs and symptoms. *JAMA* 206(5):1063–1065.

Kiriyama, S., K. Kozaka, T. Takada, S. M. Strasberg, H. A. Pitt, T. Gabata, J. Hata, K. H. Liau, F. Miura, A. Horiguchi, K. H. Liu, C. H. Su, K. Wada, P. Jagannath, T. Itoi, D. J. Gouma, Y. Mori, S. Mukai, M. E. Giménez, W. S. W. Huang, M. H. Kim, K. Okamoto, G. Belli, C. Dervenis, A. C. W. Chan, W. Y. Lau, I. Endo, H. Gomi, M. Yoshida, T. Mayumi, T. H. Baron, E. De Santibañes, A. Y. B. Teoh, T. L. Hwang, C. G. Ker, M. F. Chen, H. S. Han, Y. S. Yoon, I. S. Choi, D. S. Yoon, R. Higuchi, S. Kitano, M. Inomata, D. J. Deziel, E. Jonas, K. Hirata, Y. Sumiyama, K. Inui, and M. Yamamoto. 2018. Tokyo guidelines 2018: Diagnostic criteria and severity grading of acute cholangitis (with videos). *Journal of Hepato-Biliary-Pancreatic Sciences* 25(1):17–30.

Kisiel, M. A., S. Lee, S. Malmquist, O. Rykatkin, S. Holgert, H. Janols, C. Janson, and X. Zhou. 2023. Clustering analysis identified three long COVID phenotypes and their association with general health status and working ability. *Journal of Clinical Medicine* 12(11):3617.

Klein, J., J. Wood, J. R. Jaycox, R. M. Dhodapkar, P. Lu, J. R. Gehlhausen, A. Tabachnikova, K. Greene, L. Tabacof, A. A. Malik, V. Silva Monteiro, J. Silva, K. Kamath, M. Zhang, A. Dhal, I. M. Ott, G. Valle, M. Peña-Hernández, T. Mao, B. Bhattacharjee, T. Takahashi, C. Lucas, E. Song, D. McCarthy, E. Breyman, J. Tosto-Mancuso, Y. Dai, E. Perotti, K. Akduman, T. J. Tzeng, L. Xu, A. C. Geraghty, M. Monje, I. Yildirim, J. Shon, R. Medzhitov, D. Lutchman-singh, J. D. Possick, N. Kaminski, S. B. Omer, H. M. Krumholz, L. Guan, C. S. Dela Cruz, D. van Dijk, A. M. Ring, D. Putrino, and A. Iwasaki. 2023. Distinguishing features of long COVID identified through immune profiling. *Nature* 623(7985):139–148.

Knight, M., K. Bunch, N. Vousden, E. Morris, N. Simpson, C. Gale, P. O'Brien, M. Quigley, P. Brocklehurst, and J. J. Kurinczuk, on behalf of the UK Obstetric Surveillance System SARS-CoV-2 Infection in Pregnancy Collaborative Group. 2020. Characteristics and outcomes of pregnant women admitted to hospital with confirmed SARS-CoV-2 infection in UK: National population based cohort study. *BMJ* 369:m2107.

Kolasinski, S. L., T. Neogi, M. C. Hochberg, C. Oatis, G. Guyatt, J. Block, L. Callahan, C. Copenhaver, C. Dodge, D. Felson, K. Gellar, W. F. Harvey, G. Hawker, E. Herzig, C. K. Kwoh, A. E. Nelson, J. Samuels, C. Scanzello, D. White, B. Wise, R. D. Altman, D. DiRenzo, J. Fontanarosa, G. Giradi, M. Ishimori, D. Misra, A. A. Shah, A. K. Shmagel, L. M. Thoma, M. Turgunbaev, A. S. Turner, and J. Reston. 2020. 2019 American College of Rheumatology/Arthritis Foundation guideline for the management of osteoarthritis of the hand, hip, and knee. *Arthritis Care and Research* 72(2):149–162.

Kompaniyets, L., L. Bull-Otterson, T. K. Boehmer, S. Baca, P. Alvarez, K. Hong, J. Hsu, A. M. Harris, A. V. Gundlapalli, and S. Saydah. 2022. Post-COVID-19 symptoms and conditions among children and adolescents–United States, March 1, 2020–January 31, 2022. *MMWR Morbidity & Mortality Weekly Report* 71(31):993–999.

Kostev, K., L. Smith, A. Koyanagi, M. Konrad, and L. Jacob. 2022. Post-COVID-19 conditions in children and adolescents diagnosed with COVID-19. *Pediatric Research* 95(1):182–187.

Krupp, L. B., N. G. LaRocca, J. Muir-Nash, and A. D. Steinberg. 1989. The Fatigue Severity Scale: Application to patients with multiple sclerosis and systemic lupus erythematosus. *Archives of Neurology* 46(10):1121–1123.

Kusumoto, F. M., M. H. Schoenfeld, C. Barrett, J. R. Edgerton, K. A. Ellenbogen, M. R. Gold, N. F. Goldschlager, R. M. Hamilton, J. A. Joglar, and R. J. Kim. 2019. 2018 ACC/AHA/HRS guideline on the evaluation and management of patients with bradycardia and cardiac conduction delay: A report of the American College of Cardiology/American Heart Association Task Force on Clinical Practice Guidelines and the Heart Rhythm Society. *Journal of the American College of Cardiology* 74(7):e51–e156.

Kwo, P. Y., S. M. Cohen, and J. K. Lim. 2017. ACG clinical guideline: Evaluation of abnormal liver chemistries. *Official Journal of the American College of Gastroenterology* 112(1):18–35.

Lacy, B. E., M. Pimentel, D. M. Brenner, W. D. Chey, L. A. Keefer, M. D. Long, and B. Moshiree. 2021. ACG clinical guideline: Management of irritable bowel syndrome. *Official Journal of the American College of Gastroenterology* 116(1):17–44.

Lacy, B. E., J. Tack, and C. P. Gyawali. 2022. AGA clinical practice update on management of medically refractory gastroparesis: Expert review. *Clinical Gastroenterology and Hepatology* 20(3):491–500.

Ladlow, P., O. O'Sullivan, A. Houston, R. Barker-Davies, S. May, D. Mills, D. Dewson, R. Chamley, J. Naylor, J. Mulae, A. N. Bennett, E. D. Nicol, and D. A. Holdsworth. 2022. Dysautonomia following COVID-19 is not associated with subjective limitations or symptoms but is associated with objective functional limitations. *Heart Rhythm* 19(4):613–620.

Lai, C. C., C. K. Hsu, M. Y. Yen, P. I. Lee, W. C. Ko, and P. R. Hsueh. 2023. Long COVID: An inevitable sequela of SARS-CoV-2 infection. *Journal of Microbiology, Immunology, and Infection* 56(1):1–9.

Larsen, N. W., L. E. Stiles, and M. G. Miglis. 2021. Preparing for the long-haul: Autonomic complications of COVID-19. *Autonomic Neuroscience* 235:102841.

Larsen, N. W., L. E. Stiles, R. Shaik, L. Schneider, S. Muppidi, C. T. Tsui, L. N. Geng, H. Bonilla, and M. G. Miglis. 2022. Characterization of autonomic symptom burden in long COVID: A global survey of 2,314 adults. *Frontiers in Neurology* 13:1012668.

Larson, S. T., and J. Wilbur. 2020. Muscle weakness in adults: Evaluation and differential diagnosis. *American Family Physician* 101(2):95–108.

Leftin Dobkin, S. C., J. M. Collaco, and S. A. McGrath-Morrow. 2021. Protracted respiratory findings in children post-SARS-CoV-2 infection. *Pediatric Pulmonology* 56(12): 3682–3687.

Ley, H., Z. Skorniewska, P. J. Harrison, and M. Taquet. 2023. Risks of neurological and psychiatric sequelae 2 years after hospitalisation or intensive care admission with COVID-19 compared to admissions for other causes. *Brain, Behavior, and Immunity* 112:85–95.

Li, R., M. Shen, Q. Yang, C. K. Fairley, Z. Chai, R. McIntyre, J. J. Ong, H. Liu, P. Lu, W. Hu, Z. Zou, Z. Li, S. He, G. Zhuang, and L. Zhang. 2023. Global diabetes prevalence in COVID-19 patients and contribution to COVID-19-related severity and mortality: A systematic review and meta-analysis. *Diabetes Care* 46(4):890–897.

Lightner, D. J., A. Gomelsky, L. Souter, and S. P. Vasavada. 2019. Diagnosis and treatment of overactive bladder (non-neurogenic) in adults: AUA/SUFU guideline amendment 2019. *Journal of Urology* 202(3):558–563.

Lim, S. H., H. J. Ju, J. H. Han, J. H. Lee, W.-S. Lee, J. M. Bae, and S. Lee. 2023. Autoimmune and autoinflammatory connective tissue disorders following COVID-19. *JAMA Network Open* 6(10):e2336120.

Lindor, K. D., C. L. Bowlus, J. Boyer, C. Levy, and M. Mayo. 2022. Primary biliary cholangitis: 2021 practice guidance update from the American Association for the Study of Liver Diseases. *Hepatology* 75(4):1012–1013.

Líška, D., E. Liptaková, A. Babičová, L. Batalik, P. S. Baňárová, and S. Dobrodenková. 2022. What is the quality of life in patients with long COVID compared to a healthy control group? *Frontiers in Public Health* 10:975992.

Liu, L. W. C., C. N. Andrews, D. Armstrong, N. Diamant, N. Jaffer, A. Lazarescu, M. Li, R. Martino, W. Paterson, G. I. Leontiadis, and F. Tse. 2018. Clinical practice guidelines for the assessment of uninvestigated esophageal dysphagia. *Journal of the Canadian Association of Gastroenterology* 1(1):5–19.

Long COVID and kids: More research is urgently needed. 2022. *Nature* 602(7896):183–183.

Lopez-Leon, S., T. Wegman-Ostrosky, N. C. Ayuzo del Valle, C. Perelman, R. Sepulveda, P. A. Rebolledo, A. Cuapio, and S. Villapol. 2022. Long-COVID in children and adolescents: A systematic review and meta-analyses. *Scientific Reports* 12(1):9950.

Lott, N., C. E. Gebhard, S. Bengs, A. Haider, G. M. Kuster, V. Regitz-Zagrosek, and C. Gebhard. 2023. Sex hormones in SARS-CoV-2 susceptibility: Key players or confounders? *Nature Review Endocrinology* 19(4):217–231.

Lu, L. 2022. Guidelines for the management of cholestatic liver diseases (2021). *Journal of Clinical and Translational Hepatology* 10(4):757–769.

Lubell, J. 2022. *Long COVID: Over 200 symptoms, and a search for guidance.* American Medical Association. https://www.ama-assn.org/delivering-care/public-health/long-covid-over-200-symptoms-and-search-guidance (accessed September 6, 2023).

Luedke, J. C., G. Vargas, D. T. Jashar, A. Morrow, L. A. Malone, and R. Ng. 2024. Cognitive disengagement syndrome in pediatric patients with long COVID: Associations with mood, anxiety, and functional impairment. *Child Neuropsychology* 30(4):652–672.

Lui, D. T. W., K. H. Tsoi, C. H. Lee, C. Y. Y. Cheung, C. H. Y. Fong, A. C. H. Lee, A. R. Tam, P. Pang, T. Y. Ho, C. Y. Law, C. W. Lam, K. K. W. To, W. S. Chow, Y. C. Woo, I. F. N. Hung, K. C. B. Tan, and K. S. L. Lam. 2023. A prospective follow-up on thyroid function, thyroid autoimmunity and long COVID among 250 COVID-19 survivors. *Endocrine* 80(2):380–391.

Lynch, S., S. J. Ferrando, R. Dornbush, S. Shahar, A. Smiley, and L. Klepacz. 2022. Screening for brain fog: Is the Montreal Cognitive Assessment an effective screening tool for neurocognitive complaints post-COVID-19? *General Hospital Psychiatry* 78:80–86.

MacDonald Hull, S. P., M. L. Wood, P. E. Hutchinson, M. Sladden, and A. G. Messenger. 2003. Guidelines for the management of alopecia areata. *British Journal of Dermatology* 149(4):692–699.

Maddux, A. B., L. Berbert, C. C. Young, L. R. Feldstein, L. D. Zambrano, S. Kucukak, M. M. Newhams, K. Miller, M. M. Fitzgerald, J. He, N. B. Halasa, N. Z. Cvijanovich, L. L. Loftis, T. C. Walker, S. P. Schwartz, S. J. Gertz, K. M. Tarquinio, J. C. Fitzgerald, M. Kong, J. E. Schuster, E. H. Mack, C. V. Hobbs, C. M. Rowan, M. A. Staat, M. S. Zinter, K. Irby, H. Crandall, H. Flori, M. L. Cullimore, R. A. Nofziger, S. L. Shein, M. G. Gaspers, J. R. Hume, E. R. Levy, S. R. Chen, M. M. Patel, M. W. Tenforde, E. Weller, A. P. Campbell, and A. G. Randolph. 2022. Health impairments in children and adolescents after hospitalization for acute COVID-19 or MIS-C. *Pediatrics* 150(3):e2022057798.

Maglietta, G., F. Diodati, M. Puntoni, S. Lazzarelli, B. Marcomini, L. Patrizi, and C. Caminiti. 2022. Prognostic factors for post-COVID-19 syndrome: A systematic review and meta-analysis. *Journal of Clinical Medicine* 11(6):1541.

Maley, J. H., G. A. Alba, J. T. Barry, M. N. Bartels, T. K. Fleming, C. V. Oleson, L. Rydberg, S. Sampsel, J. K. Silver, S. Sipes, M. Verduzco-Gutierrez, J. Wood, J. Zibrak, and J. Whiteson 2022. Multi-disciplinary collaborative consensus guidance statement on the assessment and treatment of breathing discomfort and respiratory sequelae in patients with post-acute sequelae of SARS-CoV-2 infection (PASC). *PM&R* 14(1):77–95.

Malone, L. A., A. Morrow, Y. Chen, D. Curtis, S. D. de Ferranti, M. Desai, T. K. Fleming, T. M. Giglia, T. A. Hall, E. Henning, S. Jadhav, A. M. Johnston, D. R. C. Kathirithamby, C. Kokorelis, C. Lachenauer, L. Li, H. C. Lin, T. Locke, C. MacArthur, M. Mann, S. A. McGrath-Morrow, R. Ng, L. Ohlms, S. Risen, S. C. Sadreameli, S. Sampsel, S. K. S. Tejtel, J. K. Silver, T. Simoneau, R. Srouji, S. Swami, S. Torbey, M. V. Gutierrez, C. N. Williams, L. A. Zimmerman, and L. E. Vaz. 2022. Multi-disciplinary collaborative consensus guidance statement on the assessment and treatment of postacute sequelae of SARS-CoV-2 infection (PASC) in children and adolescents. *PM&R* 14(10):1241–1269.

Mariani, F., R. Morello, D. O. Traini, A. La Rocca, C. De Rose, P. Valentini, and D. Buonsenso. 2023. Risk factors for persistent anosmia and dysgeusia in children with SARS-CoV-2 infection: A retrospective study. *Children* 10(3):597.

Martora, F., A. Villani, G. Fabbrocini, and T. Battista. 2023. COVID-19 and cutaneous manifestations: A review of the published literature. *Journal of Cosmetic Dermatology* 22(1):4–10.

Maruff, P., E. Thomas, L. Cysique, B. Brew, A. Collie, P. Snyder, and R. H. Pietrzak. 2009. Validity of the CogState brief battery: Relationship to standardized tests and sensitivity to cognitive impairment in mild traumatic brain injury, schizophrenia, and AIDS dementia complex. *Archives of Clinical Neuropsychology* 24(2):165–178.

Mass General. 2022. Dermatologic manifestations of COVID-19 can become "long-hauler" symptoms. *Massachusettts General Hospital Advances in Motion.* https://advances.massgeneral.org/research-and-innovation/journal.aspx?id=1868 (accessed March 15, 2024).

Mattei, A., B. Amy de la Bretèque, S. Crestani, L. Crevier-Buchman, C. Galant, S. Hans, A. Julien-Laferrière, A. Lagier, C. Lobryeau, F. Marmouset, D. Robert, V. Woisard, and A. Giovanni. 2020. Guidelines of clinical practice for the management of swallowing disorders and recent dysphonia in the context of the COVID-19 pandemic. *European Annals of Otorhinolaryngology, Head and Neck Diseases* 137(3):173–175.

Mayo Clinic. 2022. *Fever*. https://www.mayoclinic.org/diseases-conditions/fever/diagnosis-treatment/drc-20352764 (accessed January 16, 2024).

McDonald, C., S. Koshi, L. Busner, L. Kavi, and J. L. Newton. 2014. Postural tachycardia syndrome is associated with significant symptoms and functional impairment predominantly affecting young women: A UK perspective. *BMJ Open* 4(6):e004127.

McWhirter, L., H. Smyth, I. Hoeritzauer, A. Couturier, J. Stone, and A. J. Carson. 2023. What is brain fog? *Journal of Neuroloy, Neurosurgery, and Psychiatry* 94(4):321–325.

Melamed, E., L. Rydberg, A. F. Ambrose, R. Bhavaraju-Sanka, J. S. Fine, T. K. Fleming, E. Herman, J. L. Phipps Johnson, J. R. Kucera, M. Longo, W. Niehaus, C. V. Oleson, S. Sampsel, J. K. Silver, M. M. Smith, and M. Verduzco-Gutierrez. 2023. Multidisciplinary collaborative consensus guidance statement on the assessment and treatment of neurologic sequelae in patients with post-acute sequelae of SARS-CoV-2 infection (PASC). *PM&R* 15(5):640–662.

Michael, B. D., D. Walton, E. Westenberg, D. García-Azorín, B. Singh, A. A. Tamborska, M. Netravathi, M. Chomba, G. K. Wood, and A. Easton. 2023. Consensus clinical guidance for diagnosis and management of adult COVID-19 encephalopathy patients. *Journal of Neuropsychiatry and Clinical Neurosciences* 35(1):12–27.

Michaudet, C., and J. Malaty. 2017. Chronic cough: Evaluation and management. *American Family Physician* 96(9):575–580.

Mizera, J., S. Genzor, M. Sova, L. Stanke, R. Burget, P. Jakubec, M. Vykopal, P. Pobeha, and J. Zapletalova. 2024. The effectiveness of glucocorticoid treatment in post-COVID-19 pulmonary involvement. *Pneumonia (Nathan)* 16(1):2.

Morello, R., L. Martino, and D. Buonsenso. 2023. Diagnosis and management of post-COVID (long COVID) in children: A moving target. *Current Opinion in Pediatrics* 35(2):184–192.

Morice, A. H., E. Millqvist, K. Bieksiene, S. S. Birring, P. Dicpinigaitis, C. Domingo Ribas, M. Hilton Boon, A. Kantar, K. Lai, L. McGarvey, D. Rigau, I. Satia, J. Smith, W.-J. Song, T. Tonia, J. W. K. Van Den Berg, M. J. G. Van Manen, and A. Zacharasiewicz. 2020. ERS guidelines on the diagnosis and treatment of chronic cough in adults and children. *European Respiratory Journal* 55(1):1901136.

Morrow, A. K., R. Ng, G. Vargas, D. T. Jashar, E. Henning, N. Stinson, and L. A. Malone. 2021. Postacute/Long COVID in pediatrics: Development of a multidisciplinary rehabilitation clinic and preliminary case series. *American Journal of Physical Medicine & Rehabilitation* 100(12):1140.

Morrow, A. K., L. A. Malone, C. Kokorelis, L. S. Petracek, E. F. Eastin, K. L. Lobner, L. Neuendorff, and P. C. Rowe. 2022. Long-term COVID-19 sequelae in adolescents: The overlap with orthostatic intolerance and ME/CFS. *Current Pediatrics Reports* 10(2):31–44.

Munblit, D., P. Bobkova, E. Spiridonova, A. Shikhaleva, A. Gamirova, O. Blyuss, N. Nekliudov, P. Bugaeva, M. Andreeva, A. DunnGalvin, P. Comberiati, C. Apfelbacher, J. Genuneit, S. Avdeev, V. Kapustina, A. Guekht, V. Fomin, A. A. Svistunov, P. Timashev, V. S. Subbot, V. V. Royuk, T. M. Drake, S. W. Hanson, L. Merson, G. Carson, P. Horby, L. Sigfrid, J. T. Scott, M. G. Semple, J. O. Warner, T. Vos, P. Olliaro, P. Glybochko, and D. Butnaru. 2021. Incidence and risk factors for persistent symptoms in adults previously hospitalized for COVID-19. *Clinical & Experimental Allergy* 51(9):1107–1120.

Myall, K. J., B. Mukherjee, A. M. Castanheira, J. L. Lam, G. Benedetti, S. M. Mak, R. Preston, M. Thillai, A. Dewar, P. L. Molyneaux, and A. G. West. 2021. Persistent post-COVID-19 interstitial lung disease. An observational study of corticosteroid treatment. *Annals of the American Thoracic Society* 18(5):799–806.

Nambi, G., W. K. Abdelbasset, S. M. Alrawaili, S. H. Elsayed, A. Verma, A. Vellaiyan, M. M. Eid, O. R. Aldhafian, N. B. Nwihadh, and A. K. Saleh. 2022. Comparative effectiveness study of low versus high-intensity aerobic training with resistance training in community-dwelling older men with post-COVID-19 sarcopenia: A randomized controlled trial. *Clinical Rehabilitation* 36(1):59–68.

NASEM (National Academies of Sciences, Engineering, and Medicine). 2022. *Selected heritable disorders of connective tissue and disability.* Washington, DC: The National Academies Press.

NCHS (National Center for Health Statistics). 2024. *Long COVID household pulse survey.* https://www.cdc.gov/nchs/covid19/pulse/long-covid.htm (accessed March 15, 2024).

Nehme, M., F. Chappuis, L. Kaiser, F. Assal, and I. Guessous. 2023. The prevalence, severity, and impact of post-COVID persistent fatigue, post-exertional malaise, and chronic fatigue syndrome. *Journal of General Internal Medicine* 38(3):835–839.

Ng, R., G. Vargas, D. T. Jashar, A. Morrow, and L. A. Malone. 2022. Neurocognitive and psychosocial characteristics of pediatric patients with post-acute/long-COVID: A retrospective clinical case series. *Archives of Clinical Neuropsychology* 37(8):1633–1643.

NIAMSD (National Institute of Arthritis and Musculskeletal and Skin Diseases). 2021. *Raynaud's phenomenon.* https://www.niams.nih.gov/health-topics/raynauds-phenomenon. (accessed March 13, 2024).

NICE (National Institute for Health and Care Excellence). 2017. *Idiopathic pulmonary fibrosis in adults: Diagnosis and management.* London, UK: NICE.

NICE. 2020. *Tinnitus: Assessment and management.* London, UK: NICE

NICE. 2021a. *COVID-19 rapid guideline: Managing the long-term effects of COVID-19.* London, UK: NICE.

NICE. 2021b. *Headaches in over 12s: Diagnosis and management.* London, UK: NICE.

NICE. 2021c. *Myalgic encephalomyelitis (or encephalopathy)/chronic fatigue syndrome: Diagnosis and management.* https://www.nice.org.uk/guidance/ng206 (accessed March 7, 2024).

NICE. 2021d. *NICE ME/CFS diagnostic criteria 2021.* https://me-pedia.org/wiki/NICE_ME/CFS_diagnostic_criteria_2021#Diagnostic_criteria (accessed March 7, 2024).

NICE. 2023. *Thyroid disease: Assessment and management.* London, UK: NICE.

NICE. 2023. *Venous thromboembolic diseases: Diagnosis, management and thrombophilia testing: NICE Clinical Guidelines, no. 158.* London, UK: NICE.

NIH (National Institutes of Health). n.d. Sign or symptom (Concept ID: C3540840). *MedGen.* National Library of Medicine, National Center for Biotechnology Information.

NIH. 2023. *RECOVER: Researching COVID to enhance recovery.* https://recovercovid.org/ (accessed October 13, 2023).

Núñez-Gil, I. J., G. Feltes, M. C. Viana-Llamas, S. Raposeiras-Roubin, R. Romero, E. Alfonso-Rodríguez, A. Uribarri, F. Santoro, V. Becerra-Muñoz, M. Pepe, A. F. Castro-Mejía, J. Signes-Costa, A. Gonzalez, F. Marín, J. Lopez-País, E. Cerrato, O. Vázquez-Cancela, C. Espejo-Paeres, Á. López Masjuan, L. Velicki, I. El-Battrawy, H. Ramakrishna, A. Fernandez-Ortiz, and J. Perez-Villacastín, on behalf of HOPE-2 Investigators. 2023. Post-COVID-19 symptoms and heart disease: Incidence, prognostic factors, outcomes and vaccination: Results from a multi-center international prospective registry (HOPE 2). *Journal of Clinical* Medicine 12(2):706.

Núñez-Seisdedos, M. N., I. Lázaro-Navas, L. López-González, and L. López-Aguilera. 2022. Intensive care unit-acquired weakness and hospital functional mobility outcomes following invasive mechanical ventilation in patients with COVID-19: A single-centre prospective cohort study. *Journal of Intensive Care Medicine* 37(8):1005.

Oldroyd, A. G. S., J. B. Lilleker, T. Amin, O. Aragon, K. Bechman, V. Cuthbert, J. Galloway, P. Gordon, W. J. Gregory, H. Gunawardena, M. G. Hanna, D. Isenberg, J. Jackman, P. D. W. Kiely, P. Livermore, P. M. Machado, S. Maillard, N. McHugh, R. Murphy, C. Pilkington, A. Prabu, P. Rushe, S. Spinty, J. Swan, H. Tahir, S. L. Tansley, P. Truepenny, Y. Truepenny, K. Warrier, M. Yates, C. Papadopoulou, N. Martin, L. McCann, and H. Chinoy. 2022. British society for rheumatology guideline on management of paediatric, adolescent and adult patients with idiopathic inflammatory myopathy. *Rheumatology* 61(5):1760–1768.

Oliveira, C. R., L. A. Jason, D. Unutmaz, L. Bateman, and S. D. Vernon. 2023. Improvement of long COVID symptoms over one year. *Frontiers in Medicine* 9:1065620.

Orfei, M. D., D. E. Porcari, S. D'Arcangelo, F. Maggi, D. Russignaga, and E. Ricciardi. 2022. A new look on long-COVID effects: The functional brain fog syndrome. *Journal of Clinical Medicine* 11(19).

Ortel, T. L., I. Neumann, W. Ageno, R. Beyth, N. P. Clark, A. Cuker, B. A. Hutten, M. R. Jaff, V. Manja, S. Schulman, C. Thurston, S. Vedantham, P. Verhamme, D. M. Witt, I. D. Florez, A. Izcovich, R. Nieuwlaat, S. Ross, H. J. Schünemann, W. Wiercioch, Y. Zhang, and Y. Q. Zhang. 2020. American Society of Hematology 2020 guidelines for management of venous thromboembolism: Treatment of deep vein thrombosis and pulmonary embolism. *Blood Advances* 4(19):4693–4738.

Pagen, D. M. E., M. Van Herck, C. J. A. van Bilsen, S. Brinkhues, K. Konings, C. D. J. den Heijer, M. A. Spruit, C. Hoebe, and N. Dukers-Muijrers. 2023. High proportions of post-exertional malaise and orthostatic intolerance in people living with post-COVID-19 condition: The prime post-COVID study. *Frontiers in Medicine* 10:1292446.

PCDS (Primary Care Dermatology Society). 2023. *Livedo reticularis and livedoid vasculopathy* https://www.pcds.org.uk/clinical-guidance/livedo-reticularis (accessed November 14, 2023).

Pellegrino, R., E. Chiappini, A. Licari, L. Galli, and G. L. Marseglia. 2022. Prevalence and clinical presentation of long COVID in children: A systematic review. *European Journal of Pediatrics* 181(12):3995–4009.

Penner, J., O. Abdel-Mannan, K. Grant, S. Maillard, F. Kucera, J. Hassell, M. Eyre, Z. Berger, Y. Hacohen, and K. Moshal. 2021. 6-month multidisciplinary follow-up and outcomes of patients with paediatric inflammatory multisystem syndrome (PIMS-TS) at a UK tertiary paediatric hospital: A retrospective cohort study. *The Lancet Child & Adolescent Health* 5(7):473–482.

Perlis, R. H., M. Santillana, K. Ognyanova, A. Safarpour, K. Lunz Trujillo, M. D. Simonson, J. Green, A. Quintana, J. Druckman, M. A. Baum, and D. Lazer. 2022. Prevalence and correlates of long COVID symptoms among us adults. *JAMA Network Open* 5(10):e2238804

Petersen, R. C., O. Lopez, M. J. Armstrong, T. S. Getchius, M. Ganguli, D. Gloss, G. S. Gronseth, D. Marson, T. Pringsheim, and G. S. Day. 2018. Practice guideline update summary: Mild cognitive impairment: Report of the Guideline Development, Dissemination, and Implementation Subcommittee of the American Academy of Neurology. *Neurology* 90(3):126–135.

Phillips, T. G., W. P. Slomiany, and R. Allison. 2017. Hair loss: Common causes and treatment. *American Family Physician* 96(6):371–378.

Polly, S., and A. P. Fernandez. 2022. Common skin signs of COVID-19 in adults: An update. *Cleveland Clinic Journal of Medicine* 89(3):161–167.

Powers, W. J., A. A. Rabinstein, T. Ackerson, O. M. Adeoye, N. C. Bambakidis, K. Becker, J. Biller, M. Brown, B. M. Demaerschalk, B. Hoh, E. C. Jauch, C. S. Kidwell, T. M. Leslie-Mazwi, B. Ovbiagele, P. A. Scott, K. N. Sheth, A. M. Southerland, D. V. Summers, and D. L. Tirschwell. 2019. Guidelines for the early management of patients with acute ischemic stroke: 2019 update to the 2018 guidelines for the early management of acute ischemic stroke: A guideline for healthcare professionals from the American Heart Association/American Stroke Association. *Stroke* 50(12):e440–e441.

Prabhu, M., K. Cagino, K. C. Matthews, R. L. Friedlander, S. M. Glynn, J. M. Kubiak, Y. J. Yang, Z. Zhao, R. N. Baergen, J. I. DiPace, A. S. Razavi, D. W. Skupski, J. R. Snyder, H. K. Singh, R. B. Kalish, C. M. Oxford, and L. E. Riley. 2020. Pregnancy and postpartum outcomes in a universally tested population for SARS-CoV-2 in New York City: A prospective cohort study. *BJOG* 127(12):1548–1556.

Premraj, L., N. V. Kannapadi, J. Briggs, S. M. Seal, D. Battaglini, J. Fanning, J. Suen, C. Robba, J. Fraser, and S.-M. Cho. 2022. Mid and long-term neurological and neuropsychiatric manifestations of post-COVID-19 syndrome: A meta-analysis. *Journal of the Neurological Sciences* 434:120162.

Pringsheim, T., G. S. Day, D. B. Smith, A. Rae-Grant, N. Licking, M. J. Armstrong, R. M. de Bie, E. Roze, J. M. Miyasaki, R. A. Hauser, A. J. Espay, J. P. Martello, J. A. Gurwell, L. Billinghurst, K. Sullivan, M. S. Fitts, N. Cothros, D. A. Hall, M. Rafferty, L. Hagerbrant, T. Hastings, M. D. O'Brien, H. Silsbee, G. Gronseth, and A. E. Lang, on behalf of the Guideline Subcommittee of the AAN. 2021. Dopaminergic therapy for motor symptoms in early parkinson disease practice guideline summary: A report of the AAN Guideline Subcommittee. *Neurology* 97(20):942–957.

Qaseem, A., R. M. McLean, D. O'Gurek, P. Batur, K. Lin, D. L. Kansagara, Clinical Guidelines Committee of the American College of Physicians, Commission on Health of the Public and Science of the American Academy of Family Physicians. 2020. Nonpharmacologic and pharmacologic management of acute pain from non-low back, musculoskeletal injuries in adults: A clinical guideline from the American College of Physicians and American Academy of Family Physicians. *Annals of Internal Medicine* 173(9):739–748.

Raasing, L. R. M., O. J. M. Vogels, M. Veltkamp, C. F. P. van Swol, and J. C. Grutters. 2021. Current view of diagnosing small fiber neuropathy. *Journal of Neuromuscular Diseases* 8(2):185–207.

Radtke, T., A. Ulyte, M. A. Puhan, and S. Kriemler. 2021. Long-term symptoms after SARS-CoV-2 infection in children and adolescents. *JAMA* 326(9):869–871.

Raghu, G., M. Remy-Jardin, C. J. Ryerson, J. L. Myers, M. Kreuter, M. Vasakova, E. Bargagli, J. H. Chung, B. F. Collins, E. Bendstrup, H. A. Chami, A. T. Chua, T. J. Corte, J.-C. Dalphin, S. K. Danoff, J. Diaz-Mendoza, A. Duggal, R. Egashira, T. Ewing, M. Gulati, Y. Inoue, A. R. Jenkins, K. A. Johannson, T. Johkoh, M. Tamae-Kakazu, M. Kitaichi, S. L. Knight, D. Koschel, D. J. Lederer, Y. Mageto, L. A. Maier, C. Matiz, F. Morell, A. G. Nicholson, S. Patolia, C. A. Pereira, E. A. Renzoni, M. L. Salisbury, M. Selman, S. L. F. Walsh, W. A. Wuyts, and K. C. Wilson. 2020. Diagnosis of hypersensitivity pneumonitis in adults: An official ATS/JRS/ALAT clinical practice guideline. *American Journal of Respiratory and Critical Care Medicine* 202(3):e36–e69.

Raghu, G., M. Remy-Jardin, L. Richeldi, C. C. Thomson, Y. Inoue, T. Johkoh, M. Kreuter, D. A. Lynch, T. M. Maher, F. J. Martinez, M. Molina-Molina, J. L. Myers, A. G. Nicholson, C. J. Ryerson, M. E. Strek, L. K. Troy, M. Wijsenbeek, M. J. Mammen, T. Hossain, B. D. Bissell, D. D. Herman, S. M. Hon, F. Kheir, Y. H. Khor, M. Macrea, K. M. Antoniou, D. Bouros, I. Buendia-Roldan, F. Caro, B. Crestani, L. Ho, J. Morisset, A. L. Olson, A. Podolanczuk, V. Poletti, M. Selman, T. Ewing, S. Jones, S. L. Knight, M. Ghazipura, and K. C. Wilson. 2022. Idiopathic pulmonary fibrosis (an update) and progressive pulmonary fibrosis in adults: An official ATS/ERS/JRS/ALAT clinical practice guideline. *American Journal of Respiratory and Critical Care Medicine* 205(9):e18–e47.

Rahmati, M., D. K. Yon, S. W. Lee, R. Udeh, M. McEVoy, M. S. Kim, R. M. Gyasi, H. Oh, G. F. López Sánchez, and L. Jacob. 2023. New-onset type 1 diabetes in children and adolescents as postacute sequelae of SARS-CoV-2 infection: A systematic review and meta-analysis of cohort studies. *Journal of Medical Virology* 95(6):e28833.

Raj, S. R., A. C. Arnold, A. Barboi, V. E. Claydon, J. K. Limberg, V. M. Lucci, M. Numan, A. Peltier, H. Snapper, and S. Vernino. 2021. Long-COVID postural tachycardia syndrome: An American Autonomic Society statement. *Clinical Autonomic Research* 31(3):365–368.

Raj, S. R., A. Fedorowski, and R. S. Sheldon. 2022. Diagnosis and management of postural orthostatic tachycardia syndrome. *Canadian Medical Association Journal* 194(10):E378–E385.

Raman, B., D. A. Bluemke, T. F. Lüscher, and S. Neubauer. 2022. Long COVID: Post-acute sequelae of COVID-19 with a cardiovascular focus. *European Heart Journal* 43(11): 1157–1172.

Rao, S., G. M. Lee, H. Razzaghi, V. Lorman, A. Mejias, N. M. Pajor, D. Thacker, R. Webb, K. Dickinson, L. C. Bailey, R. Jhaveri, D. A. Christakis, T. D. Bennett, Y. Chen, and C. B. Forrest. 2022. Clinical features and burden of postacute sequelae of SARS-CoV-2 infection in children and adolescents. *JAMA Pediatrics* 176(10):1000.

Rayner, D. G., E. Wang, C. Su, O. D. Patel, S. Aleluya, A. Giglia, E. Zhu, and M. Siddique. 2023. Risk factors for long COVID in children and adolescents: A systematic review and meta-analysis. *World Journal of Pediatrics* 20(2):133–142.

RCOG (Royal College of Obstetricians and Gynaecologists). 2012. *The initial management of chronic pelvic pain: Green-top Guideline 41.* https://www.rcog.org.uk/guidance/browse-all-guidance/green-top-guidelines/the-initial-management-of-chronic-pelvic-pain-green-top-guideline-no-41/ (accessed March 26, 2024).

Riera-Canales, C., and A. Llanos-Chea. 2023. COVID-19 and the gastrointestinal tract in children. *Current Opinion in Pediatrics* 35(5):585–589.

Rodriguez, B., L. Larsson, and W. J. Z'Graggen. 2022. Critical illness myopathy: Diagnostic approach and resulting therapeutic implications. *Current Treatment Options in Neurology* 24(4):173–182.

Roessler, M., F. Tesch, M. Batram, J. Jacob, F. Loser, O. Weidinger, D. Wende, A. Vivirito, N. Toepfner, F. Ehm, M. Seifert, O. Nagel, C. König, R. Jucknewitz, J. P. Armann, R. Berner, M. Treskova-Schwarzbach, D. Hertle, S. Scholz, S. Stern, P. Ballesteros, S. Baßler, B. Bertele, U. Repschläger, N. Richter, C. Riederer, F. Sobik, A. Schramm, C. Schulte, L. Wieler, J. Walker, C. Scheidt-Nave, and J. Schmitt. 2022. Post-COVID-19-associated morbidity in children, adolescents, and adults: A matched cohort study including more than 157,000 individuals with COVID-19 in Germany. *PLoS Medicine* 19(11):e1004122.

Roge, I., L. Smane, A. Kivite-Urtane, Z. Pucuka, I. Racko, L. Klavina, and J. Pavare. 2021. Comparison of persistent symptoms after COVID-19 and other non-SARS-CoV-2 infections in children. *Frontiers in Pediatrics* 9:752385.

Rogers, T. S., M. A. Noel, and B. Garcia. 2023. Dizziness: Evaluation and management. *American Family Physician* 107(5):514–523.

Rome Foundation. n.d. *Rome IV criteria.* https://theromefoundation.org/rome-iv/rome-iv-criteria/ (accessed November 14, 2023).

Rovin, B. H., S. G. Adler, J. Barratt, F. Bridoux, K. A. Burdge, T. M. Chan, H. T. Cook, F. C. Fervenza, K. L. Gibson, R. J. Glassock, D. R. W. Jayne, V. Jha, A. Liew, Z.-H. Liu, J. M. Mejía-Vilet, C. M. Nester, J. Radhakrishnan, E. M. Rave, H. N. Reich, P. Ronco, J.-S. F. Sanders, S. Sethi, Y. Suzuki, S. C. W. Tang, V. Tesar, M. Vivarelli, J. F. M. Wetzels, and J. Floege. 2021. KDIGO 2021 clinical practice guideline for the management of glomerular diseases. *Kidney International* 100(4):S1–S276.

Rowe, K. S. 2019. Long term follow up of young people with chronic fatigue syndrome attending a pediatric outpatient service. *Frontiers in Pediatrics* 7:21.

Sánchez-García, A. M., P. Martínez-López, A. M. Gómez-González, J. Rodriguez-Capitán, F. J. Pavón-Morón, R. J. Jiménez-López, J. M. García-Almeida, E. Avanesi-Molina, N. Zamboschi, C. Rueda-Molina, V. Doncel-Abad, A. I. Molina-Ramos, E. Cabrera-César, I. Ben-Abdellatif, M. Gordillo-Resina, E. Pérez-Mesa, M. Nieto-González, P. Nuevo-Ortega, C. Reina-Artacho, P. L. Sánchez-Fernández, M. F. Jiménez-Navarro, and M. A. Estecha-Foncea. 2023. Post-intensive care unit multidisciplinary approach in patients with severe bilateral SARS-CoV-2 pneumonia. *International Journal of Medical Sciences* 20(1):1–10.

Sandler, C. X., V. B. B. Wyller, R. Moss-Morris, D. Buchwald, E. Crawley, J. Hautvast, B. Z. Katz, H. Knoop, P. Little, R. Taylor, K. A. Wensaas, and A. R. Lloyd. 2021. Long COVID and post-infective fatigue syndrome: A review. *Open Forum Infectious Diseases* 8(10):ofab440.

Sansone, F., G. M. Pellegrino, A. Caronni, F. Bonazza, E. Vegni, A. Lué, T. Bocci, C. Pipolo, G. Giusti, P. Di Filippo, S. Di Pillo, F. Chiarelli, G. F. Sferrazza Papa, and M. Attanasi. 2023. Long COVID in children: A multidisciplinary review. *Diagnostics* 13(12):1990.

Satterfield, B. A., D. L. Bhatt, and B. J. Gersh. 2022. Cardiac involvement in the long-term implications of COVID-19. *Nature Review Cardiology* 19(5):332–341.

Schiffl, H., and S. M. Lang. 2023. Long-term interplay between COVID-19 and chronic kidney disease. *International Urology and Nephrology* 55(8):1977–1984.

Schild, A.-K., D. Scharfenberg, L. Kirchner, K. Klein, A. Regorius, Y. Goereci, D. Meiberth, L. Sannemann, J. Lülling, F. Schweitzer, G. R. Fink, F. Jessen, C. Franke, Ö. Onur, S. Jost, C. Warnke, and F. Maier. 2023. Subjective and objective cognitive deficits in patients with post-COVID syndrome. *Zeitschrift für Neuropsychologie* 34(2):99–110.

Schlegel, P. N., M. Sigman, B. Collura, C. De Jonge, M. L. Eisenberg, D. J. Lamb, J. P. Mulhall, C. Niederberger, J. I. Sandlow, R. Z. Sokol, S. D. Spandorfer, C. Tanrikut, J. T. Treadwell, J. T. Oristaglio, and A. Zini. 2020. Diagnosis and treatment of infertility in men: AUA/ASRM guideline part I. *Fertility and Sterility* 115(1):54–61.

Schmidt, J. 2018. Current classification and management of inflammatory myopathies. *Journal of Neuromuscular Diseases* 5(2):109–129.

Schneider, S. A., S. Desai, O. Phokaewvarangkul, E. C. Rosca, J. Sringean, P. Anand, G. Bravo, F. Cardoso, A. M. Cervantes-Arslanian, H. Chovatiya, D. Crosiers, F. Dijkstra, C. Fearon, F. Grandas, E. Guedj, A. Méndez-Guerrero, M. Hassan, J. Jankovic, A. E. Lang, K. Makhoul, L. Muccioli, S. A. O'Shea, V. R. Ostovan, J. R. Perez-Sanchez, R. Ramdhani, V. Ros-Castelló, C. Schulte, P. Shah, L. Wojtecki, and P. K. Pal. 2023. COVID-19-associated new-onset movement disorders: A follow-up study. *Journal of Neurology* 270(5):2409–2415.

Seeley, M. C., C. Gallagher, E. Ong, A. Langdon, J. Chieng, D. Bailey, A. Page, H. S. Lim, and D. H. Lau. 2023. High incidence of autonomic dysfunction and postural orthostatic tachycardia syndrome in patients with long COVID: Implications for management and health care planning. *American Journal of Medicine* (June 29): S0002-9343(23)00402-3.

Shah, S. C., M. B. Piazuelo, E. J. Kuipers, and D. Li. 2021. AGA clinical practice update on the diagnosis and management of atrophic gastritis: Expert review. *Gastroenterology* 161(4):1325–1332.e7.

Shaw, B. H., L. E. Stiles, K. Bourne, E. A. Green, C. A. Shibao, L. E. Okamoto, E. M. Garland, A. Gamboa, A. Diedrich, V. Raj, R. S. Sheldon, I. Biaggioni, D. Robertson, and S. R. Raj. 2019. The face of postural tachycardia syndrome—Insights from a large cross-sectional online community- based survey. *Journal of Internal Medicine* 286(4):438–448.

Shibata, S., Q. Fu, T. B. Bivens, J. L. Hastings, W. Wang, and B. D. Levine. 2012. Short-term exercise training improves the cardiovascular response to exercise in the postural orthostatic tachycardia syndrome. *Journal of Physiology* 590(15):3495–3505.

Shirley Ryan AbilityLab. 2019. *Neuro-QOL.* https://www.sralab.org/rehabilitation-measures/neuro-qol (accessed March 6, 2024).

Simone, C. G., and P. D. Emmady. 2020. Transverse myelitis. In *StatPearls.* Treasure Island, FL: StatPearls Publishing.

Sisó-Almirall, A., P. Brito-Zerón, L. Conangla Ferrín, B. Kostov, A. Moragas Moreno, J. Mestres, J. Sellarès, G. Galindo, R. Morera, J. Basora, A. Trilla, and M. Ramos-Casals, on behalf of the CAMFiC Long COVID-19 Study Group. 2021. Long COVID-19: Proposed primary care clinical guidelines for diagnosis and disease management. *International Journal of Environmental Research and Public Health* 18(8):4350.

Spagnuolo, R., T. Larussa, C. Iannelli, C. Cosco, E. Nisticò, E. Manduci, A. Bruno, L. Boccuto, L. Abenavoli, F. Luzza, and P. Doldo. 2020. COVID-19 and inflammatory bowel disease: Patient knowledge and perceptions in a single center survey. *Medicina* 56(8):407.

Spahic, J. M., V. Hamrefors, M. Johansson, F. Ricci, O. Melander, R. Sutton, and A. Fedorowski. 2023. Malmö POTS symptom score: Assessing symptom burden in postural orthostatic tachycardia syndrome. *Journal of Internal Medicine* 293(1):91–99.

SSA (Social Security Administration). 2020. Disability Report - Adult: Form SSA-3368-BK. Woodlawn, MD: SSA. https://www.ssa.gov/forms/ssa-3368-bk.pdf (accessed February 28, 2024).

SSA. 2021. *DI 24510.057 Sustainability and the residual functional capacity (RFC) assessment.* https://secure.ssa.gov/poms.nsf/lnx/0424510057 (accessed February 28, 2024).

SSA. n.d.-a. Disability evaluation under Social Security: 12.00 Mental disorders—Adult. https://www.ssa.gov/disability/professionals/bluebook/12.00-MentalDisorders-Adult.htm (accessed March 26, 2024).

SSA. n.d.-b. Disability evaluation under Social Security: 112.00 Mental disorders—Childhood. https://www.ssa.gov/disability/professionals/bluebook/112.00-MentalDisorders-Childhood.htm (accessed March 26, 2024).

Ssentongo, P., Y. Zhang, L. Witmer, V. M. Chinchilli, and D. M. Ba. 2022. Association of COVID-19 with diabetes: A systematic review and meta-analysis. *Scientific Reports* 12(1):20191.

Stand. n.d. *The Britannica dictionary*. https://www.britannica.com/dictionary/stand (accessed April 2, 2024).

Steenblock, C., M. Hassanein, E. G. Khan, M. Yaman, M. Kamel, M. Barbir, D. E. Lorke, J. A. Rock, D. Everett, S. Bejtullah, A. Heimerer, E. Tahirukaj, P. Beqiri, and S. R. Bornstein. 2022. Diabetes and COVID-19: Short- and long-term consequences. *Hormone and Metabolic Research* 54(8):503–509.

Štěpánek, L., M. Nakládalová, M. Janošíková, L. Štěpánek, K. Kabrhelová, and A. Boriková. 2023. Predictors and characteristics of post-acute COVID-19 syndrome in healthcare workers. *Infectious Diseases* 55(2):125–131.

Stern, Y., C. A. Barnes, C. Grady, R. N. Jones, and N. Raz. 2019. Brain reserve, cognitive reserve, compensation, and maintenance: Operationalization, validity, and mechanisms of cognitive resilience. *Neurobiology of Aging* 83:124–129.

Stevens, S., C. Snell, J. Stevens, B. Keller, and J. M. VanNess. 2018. Cardiopulmonary exercise test methodology for assessing exertion intolerance in myalgic encephalomyelitis/chronic fatigue syndrome. *Frontiers in Pediatrics* 6:242

Sudre, C. H., B. Murray, T. Varsavsky, M. S. Graham, R. S. Penfold, R. C. Bowyer, J. C. Pujol, K. Klaser, M. Antonelli, L. S. Canas, E. Molteni, M. Modat, M. Jorge Cardoso, A. May, S. Ganesh, R. Davies, L. H. Nguyen, D. A. Drew, C. M. Astley, A. D. Joshi, J. Merino, N. Tsereteli, T. Fall, M. F. Gomez, E. L. Duncan, C. Menni, F. M. K. Williams, P. W. Franks, A. T. Chan, J. Wolf, S. Ourselin, T. Spector, and C. J. Steves. 2021. Attributes and predictors of long COVID. *Nature Medicine* 27(4):626–631.

Sumantri, S., and I. Rengganis. 2023. Immunological dysfunction and mast cell activation syndrome in long COVID. *Asia Pacific Allergy* 13(1):50–53.

Sunada, N., H. Honda, Y. Nakano, K. Yamamoto, K. Tokumasu, Y. Sakurada, Y. Matsuda, T. Hasegawa, Y. Otsuka, M. Obika, Y. Hanayama, H. Hagiya, K. Ueda, H. Kataoka, and F. Otsuka. 2022. Hormonal trends in patients suffering from long COVID symptoms. *Endocrine Journal* 69(10):1173–1181.

Swarnakar, R., S. Jenifa, and S. Wadhwa. 2022. Musculoskeletal complications in long COVID-19: A systematic review. *World Journal of Virology* 11(6):485.

Tana, C., E. Bentivegna, S.-J. Cho, A. M. Harriott, D. García-Azorín, A. Labastida-Ramirez, R. Ornello, B. Raffaelli, E. R. Beltrán, R. Ruscheweyh, and P. Martelletti. 2022. Long COVID headache. *Journal of Headache and Pain* 23(1):93.

Tannis, A., J. A. Englund, A. Perez, E. J. Harker, M. A. Staat, E. P. Schlaudecker, N. B. Halasa, L. S. Stewart, J. V. Williams, M. G. Michaels, R. Selvarangan, J. E. Schuster, L. A. Sahni, J. A. Boom, G. Weinberg, P. G. Szilagyi, B. R. Clopper, Y. Zhou, M. L. McMorrow, E. J. Klein, and H. L. Moline. 2023. SARS-CoV-2 epidemiology and COVID-19 mRNA vaccine effectiveness among infants and children aged 6 months–4 years—New Vaccine Surveillance Network, United States, July 2022–September 2023. *MMWR Morbidity and Mortality Weekly Report* 72(48):1300–1306.

Taquet, M., J. R. Geddes, M. Husain, S. Luciano, and P. J. Harrison. 2021. 6-month neurological and psychiatric outcomes in 236 379 survivors of COVID-19: A retrospective cohort study using electronic health records. *The Lancet Psychiatry* 8(5):416–427.

Taquet, M., R. Sillett, L. Zhu, J. Mendel, I. Camplisson, Q. Dercon, and P. J. Harrison. 2022. Neurological and psychiatric risk trajectories after SARS-CoV-2 infection: An analysis of 2-year retrospective cohort studies including 1,284,437 patients. *The Lancet Psychiatry* 9(10):815–827.

Tarantino, S., S. Graziano, C. Carducci, R. Giampaolo, and T. Grimaldi Capitello. 2022. Cognitive difficulties, psychological symptoms, and long lasting somatic complaints in adolescents with previous SARS-CoV-2 infection: A telehealth cross-sectional pilot study. *Brain Sciences* 12(8):969.

Tenner, S., J. Baillie, J. DeWitt, and S. S. Vege. 2013. American College of Gastroenterology guideline: Management of acute pancreatitis. *Official Journal of the American College of Gastroenterology* 108(9):1400–1415, 1416.

Thaweethai, T., S. E. Jolley, E. W. Karlson, E. B. Levitan, B. Levy, G. A. McComsey, L. McCorkell, G. N. Nadkarni, S. Parthasarathy, U. Singh, T. A. Walker, C. A. Selvaggi, D. J. Shinnick, C. C. M. Schulte, R. Atchley-Challenner, L. I. Horwitz, A. S. Foulkes, and RECOVER Consortium. 2023. Development of a definition of postacute sequelae of SARS-CoV-2 infection. *JAMA* 329(22):1934–1946.

The College of Optometrists. 2022. *Clinical management guidelines.* https://www.college-optometrists.org/clinical-guidance/clinical-management-guidelines/dryeye_keratoconjunctivitissicca_kcs (accessed November 10, 2023).

Treskova-Schwarzbach, M., L. Haas, S. Reda, A. Pilic, A. Borodova, K. Karimi, J. Koch, T. Nygren, S. Scholz, V. Schönfeld, S. Vygen-Bonnet, O. Wichmann, and T. Harder. 2021. Pre-existing health conditions and severe COVID-19 outcomes: An umbrella review approach and meta-analysis of global evidence. *BMC Medicine* 19(1):212.

Tsampasian, V., H. Elghazaly, R. Chattopadhyay, M. Debski, T. K. P. Naing, P. Garg, A. Clark, E. Ntatsaki, and V. S. Vassiliou. 2023. Risk factors associated with post-COVID-19 condition: A systematic review and meta-analysis. *JAMA Internal Medicine* 183(6):566–580.

Tsuchida, T., N. Yoshimura, K. Ishizuka, K. Katayama, Y. Inoue, M. Hirose, Y. Nakagama, Y. Kido, H. Sugimori, T. Matsuda, and Y. Ohira. 2023. Five cluster classifications of long COVID and their background factors: A cross-sectional study in Japan. *Clinical and Experimental Medicine* 23(7):3663–3670.

Tunkel, D. E., C. A. Bauer, G. H. Sun, R. M. Rosenfeld, S. S. Chandrasekhar, E. R. Cunningham, S. M. Archer, B. W. Blakley, J. M. Carter, E. C. Granieri, J. A. Henry, D. Hollingsworth, F. A. Khan, S. Mitchell, A. Monfared, C. W. Newman, F. S. Omole, C. D. Phillips, S. K. Robinson, M. B. Taw, R. S. Tyler, R. Waguespack, and E. J. Whamond. 2014. Clinical practice guideline: Tinnitus. *Otolaryngology–Head and Neck Surgery* 151(S2): S1–S40.

Twomey, R., J. DeMars, K. Franklin, S. N. Culos-Reed, J. Weatherald, and J. G. Wrightson. 2022. Chronic fatigue and postexertional malaise in people living with long COVID: An observational study. *Physical Therapy* 102(4):pzac005.

U.S. Preventive Services Task Force. 2020. Screening for cognitive impairment in older adults: U.S. Preventive Services Task Force recommendation statement. *JAMA* 323(8):757–763.

Vahratian, A., D. Adjaye-Gbewonyo, J.-M. S. Lin, and S. Saydah. 2023. Long COVID in children: United States, 2022. *NCHS Data Brief* 479:1–6.

Valdes, E., B. Fuchs, C. Morrison, L. Charvet, A. Lewis, S. Thawani, L. Balcer, S. L. Galetta, T. Wisniewski, and J. A. Frontera. 2022. Demographic and social determinants of cognitive dysfunction following hospitalization for COVID-19. *Journal of the Neurological Sciences* 438:120146.

Valent, P., C. Akin, B. Nedoszytko, P. Bonadonna, K. Hartmann, M. Niedoszytko, K. Brockow, F. Siebenhaar, M. Triggiani, M. Arock, J. Romantowski, A. Górska, L. B. Schwartz, and D. D. Metcalfe. 2020. Diagnosis, classification and management of Mast Cell Activation Syndromes (MCAS) in the era of personalized medicine. *International Journal of Molecular Sciences* 21(23):9030.

Valent, P., C. Akin, K. Hartmann, I. Alvarez-Twose, K. Brockow, O. Hermine, M. Niedoszytko, J. Schwaab, J. J. Lyons, M. C. Carter, H. O. Elberink, J. H. Butterfield, T. I. George, G. Greiner, C. Ustun, P. Bonadonna, K. Sotlar, G. Nilsson, M. Jawhar, F. Siebenhaar, S. Broesby-Olsen, S. Yavuz, R. Zanotti, M. Lange, B. Nedoszytko, G. Hoermann, M. Castells, D. H. Radia, J. I. Muñoz-Gonzalez, W. R. Sperr, M. Triggiani, H. C. Kluin-Nelemans, S. J. Galli, L. B. Schwartz, A. Reiter, A. Orfao, J. Gotlib, M. Arock, H. P. Horny, and D. D. Metcalfe. 2021. Updated diagnostic criteria and classification of mast cell disorders: A consensus proposal. *Hemasphere* 5(11):e646.

Van Doorn, P. A., P. Y. K. Van Den Bergh, R. D. M. Hadden, B. Avau, P. Vankrunkelsven, S. Attarian, P. H. Blomkwist-Markens, D. R. Cornblath, H. S. Goedee, T. Harbo, B. C. Jacobs, S. Kusunoki, H. C. Lehmann, R. A. Lewis, M. P. Lunn, E. Nobile-Orazio, L. Querol, Y. A. Rajabally, T. Umapathi, H. A. Topaloglu, and H. J. Willison. 2023. European Academy of Neurology/Peripheral Nerve Society guideline on diagnosis and treatment of Guillain-Barré syndrome. *Journal of the Peripheral Nervous System* 28(4):535–563.

Varni, J. W., and C. A. Limbers. 2008. The PedsQL multidimensional fatigue scale in young adults: Feasibility, reliability and validity in a university student population. *Quality of Life Research* 17(1):105–114.

Varni, J. W., M. Seid, and P. S. Kurtin. 2001. PedsQL 4.0: Reliability and validity of the Pediatric Quality of Life Inventory version 4.0 generic core scales in healthy and patient populations. *Medical Care* 39(8):800–812.

Venkatesan, A., and R. G. Geocadin. 2014. Diagnosis and management of acute encephalitis: A practical approach. *Neurology Clinical Practice* 4(3):206–215.

Vernino, S., K. M. Bourne, L. E. Stiles, B. P. Grubb, A. Fedorowski, J. M. Stewart, A. C. Arnold, L. A. Pace, J. Axelsson, J. R. Boris, J. P. Moak, B. P. Goodman, K. R. Chemali, T. H. Chung, D. S. Goldstein, A. Diedrich, M. G. Miglis, M. M. Cortez, A. J. Miller, R. Freeman, I. Biaggioni, P. C. Rowe, R. S. Sheldon, C. A. Shibao, D. M. Systrom, G. A. Cook, T. A. Doherty, H. I. Abdallah, A. Darbari, and S. R. Raj. 2021. Postural orthostatic tachycardia syndrome (POTS): State of the science and clinical care from a 2019 National Institutes of Health Expert Consensus Meeting—Part 1. *Autonomic Neuroscience* 235:102828.

Vernon, S. D., M. Hartle, K. Sullivan, J. Bell, S. Abbaszadeh, D. Unutmaz, and L. Bateman. 2023. Post-exertional malaise among people with long COVID compared to myalgic encephalomyelitis/chronic fatigue syndrome (ME/CFS). *Work* 74(4):1179–1186.

Virani, S. S., L. K. Newby, S. V. Arnold, V. Bittner, L. C. Brewer, S. H. Demeter, D. L. Dixon, W. F. Fearon, B. Hess, H. M. Johnson, D. S. Kazi, D. Kolte, D. J. Kumbhani, J. Lofaso, D. Mahtta, D. B. Mark, M. Minissian, A. M. Navar, A. R. Patel, M. R. Piano, F. Rodriguez, A. W. Talbot, V. R. Taqueti, R. J. Thomas, S. Van Diepen, B. Wiggins, and M. S. Williams; Peer Review Committee Members. 2023. 2023 AHA/ACC/ACCP/ASPC/NLA/PCNA guideline for the management of patients with chronic coronary disease: A report of the American Heart Association/American College of Cardiology Joint Committee on Clinical Practice Guidelines. *Circulation* 148(9):e9–e119.

Von Knobelsdorff-Brenkenhoff, F., and J. Schulz-Menger. 2023. Cardiovascular magnetic resonance in the guidelines of the European Society of Cardiology: A comprehensive summary and update. *Journal of Cardiovascular Magnetic* Resonance 25(1):42.

Walker, L. S., and J. W. Greene. 1991. The functional disability inventory: Measuring a neglected dimension of child health status. *Journal of Pediatric Psychology* 16(1):39-58.

Walker, S., H. Goodfellow, P. Pookarnjanamorakot, E. Murray, J. Bindman, A. Blandford, K. Bradbury, B. Cooper, F. L. Hamilton, J. R. Hurst, H. Hylton, S. Linke, P. Pfeffer, W. Ricketts, C. Robson, F. A. Stevenson, D. Sunkersing, J. Wang, M. Gomes, W. Henley, and Living with COVID Recovery Collaboration. 2023. Impact of fatigue as the primary determinant of functional limitations among patients with post-COVID-19 syndrome: A cross-sectional observational study. *BMJ Open* 13(6):e069217.

Ware, J. E., Jr., and C. D. Sherbourne. 1992. The MOS 36-item short-form health survey (SF-36). I. Conceptual framework and item selection. *Medical Care* 30(6):473–483.

Weinstock, L. B., J. B. Brook, A. S. Walters, A. Goris, L. B. Afrin, and G. J. Molderings. 2021. Mast cell activation symptoms are prevalent in long-COVID. *International Journal of Infectious Diseases* 112:217–226.

Wernhart, S., E. Weihe, M. Totzeck, B. Balcer, T. Rassaf, and P. Luedike. 2023. Cardiopulmonary profiling of athletes with post-exertional malaise after COVID-19 infection—A single-center experience. *Journal of Clinical Medicine* 12(13):4348.

Whitcroft, K. L., and T. Hummel. 2019. Clinical diagnosis and current management strategies for olfactory dysfunction: A review. *JAMA Otolaryngology–Head & Neck Surgery* 145(9):846–853.

Whiteson, J. H., A. Azola, J. T. Barry, M. N. Bartels, S. Blitshteyn, T. K. Fleming, M. D. McCauley, J. D. Neal, J. Pillarisetti, and S. Sampsel. 2022. Multi-disciplinary collaborative consensus guidance statement on the assessment and treatment of cardiovascular complications in patients with post-acute sequelae of SARS-CoV-2 infection (PASC). *PM&R* 14(7):855878.

WHO (World Health Organization). 2023a. *Clinical management of COVID-19: Living guideline.* Geneva, Switzerland: WHO.

WHO. 2023b. *International statistical classification of diseases and related health problems, 11th revision.* Geneva, Switzerland: WHO.

Wilkinson, J. M., D. C. Codipilly, and R. P. Wilfahrt. 2021. Dysphagia: Evaluation and collaborative management. *American Family Physician* 103(2):97-106.

Winstein, C. J., J. Stein, R. Arena, B. Bates, L. R. Cherney, S. C. Cramer, F. Deruyter, J. J. Eng, B. Fisher, and R. L. Harvey. 2016. Guidelines for adult stroke rehabilitation and recovery: A guideline for healthcare professionals from the American Heart Association/American Stroke Association. *Stroke* 47(6):e98–e169.

Wong, M. C., J. Huang, Y. Y. Wong, G. L. Wong, T. C. Yip, R. N. Chan, S. W. Chau, S. C. Ng, Y. K. Wing, and F. K. Chan. 2023. Epidemiology, symptomatology, and risk factors for long COVID symptoms: Population-based, multicenter study. *JMIR Public Health and Surveillance* 9:e42315.

Wood, G. C., R. P. Bentall, M. Gopfert, and R. H. Edwards. 1991. A comparative psychiatric assessment of patients with chronic fatigue syndrome and muscle disease. *Psychological Medicine* 21(3):619–628.

Wulf Hanson, S., C. Abbafati, J. G. Aerts, Z. Al-Aly, C. Ashbaugh, T. Ballouz, O. Blyuss, P. Bobkova, G. Bonsel, S. Borzakova, D. Buonsenso, D. Butnaru, A. Carter, H. Chu, C. De Rose, M. M. Diab, E. Ekbom, M. El Tantawi, V. Fomin, R. Frithiof, A. Gamirova, P. V. Glybochko, J. A. Haagsma, S. Haghjooy Javanmard, E. B. Hamilton, G. Harris, M. H. Heijenbrok-Kal, R. Helbok, M. E. Hellemons, D. Hillus, S. M. Huijts, M. Hultström, W. Jassat, F. Kurth, I. M. Larsson, M. Lipcsey, C. Liu, C. D. Loflin, A. Malinovschi, W. Mao, L. Mazankova, D. McCulloch, D. Menges, N. Mohammadifard, D. Munblit, N. A. Nekliudov, O. Ogbuoji, I. M. Osmanov, J. L. Peñalvo, M. S. Petersen, M. A. Puhan, M. Rahman, V. Rass, N. Reinig, G. M. Ribbers, A. Ricchiuto, S. Rubertsson, E. Samitova, N. Sarrafzadegan, A. Shikhaleva, K. E. Simpson, D. Sinatti, J. B. Soriano, E. Spiridonova, F. Steinbeis, A. A. Svistunov, P. Valentini, B. J. van de Water, R. van den Berg-Emons, E. Wallin, M. Witzenrath, Y. Wu, H. Xu, T. Zoller, C. Adolph, J. Albright, J. O. Amlag, A. Y. Aravkin, B. L. Bang-Jensen, C. Bisignano, R. Castellano, E. Castro, S. Chakrabarti, J. K. Collins, X. Dai, F. Daoud, C. Dapper, A. Deen, B. B. Duncan, M. Erickson, S. B. Ewald, A. J. Ferrari, A. D. Flaxman, N. Fullman, A. Gamkrelidze, J. R. Giles, G. Guo, S. I. Hay, J. He, M. Helak, E. N. Hulland, M. Kereselidze, K. J. Krohn, A. Lazzar-Atwood, A. Lindstrom, R. Lozano, D. C. Malta, J. Månsson, A. M. Mantilla Herrera, A. H. Mokdad, L. Monasta, S. Nomura, M. Pasovic, D. M. Pigott, R. C. Reiner, Jr., G. Reinke, A. L. P. Ribeiro, D. F. Santomauro, A. Sholokhov, E. E. Spurlock, R. Walcott, A. Walker, C. S. Wiysonge, P. Zheng, J. P. Bettger, C. J. L. Murray, and T. Vos; Global Burden of Disease Long COVID Collaborators. 2022. Estimated global proportions of individuals with persistent fatigue, cognitive, and respiratory symptom clusters following symptomatic COVID-19 in 2020 and 2021. *JAMA* 328(16):1604–1615.

Xie, Y., and Z. Al-Aly. 2022. Risks and burdens of incident diabetes in long COVID: a cohort study. *The Lancet Diabetes & Endocrinology* 10(5):311–321.

Xie, Y., E. Xu, and Z. Al-Aly. 2022a. Risks of mental health outcomes in people with COVID-19: Cohort study. *BMJ*:e068993.

Xie, Y., E. Xu, B. Bowe, and Z. Al-Aly. 2022b. Long-term cardiovascular outcomes of COVID-19. *Nature Medicine* 28(3):583–590.

Xu, E., Y. Xie, and Z. Al-Aly. 2022. Long-term neurologic outcomes of COVID-19. *Nature Medicine* 28(11):2406–2415.

Xu, E., Y. Xie, and Z. Al-Aly. 2023. Long-term gastrointestinal outcomes of COVID-19. *Nature Communications* 14(1):983.

Yong, S. J., and S. Liu. 2022. Proposed subtypes of post-COVID-19 syndrome (or long-COVID) and their respective potential therapies. *Reviews in Medical Virology* 32(4):e2315.

Yousaf, A. R., J. Mak, L. Gwynn, R. Bloodworth, R. Rai, Z. Jeddy, L. B. Leclair, L. Edwards, L. E. W. Olsho, G. Newes-Adeyi, A. F. Dalton, M. Gaglani, S. K. Yoon, K. Hegmann, K. Ellingson, L. R. Feldstein, A. P. Campbell, A. Britton, and S. Saydah. 2023. 1935. CO-VID-19 mRNA vaccination reduces the occurrence of post-COVID conditions in U.S. children aged 5–17 years following Omicron SARS-CoV-2 infection, July 2021–September 2022. *Open Forum Infectious Diseases* 10(Supplement 2):ofad500.2466.

Zambrano, L. D., M. M. Newhams, S. M. Olson, N. B. Halasa, A. M. Price, J. A. Boom, L. C. Sahni, S. Kamidani, K. M. Tarquinio, A. B. Maddux, S. M. Heidemann, S. S. Bhumbra, K. E. Bline, R. A. Nofziger, C. V. Hobbs, T. T. Bradford, N. Z. Cvijanovich, K. Irby, E. H. Mack, M. L. Cullimore, P. S. Pannaraj, M. Kong, T. C. Walker, S. J. Gertz, K. N. Michelson, M. A. Cameron, K. Chiotos, M. Maamari, J. E. Schuster, A. O. Orzel, M. M. Patel, A. P. Campbell, and A. G. Randolph, for the Overcoming COVID-19 Investigators. 2022. Effectiveness of BNT162b2 (Pfizer-BioNTech) mRNA vaccination against multisystem inflammatory syndrome in children among persons aged 12–18 years — United States, July–December 2021. *MMWR Morbidity and Mortality Weekly Report* 71(2):52–58.

Zambrano, L. D., M. M. Newhams, R. M. Simeone, K. E. Fleming-Dutra, N. Halasa, M. Wu, A. O. Orzel-Lockwood, S. Kamidani, P. S. Pannaraj, K. Chiotos, M. A. Cameron, A. B. Maddux, J. E. Schuster, H. Crandall, M. Kong, R. A. Nofziger, M. A. Staat, S. S. Bhumbra, K. Irby, J. A. Boom, L. C. Sahni, J. R. Hume, S. J. Gertz, M. Maamari, C. Bowens, E. R. Levy, T. T. Bradford, T. C. Walker, S. P. Schwartz, E. H. Mack, J. A. Guzman-Cottrill, C. V. Hobbs, M. S. Zinter, N. Z. Cvijanovich, K. E. Bline, S. R. Hymes, A. P. Campbell, and A. G. Randolph, for the Overcoming COVID-19 Investigators. 2024. Characteristics and clinical outcomes of vaccine-eligible US children under-5 years hospitalized for acute COVID-19 in a national network. *Pediatric Infectious Disease Journal* 43(3):242–249.

Zang, C., Y. Zhang, J. Xu, J. Bian, D. Morozyuk, E. J. Schenck, D. Khullar, A. S. Nordvig, E. A. Shenkman, R. L. Rothman, J. P. Block, K. Lyman, M. G. Weiner, T. W. Carton, F. Wang, and R. Kaushal. 2023. Data-driven analysis to understand long COVID using electronic health records from the recover initiative. *Nature Communications* 14(1):1948.

Zesiewicz, T. A., R. J. Elble, E. D. Louis, G. S. Gronseth, W. G. Ondo, R. B. Dewey, M. S. Okun, K. L. Sullivan, and W. J. Weiner. 2011. Evidence-based guideline update: Treatment of essential tremor: Report of the Quality Standards Subcommittee of the American Academy of Neurology. *Neurology* 77(19):1752–1755.

Zheng, Y. B., N. Zeng, K. Yuan, S. S. Tian, Y. B. Yang, N. Gao, X. Chen, A. Y. Zhang, A. L. Kondratiuk, P. P. Shi, F. Zhang, J. Sun, J. L. Yue, X. Lin, L. Shi, A. Lalvani, J. Shi, Y. P. Bao, and L. Lu. 2023. Prevalence and risk factor for long COVID in children and adolescents: A meta-analysis and systematic review. *Journal of Infection and Public Health* 16(5):660–672.

ANNEX TABLE 3-1 Selected Respiratory Conditions Associated with Long COVID

Health Effects	Potential Functional Limitations	Selected Diagnostic and Management Guidelines	Potential Social Security Administration Listings
Pulmonary fibrosis	Standing, walking, strenuous physical activity, lifting, carrying, pushing/pulling, climbing, low work, speaking	• Idiopathic pulmonary fibrosis (an update) and progressive pulmonary fibrosis in adults: An official ATS/ERS/JRS/ALAT clinical practice guideline (Raghu et al., 2022) • Idiopathic pulmonary fibrosis in adults: Diagnosis and management (NICE, 2017)	3.02
Hypoxemia	Standing; walking; strenuous physical activity; lifting; carrying; pushing/pulling; overhead reaching; climbing; low work; understanding, remembering, and applying information; concentrating, persisting, or maintaining pace	N/A	None
Pneumonitis	Walking, strenuous physical activity, lifting, carrying, pushing/pulling, overhead reaching, climbing, low work	• Diagnosis of hypersensitivity pneumonitis in adults: An official ATS/JRS/ALAT clinical practice guideline (Raghu et al., 2020)	None
Chronic cough	Strenuous physical activity, speaking	• ERS guidelines on the diagnosis and treatment of chronic cough in adults and children (Morice et al., 2020) • Chronic cough: Evaluation and management (Michaudet and Malaty, 2017)	None

ANNEX TABLE 3-1 Continued

Health Effects	Potential Functional Limitations	Selected Diagnostic and Management Guidelines	Potential Social Security Administration Listings
Chronic pulmonary hypertension	Standing; walking; strenuous physical activity; lifting; carrying; pushing/pulling; overhead reaching; climbing; low work; understanding, remembering, and applying information; concentrating, persisting, or maintaining pace	• 2022 ESC/ERS guidelines for the diagnosis and treatment of pulmonary hypertension (Humbert et al., 2022)	3.09
Asthma	Walking, strenuous physical activity, carrying, pushing/pulling, overhead reaching, climbing, low work, speaking	• 2020 Focused updates to the asthma management guidelines: A report from the National Asthma Education and Prevention Program Coordinating Committee Expert Panel Working Group (Expert Panel Working Group, 2020) • Management of severe asthma: A European Respiratory Society/ American Thoracic Society guideline (Holguin et al., 2020)	None
Dyspnea	Walking, strenuous physical activity, carrying, pushing/pulling, overhead reaching, climbing, low work, speaking	• Chronic dyspnea: Diagnosis and evaluation (Badhwar and Syed, 2020)	None

SOURCES: Maley et al., 2022; Zang et al., 2023.

ANNEX TABLE 3-2 Selected Cardiovascular Conditions Associated with Long COVID

Health Effects	Potential Functional Limitations	Selected Diagnostic and Management Guidelines	Potential Social Security Administration Listings
Heart failure	Standing, walking, strenuous physical activity, lifting, carrying, pushing/pulling, reaching, foot/leg controls, climbing, low work, speaking	• 2022 AHA/ACC/HFSA guideline for the management of heart failure: A report of the American College of Cardiology/American Heart Association Joint Committee on Clinical Practice Guidelines (Heidenreich et al., 2022)	4.02
Coronary disease	Walking, strenuous physical activity, lifting, carrying, pushing/pulling, reaching, climbing, low work	• 2023 AHA/ACC/ACCP/ASPC/NLA/PCNA guideline for the management of patients with chronic coronary disease: A report of the American Heart Association/American College of Cardiology Joint Committee on Clinical Practice Guidelines (Virani et al., 2023)	4.04
Dysrhythmia (tachycardia and bradyarrhythmia)	Standing, walking, strenuous physical activity, lifting, carrying, pushing/pulling, reaching, climbing, low work	• 2018 ACC/AHA/HRS guideline on the evaluation and management of patients with bradycardia and cardiac conduction delay: A report of the American College of Cardiology/American Heart Association Task Force on Clinical Practice Guidelines and the Heart Rhythm Society (Kusumoto et al., 2019)	4.05
Pulmonary embolism	Walking, strenuous physical activity, lifting, carrying, pushing/pulling, overhead reaching, climbing, low work	• American Society of Hematology 2020 guidelines for management of venous thromboembolism: Treatment of deep vein thrombosis and pulmonary embolism (Ortel et al., 2020)	7.08

ANNEX TABLE 3-2 Continued

Health Effects	Potential Functional Limitations	Selected Diagnostic and Management Guidelines	Potential Social Security Administration Listings
Venous thrombosis	Standing, walking, strenuous physical activity, foot/leg controls	• Venous thromboembolic diseases: Diagnosis, management and thrombophilia testing: NICE Clinical Guidelines, no. 158 (NICE, 2023b) • American Society of Hematology 2020 guidelines for management of venous thromboembolism: Treatment of deep vein thrombosis and pulmonary embolism (Ortel et al., 2020)	4.11
Vasculitis	Strenuous physical activity, lifting, carrying, pushing/pulling, reaching, overhead reaching	• Vasculitis clinical practice guidelines (ACR, 2021)	14.03
Cardiac inflammatory disease (myocarditis and/or pericarditis)	Walking, strenuous physical activity, lifting, carrying, pushing/pulling, reaching, foot/leg controls, climbing, low work	• Management of acute myocarditis and chronic inflammatory cardiomyopathy: An Expert Consensus Document (Ammirati et al., 2020) • Management of acute and recurrent pericarditis (Chiabrando et al., 2020)	None

SOURCES: Whiteson et al., 2022; Xie et al., 2022b; Zang et al., 2023.

ANNEX TABLE 3-3 Selected Neurological Conditions Associated with Long COVID

Health Effects	Potential Functional Limitations	Selected Diagnostic and Management Guidelines	Potential Social Security Administration Listings
Autonomic dysfunction/ Postural orthostatic tachycardia syndrome	Sitting; standing; walking; strenuous physical activity; lifting; carrying; pushing/ pulling; reaching; climbing; low work; near visual acuity; understanding, remembering, and applying information; concentrating, persisting, or maintaining pace; problem solving	• Multi-disciplinary collaborative consensus guidance statement on the assessment and treatment of autonomic dysfunction in patients with post-acute sequelae of SARS-CoV-2 infection (PASC) (Blitshteyn, 2022) • Diagnosis and management of postural orthostatic tachycardia syndrome (Raj et al., 2021)	None
Dizziness (vestibular/ orthostatic)	Sitting; standing; walking; strenuous physical activity; lifting; carrying; pushing/ pulling; reaching; climbing; low work; near visual acuity; understanding, remembering, and applying information; concentrating, persisting, or maintaining pace; problem solving	• Dizziness: Evaluation and management (Rogers et al., 2023)	2.07
Encephalitis/ Encephalopathy	Sitting; standing; walking; strenuous physical activity; lifting; carrying; pushing/ pulling; reaching; gross and fine manipulation; foot/leg controls; climbing; low work; vision; hearing; speaking; understanding, remembering, and applying information; concentrating, persisting, or maintaining pace; problem solving; adapting or managing oneself; interacting with others	• Autoimmune encephalitis (Gole and Anand, 2023) • Diagnosis and management of acute encephalitis: A practical approach (Venkatesan and Geocadin, 2014) • Consensus clinical guidance for diagnosis and management of adult COVID-19 encephalopathy patients (Michael et al., 2023)	None

ANNEX TABLE 3-3 Continued

Health Effects	Potential Functional Limitations	Selected Diagnostic and Management Guidelines	Potential Social Security Administration Listings
Neurodegenerative disease	Sitting; standing; walking; strenuous physical activity; lifting; climbing; low work; speaking; understanding, remembering, and applying information; concentrating, persisting, or maintaining pace; problem solving; adapting or managing oneself; interacting with others	• Dopaminergic therapy for motor symptoms in early Parkinson disease practice guideline summary: A report of the AAN Guideline Subcommittee (Pringsheim et al., 2021) • Aducanumab use in symptomatic Alzheimer disease evidence in focus: A report of the AAN Guidelines Subcommittee (Day et al., 2022)	11.17
Neurocognitive disorders/post-COVID cognitive impairment	Speaking; understanding, remembering, and applying information; concentrating, persisting, or maintaining pace; problem solving; adapting or managing oneself; interacting with others	• Multi-disciplinary collaborative consensus guidance statement on the assessment and treatment of cognitive symptoms in patients with post-acute sequelae of SARS-CoV-2 infection (PASC) (Fine et al., 2022) • Practice guideline update summary: Mild cognitive impairment: Report of the Guideline Development, Dissemination, and Implementation Subcommittee of the American Academy of Neurology (Petersen et al., 2018)	None

continued

ANNEX TABLE 3-3 Continued

Health Effects	Potential Functional Limitations	Selected Diagnostic and Management Guidelines	Potential Social Security Administration Listings
Abnormal movements/ Tremors	Standing, walking, strenuous physical activity, lifting, carrying, reaching, gross and fine manipulation, foot/leg controls, climbing, low work, speaking	• Evidence-based guideline update: Treatment of essential tremor: Report of the Quality Standards Subcommittee of the American Academy of Neurology (Zesiewicz et al., 2011) • Differentiation and diagnosis of tremor (Crawford and Zimmerman, 2011) • Movement Disorder Society's evidence-based review of treatments for essential tremor (Ferreira et al., 2019) • COVID-19-associated new-onset movement disorders: A follow-up study (Schneider et al., 2023)	12.07
Dysphagia	Eating, drinking, swallowing	• Dysphagia: Evaluation and collaborative management (Wilkinson et al., 2021) • Clinical practice guidelines for the assessment of uninvestigated esophageal dysphagia (Liu et al., 2018)	None

ANNEX TABLE 3-3 Continued

Health Effects	Potential Functional Limitations	Selected Diagnostic and Management Guidelines	Potential Social Security Administration Listings
Guillain-Barré	Sitting, standing, walking, lifting, low work, reaching, gross and fine manipulation, climbing, foot/leg controls, strenuous physical activity, speaking, vision	• Practice parameter: Immunotherapy for Guillain-Barré syndrome: Report of the Quality Standards Subcommittee of the American Academy of Neurology (Hughes et al., 2003) • European Academy of Neurology/Peripheral Nerve Society guideline on diagnosis and treatment of Guillain-Barré syndrome (Van Doorn et al., 2023)	11.14
Stroke	Sitting; standing; walking; strenuous physical activity; lifting; carrying; pushing/pulling; reaching; gross and fine manipulation; foot/leg controls; climbing; low work; vision; hearing; speaking; understanding, remembering, and applying information; concentrating, persisting, or maintaining pace; problem solving; adapting or managing oneself; interacting with others	• Guidelines for the early management of patients with acute ischemic stroke: 2019 update to the 2018 guidelines for the early management of acute ischemic stroke: A guideline for healthcare professionals from the American Heart Association/American Stroke Association (Powers et al., 2019) • Guidelines for adult stroke rehabilitation and recovery: A guideline for healthcare professionals from the American Heart Association/American Stroke Association (Winstein et al., 2016)	11.04

continued

ANNEX TABLE 3-3 Continued

Health Effects	Potential Functional Limitations	Selected Diagnostic and Management Guidelines	Potential Social Security Administration Listings
Spinal cord infarction	Standing, sitting, walking, strenuous physical activity, lifting, carrying, pushing/pulling, reaching, gross and fine manipulation, foot/leg controls, climbing, low work	N/A	None
Peripheral/small fiber neuropathy	Standing, walking, strenuous physical activity, carrying, reaching, gross and fine manipulation, foot/leg controls, climbing	• Current view of diagnosing small fiber neuropathy (Raasing et al., 2021) • Small fiber neuropathy: A clinical and practical approach (Geerts et al., 2023)	11.14
Bell's palsy/cranial neuropathies	Vision, hearing, speaking	• Bell palsy: Rapid evidence review (Dalrymple et al., 2023) • Clinical practice guideline: Bell's palsy (Baugh et al., 2013)	11.14
Migraine and other chronic headaches	Strenuous physical activity; vision; understanding, remembering, and applying information; concentrating, persisting, or maintaining pace; interacting with others	• Outpatient primary care management of headaches: Guidelines from the VA/DoD (Ford et al., 2021) • Headaches in over 12s: Diagnosis and management (NICE, 2021b)	None
Pain	Standing; walking; strenuous physical activity; lifting; carrying; pushing/pulling; climbing; low work; understanding, remembering, and applying information; concentrating, persisting, or maintaining pace	• Clinical guidelines (AAPM, 2023)	None

ANNEX TABLE 3-3 Continued

Health Effects	Potential Functional Limitations	Selected Diagnostic and Management Guidelines	Potential Social Security Administration Listings
Proprioception and balance disorders	Standing, walking, lifting, carrying, pushing/pulling, reaching, gross and fine manipulation, foot/leg controls, climbing, low work	• Diagnosis and management of balance vestibular disorder (ASHA, 2016)	None
Seizure	Climbing; strenuous physical activity; understanding, remembering, and applying information; concentrating, persisting, or maintaining pace	• AES clinical practice guideline development manual (American Epilepsy Society, 2019)	11.02
Transverse myelitis or other demyelinating disease	Sitting, standing, walking, strenuous physical activity, lifting, carrying, pushing/pulling, reaching, gross and fine manipulation, foot/leg controls, climbing, low work, vision	• Transverse myelitis (Simone and Emmady, 2020	11.08
Raynaud's	Fine manipulation	• Raynaud's phenomenon (NIAMSD, 2021)	114.04
Paresthesia	Fine manipulation, foot/leg controls	• A comprehensive algorithm for management of neuropathic pain (Bates et al., 2019)	None
Critical illness myopathy and/or neuropathy	Standing, walking, strenuous physical activity, lifting, carrying, pushing/pulling, reaching, gross and fine manipulation, foot/leg controls, low work	• Critical illness myopathy: Diagnostic approach and resulting therapeutic implications (Rodriguez et al., 2022)	None

SOURCES: Melamed et al., 2023; Premraj et al., 2022; Xu et al., 2022; Zang et al., 2023.

ANNEX TABLE 3-4 Selected Special Senses and Speech Conditions Associated with Long COVID

Health Effects	Potential Functional Limitations	Selected Diagnostic and Management Guidelines	Potential Social Security Administration Listings
Anosmia/dysnosmia	N/A	• Clinical diagnosis and current management strategies for olfactory dysfunction: A review (Whitcroft and Hummel, 2019) • Management of new onset loss of sense of smell during the COVID-19 pandemic—BRS consensus guidelines (Hopkins et al., 2021)	None
Ageusia/dysgeusia	N/A	• Dysgeusia (ENT Health, 2020)	None
Dysarthria/dysphonia	Speaking	• Guidelines of clinical practice for the management of swallowing disorders and recent dysphonia in the context of the COVID-19 pandemic (Mattei et al., 2020)	2.09
Visual, ocular symptoms (changes in vision/dry eye)	Near or far visual acuity, peripheral vision	• Clinical management guidelines (The College of Optometrists, 2022)	2.02, 2.03, 2.04
Tinnitus	Hearing	• Clinical practice guideline: Tinnitus (Tunkel et al., 2014) • Tinnitus: Assessment and management (NICE, 2020) • Hearing loss, tinnitus, and dizziness in COVID-19: A systematic review and meta-analysis (Jafari et al., 2022) • Self-reported tinnitus and vertigo or dizziness in a cohort of adult Long COVID patients (Degen et al., 2022)	2.07

SOURCES: Melamed et al., 2023; Premraj et al., 2022; Xu et al., 2022.

ANNEX TABLE 3-5 Selected Musculoskeletal Conditions Associated with Long COVID

Health Effects	Potential Functional Limitations	Selected Diagnostic and Management Guidelines	Potential Social Security Administration Listings
Myopathy	Standing, walking, strenuous physical activity, lifting, pushing/pulling, overhead reaching, gross and fine manipulation, climbing, low work, vision	• Current classiciation and mangement of inflammatory myopathies (Schmidt, 2018)	None
Muscle weakness	Standing, walking, strenuous physical activity, lifting, pushing/pulling, reaching, gross and fine manipulation, climbing, low work	• Muscle weakness in adults: Evaluation and differential diagnosis (Larson and Wilbur, 2020) • Musculoskeletal complications in long COVID-19: A systematic review (Swarnakar et al., 2022)	None
Sarcopenia	Standing, walking, strenuous physical activity, lifting, pushing/pulling, reaching, gross and fine manipulation, climbing, low work	• International clinical practice guidelines for sarcopenia (ICFSR): Screening, diagnosis and management (Dent et al., 2018)	None
Myositis	Standing, walking, strenuous physical activity, lifting, pushing/pulling, reaching, gross and fine manipulation, climbing, low work	• British Society for Rheumatology guideline on management of paediatric, adolescent and adult patients with idiopathic inflammatory myopathy (Oldroyd et al., 2022)	14.05
Myalgia	Standing, walking, strenuous physical activity, lifting, pushing/pulling, reaching, gross and fine manipulation, climbing, low work	• Nonpharmacologic and pharmacologic management of acute pain from non-low back, musculoskeletal injuries in adults: A clinical guideline from the American College of Physicians and American Academy of Family Physicians (Qaseem et al., 2020)	None

continued

ANNEX TABLE 3-5 Continued

Health Effects	Potential Functional Limitations	Selected Diagnostic and Management Guidelines	Potential Social Security Administration Listings
Arthralgia	Standing, walking, strenuous physical activity, lifting, pushing/pulling, reaching, gross and fine manipulation, climbing, low work	• 2019 American College of Rheumatology/Arthritis Foundation guideline for the management of osteoarthritis of the hand, hip, and knee (Kolasinski et al., 2020)	None
Arthritis	Sitting, standing, walking, strenuous physical activity, lifting, pushing/pulling, reaching, gross and fine manipulation, climbing, low work	• American College of Rheumatology guideline for the treatment of rheumatoid arthritis (Fraenkel et al., 2021)	14.09

SOURCES: Swarnakar et al., 2022; Zang et al., 2023.

ANNEX TABLE 3-6 Selected Endocrine Conditions Associated with Long COVID

Health Effects	Potential Functional Limitations	Selected Diagnostic and Management Guidelines	Potential Social Security Administration Listings
Diabetes type 1	Standing; walking; strenuous physical activity; lifting; pushing/pulling; reaching; gross and fine manipulation; climbing; low work; vision; understanding, remembering, and applying information; concentrating, persisting, or maintaining pace	• Classification and diagnosis of diabetes: Standards of care in diabetes—2023 (ElSayed et al., 2023)	None (diabetes complications are included under organ-specific listings)
Diabetes type 2	Standing; walking; strenuous physical activity; lifting; pushing/pulling; reaching; gross and fine manipulation; climbing; low work; vision; understanding, remembering, and applying information; concentrating, persisting, or maintaining pace	• Classification and diagnosis of diabetes: Standards of care in diabetes—2023 (ElSayed et al., 2023)	None (diabetes complications are included under organ-specific listings)
Dyslipidemia	Vision	• American Heart Association/American College of Cardiology/American Association of Cardiovascular and Pulmonary Rehabilitation/American Academy of Physician Assistants/Association of Black Cardiologists/American College of Preventive Medicine/American Diabetes Association/American Geriatrics Society/American Pharmacists Association/American Society for Preventative Cardiology/National Lipid Association/Preventive Cardiovascular Nurses Association guideline on the management of blood cholesterol: A report of the American College of Cardiology/American Heart Association Task Force on Clinical Practice Guidelines (Grundy et al., 2019)	None

continued

ANNEX TABLE 3-6 Continued

Health Effects	Potential Functional Limitations	Selected Diagnostic and Management Guidelines	Potential Social Security Administration Listings
Thyroid gland disorders	Standing; walking; strenuous physical activity; lifting; pushing/pulling; reaching; gross and fine manipulation; climbing; low work; understanding, remembering, and applying information; concentrating, persisting, or maintaining pace; problem solving; interacting with others	• Thyroid disease: Assessment and management (NICE, 2023a)	None
Hypothalamic, pituitary, adrenal axis dysfunction	Standing; walking; strenuous physical activity; lifting; pushing/pulling; reaching; gross and fine manipulation; climbing; low work; understanding, remembering, and applying information; concentrating, persisting, or maintaining pace; problem solving; interacting with others	• Diagnosis and treatment of primary adrenal insufficiency: An Endocrine Society clinical practice guideline (Bornstein et al., 2016)	None
Reproductive hormone dysfunction	Low testosterone: Understanding, remembering, and applying information; concentrating, persisting, or maintaining pace; problem solving	• Sex hormones in SARS-CoV-2 susceptibility: Key players or confounders? (Lott et al., 2023)	None

SOURCES: Xie and Al-Aly, 2022; Xu et al., 2023; Zang et al., 2023.

ANNEX TABLE 3-7 Selected Immune Conditions Associated with Long COVID

Health Effects	Potential Functional Limitations	Selected Diagnostic and Management Guidelines	Potential Social Security Administration Listings
Mast cell activation syndrome	Strenuous physical activity; low work; understanding, remembering, and applying information; concentrating, persisting, or maintaining pace; problem solving; adapting or managing oneself	• Selecting the right criteria and proper classification to diagnose mast cell activation syndromes: A critical review (Gülen et al., 2021) • Diagnosis, classification and management of mast cell activation syndromes (MCAS) in the era of personalized medicine (Valent et al., 2020)	None
Autoimmune disorders (including rheumatoid arthritis, ankylosing spondylitis, systemic lupus erythematosus, myositis, systemic sclerosis, Sjögren's syndrome, mixed connective tissue disease, and inflammatory bowel disease)	Sitting; standing; walking; strenuous physical activity; lifting; carrying; pushing/pulling; reaching; gross and fine manipulation; foot/leg controls; climbing; low work; vision; hearing; speaking; understanding, remembering, and applying information; concentrating, persisting, or maintaining pace; problem solving; interacting with others; adapting or managing oneself	• Diagnostic testing and interpretation of tests for autoimmunity (Castro and Gourley, 2010)	14.00D

NOTE: Myositis and rheumatoid arthritis are discussed in Annex Table 3-5 (musculoskeletal conditions).
SOURCES: Chang et al., 2023; Lim et al., 2023; Sumantri and Rengganis, 2023; Weinstock et al., 2021.

ANNEX TABLE 3-8 Selected Gastrointestinal Conditions Associated with Long COVID

Health Effects	Potential Functional Limitations	Selected Diagnostic and Management Guidelines	Potential Social Security Administration Listings
Gastroesophageal reflux and peptic ulcer disease	N/A	• American College of Gastroenterology's gastroenterology guidelines (American College of Gastroenterology, 2023)	None
Gastritis/enteritis	Strenuous physical activity	• American Gastroenterological Association clinical practice update on the diagnosis and management of atrophic gastritis: Expert review (Shah et al., 2021)	None
Ischemic colitis	Strenuous physical activity	• ACG clinical guideline: Epidemiology, risk factors, patterns of presentation, diagnosis, and management of colon ischemia (CI) (Brandt et al., 2015)	None
Irritable bowel syndrome/ motility disorders	Strenuous physical activity; lifting; carrying; pushing/pulling; reaching; gross and fine manipulation; foot/leg controls; climbing; low work; vision; hearing; speaking; understanding, remembering, and applying information; concentrating, persisting, or maintaining pace; problem solving; interacting with others; adapting or managing oneself	• ACG clinical guideline: Management of irritable bowel syndrome (Lacy et al., 2021)	None
Gut dysbiosis	N/A	N/A	None

ANNEX TABLE 3-8 Continued

Health Effects	Potential Functional Limitations	Selected Diagnostic and Management Guidelines	Potential Social Security Administration Listings
Cholestasis	N/A	• Guidelines for the management of cholestatic liver diseases (2021) (Lu, 2022) • ACG clinical guideline: Diagnosis and management of biliary strictures (Elmunzer et al., 2023) • ACG clinical guideline: Evaluation of abnormal liver chemistries (Kwo et al., 2017) • EASL clinical practice guidelines: Management of cholestatic liver diseases (EASL, 2009)	5.05
Chronic liver disease	Standing, walking, strenuous physical activity	• EASL clinical practice guidelines for the management of patients with decompensated cirrhosis (Angeli et al., 2018)	5.05
Cholangitis	N/A	• Tokyo guidelines 2018: Diagnostic criteria and severity grading of acute cholangitis (with videos) (Kiriyama et al., 2018) • Primary biliary cholangitis: 2021 practice guidance update from the American Association for the Study of Liver Diseases (Lindor et al., 2022)	None

continued

ANNEX TABLE 3-8 Continued

Health Effects	Potential Functional Limitations	Selected Diagnostic and Management Guidelines	Potential Social Security Administration Listings
Pancreatitis	N/A	• American Gastroenterological Association institute guideline on initial management of acute pancreatitis (Crockett et al., 2018) • American College of Gastroenterology guideline: Management of acute pancreatitis (Tenner et al., 2013)	None
Weight loss due to gastrointestinal disease	Strenuous physical activity	N/A	5.08
Chronic abdominal pain	Strenuous physical activity, overhead reaching	• Evaluation of acute abdominal pain in adults (Cartwright and Knudson, 2008) • Rome IV criteria (Rome Foundation, n.d.)	None
Nausea or vomiting	Strenuous physical activity, climbing	• AGA clinical practice update on management of medically refractory gastroparesis: Expert review (Lacy et al., 2022)	None

SOURCES: Xu et al., 2023; Zang et al., 2023.

ANNEX TABLE 3-9 Selected Genitourinary Conditions Associated with Long COVID

Health Effects	Potential Functional Limitations	Selected Diagnostic and Management Guidelines	Potential Social Security Administration Listings
Sexual dysfunction	N/A	• Clinical practice guidelines for management of sexual dysfunction (Avasthi et al., 2017)	None
Dysmenorrhea/ menstrual irregularities (with moderate to severe pain)	Standing, walking, strenuous physical activity, lifting, carrying, pushing/pulling, foot/leg controls, climbing, low work	• Dysmenorrhea and endometriosis in the adolescent – Committee opinion number 760 (ACOG, 2018) • The initial management of chronic pelvic pain: Green Top Guideline 41 (RCOG, 2012)	None
Oligospermia	N/A	• Diagnosis and treatment of infertility in men: AUA/ASRM guideline part I (Schlegel et al., 2020)	None
Orchitis/ epididymitis (with moderate to severe pain)	Standing, walking, strenuous physical activity, lifting, carrying, pushing/pulling, climbing, low work	• Sexually transmitted infections treatment guidelines, 2021 (CDC, 2021c)	None
Acute kidney injury (<12 months)	N/A	• Kidney Disease Improving Global Outcomes (KDIGO) clinical practice guideline for acute kidney injury (KDIGO, 2012) • KDIGO 2021 clinical practice guideline for the management of glomerular diseases (Rovin et al., 2021)	None

continued

ANNEX TABLE 3-9 Continued

Health Effects	Potential Functional Limitations	Selected Diagnostic and Management Guidelines	Potential Social Security Administration Listings
Chronic kidney disease (>12 months)	Standing; walking; strenuous physical activity; lifting; carrying; pushing/pulling; reaching; fine manipulation; foot/leg controls; climbing; low work; understanding, remembering, and applying information; concentrating, persisting, or maintaining pace; problem solving	• KDIGO clinical practice guideline for the evaluation and management of chronic kidney disease (KDIGO, 2013)	6.05
Overactive bladder syndrome	Sitting; standing; walking; strenuous physical activity; lifting; carrying; pushing/pulling; climbing; low work; concentrating, persisting, or maintaining pace; adapting or managing oneself	• Diagnosis and treatment of overactive bladder (non-neurogenic) in adults: AUA/SUFU guideline amendment 2019 (Lightner et al., 2019)	None

SOURCES: Bowe et al., 2021; Schiffl et al., 2023; Zang et al., 2023.

ANNEX TABLE 3-10 Selected Skin Conditions Associated with Long COVID

Health Effects	Potential Functional Limitations	Selected Diagnostic and Management Guidelines	Potential Social Security Administration Listings
Hair loss	N/A	• Hair loss: Common causes and treatment (Phillips et al., 2017) • Guidelines for the management of alopecia areata (MacDonald Hull et al., 2003)	None
Livedo reticularis	N/A	• Livedo reticularis and livedoid vasculopathy (Primary Care Dermatology Society, 2023) • Livedo reticularis: An update (Gibbs et al., 2005)	None
Pernio	Sitting, strenuous physical activity, lifting, carrying, pushing/pulling, reaching, gross and fine manipulation, foot/leg controls, low work	• Clinical characteristics, etiologic associations, laboratory findings, treatment, and proposal of diagnostic criteria of pernio (chilblains) in a series of 104 patients at Mayo Clinic, 2000 to 2011 (Cappel and Wetter, 2014)	8.05
Retiform purpura	Sitting, strenuous physical activity, lifting, carrying, pushing/pulling, reaching, gross and fine manipulation, foot/leg controls, low work	• Retiform purpura: A diagnostic approach (Georgesen et al., 2020)	8.05
Chronic urticaria	Sitting, strenuous physical activity, lifting, carrying, pushing/pulling, reaching, gross and fine manipulation, foot/leg controls, low work	• The diagnosis and management of acute and chronic urticaria: 2014 update (Bernstein et al., 2014)	None

SOURCES: Grover et al., 2022; Zang et al., 2023.

ANNEX TABLE 3-11 Selected Neuropsychiatric Conditions Associated with Long COVID

Health Effects	Potential Functional Limitations	Selected Diagnostic and Management Guidelines	Potential Social Security Administration Listings
Loss of sexual desire	N/A	• *Diagnostic and statistical manual of mental disorders, fifth edition, text revision* (DSM-5-TR) (APA, 2022)	None
Attention deficit/ hyperactivity disorder	Sitting; concentrating, persisting, or maintaining pace; interacting with others; adapting or managing oneself	• DSM-5-TR (APA, 2022)	None
Anxiety/panic disorders	Speaking; concentrating, persisting, or maintaining pace; interacting with others; adapting or managing oneself	• DSM-5-TR (APA, 2022)	12.06
Depression	Speaking; concentrating, persisting, or maintaining pace; interacting with others; adapting or managing oneself	• DSM-5-TR (APA, 2022)	12.04
Post-traumatic stress disorder	Speaking; concentrating, persisting, or maintaining pace; interacting with others; adapting or managing oneself	• DSM-5-TR (APA, 2022)	12.15
Psychotic disorder	Speaking; understanding, remembering, and applying information; concentrating, persisting, or maintaining pace; problem solving; interacting with others; adapting or managing oneself	• DSM-5-TR (APA, 2022)	12.03
Stress	Concentrating, persisting, or maintaining pace; interacting with others; adapting or managing oneself	• DSM-5-TR (APA, 2022)	12.06

ANNEX TABLE 3-11 Continued

Health Effects	Potential Functional Limitations	Selected Diagnostic and Management Guidelines	Potential Social Security Administration Listings
Adjustment disorder	Concentrating, persisting, or maintaining pace; interacting with others; adapting or managing oneself	• DSM-5-TR (APA, 2022)	12.15
Eating disorder	Standing; strenuous physical activity; climbing; concentrating, persisting, or maintaining pace; interacting with others; adapting or managing oneself	• DSM-5-TR (APA, 2022)	None
Obsessive compulsive disorder	Concentrating, persisting, or maintaining pace; interacting with others; adapting or managing oneself	• DSM-5-TR (APA, 2022)	None
Disordered sleep	Understanding, remembering, and applying information; concentrating, persisting, or maintaining pace; problem solving; interacting with others; adapting or managing oneself	• DSM-5-TR (APA, 2022)	None

SOURCES: Cheng et al., 2023; Premraj et al., 2022; Xie et al., 2022a; Zang et al., 2023.

ANNEX TABLE 3-12 Multisystem Conditions Associated with Long COVID

Health Effects	Potential Functional Limitations	Selected Diagnostic and Management Guidelines	Potential Social Security Administration Listings
Chronic fatigue/post-exertional malaise	Walking; strenuous physical activity; lifting; carrying; pushing/pulling; reaching; climbing; low work; understanding, remembering, and applying information; adapting or managing oneself	• Multidisciplinary collaborative consensus guidance statement on the assessment and treatment of fatigue in post-acute sequelae of SARS-CoV-2 infection (PASC) patients (Herrera et al., 2021)	None
Myalgic encephalitis/chronic fatigue syndrome	Sitting; standing; walking; strenuous physical activity; lifting; carrying; pushing/pulling; reaching; gross and fine manipulation; foot/leg controls; climbing; low work; vision; hearing; speaking; understanding, remembering, and applying information; concentrating, persisting, or maintaining pace; problem solving; interacting with others; adapting or managing oneself	• *Beyond myalgic encephalomyelitis/chronic fatigue syndrome: Redefining an illness* (IOM, 2015) • Myalgic encephalomyelitis/chronic fatigue syndrome: Essentials of diagnosis and management (Bateman et al., 2021) • Myalgic encephalomyelitis (or encephalopathy)/chronic fatigue syndrome: Diagnosis and management (NICE, 2021c) • Diagnosis and management of myalgic encephalomyelitis/chronic fatigue syndrome (Grach et al., 2023)	None
Fever	N/A	• Fever (Mayo Clinic, 2022)	None

SOURCE: Zang et al., 2023.

ANNEX TABLE 3-13 Physical Activities; Vision, Hearing, and Speech; and Mental Activities

Activity	Definition
Physical Activities	
Sitting	For the purpose of collecting occupational data, the U.S. Bureau of Labor Statistics considers sitting to be present when any of the following conditions exists:
	• Workers remain in a seated position. This includes active sitting. For example, bicyclists sit but push/pull with their feet/legs. • Workers are lying down. This includes active lying down. For example, a mechanic lying on a dolly working underneath a vehicle is sitting. • Workers may choose between sitting and standing for a given task. For example, office workers can choose a standing desk. (BLS, 2020, p. 112)
	From a functional perspective, however, sitting as a physical activity involves resting one's lower body (buttocks) on a seat or the ground, while maintaining one's upper body (torso, neck, head) in an upright position. In addition to strong neck, shoulder, and core muscles, sitting requires balance and good proprioception. Although lying on a raised surface (e.g., a bed) may be grouped with sitting, sitting is distinct from lying down on the ground (e.g., lying on a dolly underneath a vehicle), which this report groups under low work.
Standing	For the purpose of collecting occupational data, the Occupational Requirements Survey distinguishes only between sitting (as defined previously) and standing/walking defined as "whenever workers are not sitting or lying down," including "time spent stooping, crawling, kneeling, crouching, or climbing" (BLS, 2020, p. 112). In other words, "a worker is always either sitting or standing/walking" (BLS, 2020, p. 112).
	From a functional perspective, standing is distinct from walking, which in turn is distinct from low work (stooping, crawling, kneeling, crouching), or climbing. For the purpose of this report, standing is defined as being "in an upright position with all of [one's] weight on [one's] feet" (*Stand*, n.d.).
Walking	Moving along on foot or advancing by steps, with one foot always on the ground.
	Distance (long or short) and surface type (uneven, rough) can affect an individual's ability to walk.
Strenuous physical activity	Strenuous physical activity captures activities that require exertion and stamina—for example, running, jumping, swimming, throwing, catching, and the like. It potentially includes all other physical activities, in addition to running and other impact activities.
Lifting (floor to waist and overhead)	Use of upper and/or lower extremities to raise or lower an object from one level to another, including upward pulling (BLS, 2020, p. 118).

continued

ANNEX TABLE 3-13 Continued

Activity	Definition
Carrying	"Transporting an object, usually by holding it in the hands or arms, or wearing it on the body, usually around the waist or upper torso" (BLS, 2020, p.118). Carrying usually also requires the ability to stand, lift, and walk.
Pushing/pulling	Use of upper and/or lower extremities to exert force upon an object so that the object moves away from or toward the origin of the force (BLS, 2020, p. 125).
Reaching	"Extending the hand(s) and arm(s) in any direction, requiring the straightening and extending of the arm(s) and elbow(s) and the engagement of the shoulder(s)" (BLS, 2020, p. 130). Reaching may require standing.
Overhead reaching	Extending the arm(s) with the hand(s) higher than the head and (1) the elbow is bent and the angle at the shoulders is about 90 degrees or more or (2) the elbow is extended and the angle at the shoulder is about 120 degrees or more (BLS, 2020, p. 130). Overhead reaching requires neck extension and may require standing.
At/below the shoulder reaching	Reaching that does not meet the threshold for overhead reaching described above (BLS, 2020, p. 130). At/below the shoulder reaching may require standing.
Gross manipulation	Gross manipulation involves "seizing, holding, grasping, turning, or otherwise working with the hand(s). Fingers are involved only to the extent that they are an extension of the hand to hold or operate an object or tool, such as hammer" (BLS, 2020, p. 187). It includes handling of large objects.
Fine manipulation	Fine manipulation involves "touching, picking, pinching, or otherwise working primarily with fingers rather than with the whole hand or arm" (BLS, 2020, p. 133). It includes writing, typing, or handling small objects (fingering).
Foot/leg controls	Refers to the "use of one or both feet or legs to move controls on machinery or equipment. Controls include, but are not limited to, pedals, buttons, levers, and cranks" (BLS, 2020, p. 133).
Climbing	"The act of ascending or descending stairs, ramps, ladders, ropes or scaffolding and similar structures using feet, legs, hands, and/or arms" (BLS, 2020, p. 142).

ANNEX TABLE 3-13 Continued

Activity	Definition
Low work	Low work is a group of activities that includes stooping, crouching, kneeling, crawling, and lying on the ground.
	Stooping is the act of "bending the body forward and down while bending the spine at the waist 45 degrees or more either over something below waist level or down towards an object on or near the ground" (BLS, 2020, p. 193). Must be performed standing.
	Crouching is "bending the body downward and forward by bending the legs and spine" (BLS, 2020, p. 138).
	Kneeling is "bending the legs at the knees to come to rest on the knee or knees" (BLS, 2020, p. 139).
	Crawling is "moving about on hands and knees or hands and feet" (BLS, 2020, p. 139).
	Lying on the ground includes the need to get down and up from the ground (e.g., lying down on a trolley on the ground).
	Clustering the low work activities is appropriate because one generally has to be able to stoop, crouch, and kneel to be able to crawl. There might be an occasion when someone only has to kneel momentarily (e.g., to lift a child) that might be less difficult for some people, but most of the difficulties are shared among these activities.
	From a functional perspective, lying on the ground has more in common with other low work activities in that it includes the need to get up and down from the ground and potentially squirming around to do work while on the ground. These are difficult tasks that are equivalent to the other low work activities.

Vision, Hearing, and Speaking Activities

Activity	Definition
Near visual acuity	"Clarity of vision at approximately 20 inches or less, as when working with small objects or reading small print" (BLS, 2020, p. 154), including the use of a computer in support of a critical job function, regardless of distance.
Far visual acuity	"Clarity of vision at a distance of 20 feet or more, involving the ability to distinguish features of a person or objects at a distance" (BLS, 2020, p. 154).
Peripheral vision	"What is seen above, below, to the left or right by the eye while staring straight ahead" (BLS, 2020, p. 154).
Hearing	"Ability to hear, understand, and distinguish speech and/or other sounds" (BLS, 2020, p. 149). Includes hearing in-person one-on-one and group or conference communication; telephones and similar devices, such as radios, walkie-talkies, intercoms, and public address systems; and other such sounds as machinery alarms and equipment sounds. Passing a hearing test may be required for certain jobs.
Speaking	"Expressing or exchanging ideas by means of the spoken word to impart oral information to clients or the public and to convey detailed spoken instructions to other workers accurately, loudly, or quickly" (BLS, 2020, p. 149).

continued

ANNEX TABLE 3-13 Continued

Activity	Definition
Mental Activities	
Understand, remember, and apply information	The abilities to learn, recall, and use (apply) information (SSA, n.d.-a, n.d.-b).
Concentrate, persist, or maintain pace	The abilities to focus attention on work/school activities and stay on task at a sustained rate (SSA, n.d.-a, n.d.-b).
Problem solve	"Analyze issues and make decisions that have a moderate to significant level of difficulty (e.g., the full extent of issues may not be readily apparent and requires independent judgment and research or investigation). The defining characteristics of problem solving are that there is no obvious, immediate solution to a problem or issue, and the worker must identify and weigh alternatives to arrive at a solution" (BLS, 2020, p. 99).
Interact with others	The abilities to relate to and work with supervisors, coworkers, the public, teachers, peers, and others—for example, cooperating with others; asking for help when needed; handling conflicts with others; stating [one's] point of view; initiating or sustaining conversation; understanding and responding to social cues (physical, verbal, emotional); responding to requests, suggestions, criticism, correction, and challenges; and keeping social interactions free of excessive irritability, sensitivity, argumentativeness, or suspiciousness. (SSA, n.d.-a; see also SSA, n.d.-b)
Adapt or manage oneself	The abilities to "regulate emotions, control behavior, and maintain well-being" in a work or school setting—for example, responding to demands; adapting to changes; managing [one's] psychologically based symptoms; distinguishing between acceptable and unacceptable work performance; setting realistic goals; making plans for [oneself] independently of others; maintaining personal hygiene and [appropriate attire]; and being aware of normal hazards and taking appropriate precautions. (SSA, n.d.-a; see also SSA, n.d.-b)

SOURCES: BLS, 2020; SSA, n.d.-a, n.d.-b; table reprinted from NASEM, 2022, p. 197.

4

Global Functioning in Long COVID

For many individuals, the effects of SARS-CoV-2 infection persist well beyond the acute phase and can result in considerable disability. A 2-year prospective cohort study of 548 individuals meeting the World Health Organization's definition of Post–COVID-19 Condition found that at the end of the 23-month follow-up period, only 7.6 percent of the subjects (38 percent hospitalized) had recovered (Mateu et al., 2023). The U.S. Household Pulse Survey revealed that 26.4 percent of adults with Long COVID experienced substantial activity limitations (Ford et al., 2023). Similarly, the Public Health Agency of Canada reported that 21.3 percent of adults with the condition "often" or "always" experienced substantial activity limitations (Public Health Agency of Canada, 2023), and the UK Office for National Statistics reported that 20 percent indicated their daily activity performance had been "limited a lot" (Rea et al., 2023). Additionally, a study of U.S. veterans (older, male population) followed for 2 years found that Long COVID contributed 80.4 disability-adjusted life years (DALYs) per 1,000 persons, compared with 50 and 52 DALYs for cancer and heart disease, respectively (Bowe et al., 2023).

This chapter provides an overview of the literature on patterns and trends of work- or school-related functional changes associated with Long COVID in adults and children. The chapter addresses global functioning, meaning an individual's overall ability to function, in people with Long COVID. The committee reviewed prospective cohort studies that followed Long COVID patients and assessed their functioning for 6 months or more.

For less well-studied topics, cohorts followed for a shorter duration and cross-sectional studies were also reviewed (the committee did not conduct a systematic review; see Appendix A for the literature search strategy). Functional disability post–COVID-19 has been characterized as inability to return to work, poor quality of life, diminished ability to perform activities of daily living (ADLs), decreased physical and cognitive function, and overall disability (Ahmad et al., 2023; Becker et al., 2021b; Frontera et al., 2022, 2021; Ghossein-Doha et al., 2022; Hartung et al., 2022; Rass et al., 2022). The committee notes that outcomes differ for people hospitalized for COVID-19 and those with milder cases; those with more severe initial infection who were admitted to the intensive care unit (ICU) may have different outcomes still. Thus, this chapter groups studies by nonhospitalized, hospitalized, and ICU patients. The committee notes that it recognizes the need to separate the effects of hospitalization or critical illness from effects unique to COVID-19, as their recovery trajectories and pathophysiologies may differ. The chapter also provides a table of selected assessment measures used to quantify the impact of Long COVID, sections on unique considerations for children and other special populations with Long COVID, and a summary of how rehabilitation can affect functioning in individuals with the condition.

LONG-TERM FUNCTIONAL OUTCOMES IN PATIENTS NOT HOSPITALIZED FOR COVID-19

Although severe initial infection with SARS-CoV-2 is one of the strongest predictors of poor long-term functional outcomes, individuals with mild initial illness make up the great majority of the population with long-term functional impairments, simply because of their greater numbers relative to those with severe infection (Ahmad et al., 2023; Banic et al., 2022; Hodgson et al., 2021). A large Scottish population-based study, for example, found that 5 percent of those with mild COVID-19 had not recovered at least 6 months following infection, compared with 16 percent of those who required hospitalization—a ratio of approximately 1:3 (Hastie et al., 2022). Other studies have found a similar degree of increased risk among those hospitalized for COVID-19 (Jassat et al., 2023). However, the proportion of people not hospitalized for acute SARS-CoV-2 infection compared with those hospitalized is approximately 95–98:1, dwarfing the increased risk of Long COVID conveyed by hospitalization (Angulo et al., 2021; Mahajan et al., 2021; Menachemi et al., 2021). Thus, consideration of functional impairment from Long COVID must include those with mild initial illness.

Symptom burden is closely associated with functional impairment, with numerous studies demonstrating a correlation between an increased number and severity of long-term symptoms and decreased quality of life, physical functioning, and ability to work (Bahmer et al., 2022; Cazé et al., 2023; Chatys-Bogacka et al., 2022; Dennis et al., 2021, 2023; Graham et al., 2021; Gutiérrez-Canales et al., 2022; Han et al., 2022; Hastie et al., 2022; Hossain et al., 2021; Kenny et al., 2022; O'Kelly et al., 2022; Perlis et al., 2023; Seeßle et al., 2022). People not hospitalized for COVID-19 are less likely to experience severe organ dysfunction (e.g., kidney failure requiring dialysis, disabling stroke, or measurable reduction in lung function) compared with those initially hospitalized. In one study of 337 patients, for example, 20 percent of individuals initially hospitalized had reduced diffusing capacity of the lungs for carbon monoxide (DLCO) after 3–6 months compared with only 4 percent of those not requiring hospitalization (Björsell et al., 2023). Instead, the population with mild initial illness more typically experiences long-term symptoms such as fatigue, sleep disturbance, brain fog, headaches, and muscle pains. Breathlessness is common, often despite the lack of measurable abnormalities in lung function (Bahmer et al., 2022; Björsell et al., 2023; Dennis et al., 2021; Graham et al., 2021; Gutiérrez-Canales et al., 2022; Hossain et al., 2021; Kim et al., 2022b; Perez Giraldo et al., 2023; Seeßle et al., 2022).

Long-term loss of smell or taste is particularly disproportionate in the population with mild infection compared with those hospitalized (Graham et al., 2021; Hossain et al., 2021; Perez Giraldo et al., 2023). While sometimes dismissed as a minor impairment, loss of smell or taste can have important functional consequences and decrease quality of life. In a study of 322 people with COVID-19–related olfactory loss, 96 percent reported at least one quality-of-life impact, including reduced enjoyment of food (87 percent) and reduced enjoyment of life (56 percent) (Coelho et al., 2021). More than 57 percent reported at least one safety-related event, such as inability to smell smoke (45 percent), burning food (28 percent), ingesting spoiled food (15 percent), and being unable to detect a gas leak (7 percent). Moreover, loss of olfactory function may correlate with other neurological abnormalities (Coelho et al., 2021). A study of 23 patients with persistent olfactory dysfunction found that the degree of that sensory loss was correlated with impaired visuospatial memory and executive function (Muccioli et al., 2023).

Risk Factors

Risk factors for long-term symptoms in the nonhospitalized population are similar to those for the hospitalized population. They include female sex, lack of vaccination against SARS-CoV-2, baseline disability or comorbidities, and smoking (Ayoubkhani et al., 2022; Björsell et al., 2023; Dennis et al., 2023; Gutiérrez-Canales et al., 2022; Jassat et al., 2023; Kim et al.,

2022b; Mateu et al., 2023; Mohamed Hussein et al., 2021; Tanguay et al., 2023). People with elevated heart rate at 3 months are more likely still to have symptoms at 1 year (O'Kelly et al., 2022). Some work suggests that people suffering specific symptoms in the acute phase are more likely to suffer those symptoms long term (Golla et al., 2023; Tanguay et al., 2023; Thronicke et al., 2022). In contrast with hospitalized patients, however, older age is less consistently a risk factor for Long COVID symptoms in the nonhospitalized population. Some studies have found higher rates of Long COVID in older nonhospitalized patients compared with younger patients (Kim et al., 2022b). However, a study of 2,198 people in Bangladesh found that Long COVID was associated with younger age, while two studies collectively involving 427 people in the United Kingdom and Germany, mostly with mild disease, found that cognitive dysfunction and dyspnea were more common in younger than in older patients (Dennis et al., 2023; Hossain et al., 2021; Seeßlle et al., 2022). Other studies similarly have found dyspnea to be more common in people <60 years of age compared with those that are older (Björsell et al., 2023). Finally, a study of 1,173 nonhospitalized patients in Canada found that age was not a significant predictor of the development of Long COVID, whereas older age was a predictor among hospitalized patients (Tanguay et al., 2023). Additionally, environmental exposures including certain air pollutants and toxicants have been found to be associated with increased risk of Long COVID, though data vary regionally (Zhang et al., 2023).

Recovery Trajectories

Many nonhospitalized people with persistent symptoms following acute SARS-CoV-2 infection improve over time. In one study of 331 people with persistent symptoms at about 6 months following infection, symptom prevalence was found to be reduced at 1 year: fatigue decreased from 98 to 64 percent, myalgia from 89 to 35 percent, shortness of breath from 90 to 47 percent, headache from 85 to 34 percent, chest pain from 81 to 38 percent, fever from 73 to 2 percent, cough from 75 to 11 percent, and sore throat from 71 to 11 percent (Dennis et al., 2023). However, only 18 percent had fully recovered by 1 year (Dennis et al., 2023). Similarly, a study of 96 people with symptoms at 5 months found that only 22 percent had fully recovered by 1 year (Seeßle et al., 2022). Another study found that approximately one-quarter of those who initially lost the sense of smell or taste had not regained those functions by 1 year (Fortunato et al., 2022), and in another study, objective measures of lung function were found to improve only slightly between 3 months and 1 year after mild infection (Lenoir et al., 2023). In the NIH RECOVER study, approximately two-thirds of 409 adults who met criteria for persistent symptoms at 6 months still met those criteria at 9 months (Thaweethai et al., 2023).

Among those who do not improve, most remain stable, but some worsen. In one study, for example, 13 percent of Long COVID patients who had mild initial disease experienced worsening quality of life scores between 3 and 12 months following infection (Tanguay et al., 2023). A survey of 4,510 U.S. adults found that Long COVID patients with disabilities were not significantly more likely to experience long-term symptoms compared with respondents without disabilities (adjusted odds ratio [aOR]=1.65 [0.78–3.50]) (Miller et al., 2023). Seeking health care for reported symptoms was higher among respondents with disabilities (40 percent) than among those without disabilities (18 percent) (Miller et al., 2023).

LONG-TERM FUNCTIONAL OUTCOMES IN PATIENTS HOSPITALIZED FOR COVID-19

Functional disability is highly prevalent in individuals surviving hospitalization for COVID-19. In the majority of the studies summarized here, hospitalization for COVID-19 is defined as a hospital stay with a symptomatic PCR-confirmed COVID-19 test. A few studies define it as discharge from the hospital with a diagnosis of confirmed or suspected COVID-19. One prospective longitudinal study of adults hospitalized for COVID-19 in 44 hospitals across the United States found that approximately 75 percent of survivors experienced cardiopulmonary, financial, and functional problems 6 months after hospitalization (Admon et al., 2023). Other cohort studies have similarly suggested that approximately 50–87 percent of patients hospitalized for COVID-19 may continue to experience functional disability through 6- to 12-month follow-up periods (D'Ettorre et al., 2022; Kim et al., 2022a; McAuley et al., 2023; Menges et al., 2021; Rass et al., 2022; Sahanic et al., 2023; Schlemmer et al., 2023; Shirakawa et al., 2023; Sonnweber et al., 2022; Steinbeis et al., 2022; Taboada et al., 2022; Valdes et al., 2022; Weber et al., 2022).

Emerging evidence indicates that once established, symptoms can persist even longer than 1 year. In a prospective study, 54 percent of 1,359 hospitalized patients in China still had at least one symptom at 3 years postinfection, and 13 percent of those who were employed prior to infection were still unable to work after 3 years (Zhang et al., 2024). The high symptom burden of Long COVID is particularly contributory (Kersten et al., 2022). One study found that 44 percent of patients hospitalized for COVID-19 reported three or more persistent symptoms at 6 months follow-up, and that disability was widespread across all areas of functioning in these patients (Hodgson et al., 2021). This finding is echoed across studies, encompassing significant decreases in health-related quality of life, significant physical limitations, impairing fatigue, difficulties performing ADLs, changes in occupation, and cognitive impairment (Becker et al., 2021a, 2021b;

Bellan et al., 2022; Daher et al., 2020; Damanti et al., 2022; Evans et al., 2021; Miskowiak et al., 2023; Stavem et al., 2022).

Risk Factors

COVID-19 severity is among the greatest risk factors for poor functional outcomes following recovery from acute infection (Ahmad et al., 2023; Banic et al., 2022; Hodgson et al., 2021). Studies have shown that patients hospitalized for COVID-19 are more likely to have more severe symptoms and worse functional outcomes on average compared with those who were not hospitalized (Björsell et al., 2023; Jassat et al., 2023; Krysa et al., 2023; Niedziela et al., 2022; Xie et al., 2022; Xu et al., 2022). In a cross-sectional study conducted in Alberta, Canada, that included 330 respondents, Krysa and colleagues (2023) found that twice as many previously hospitalized than nonhospitalized patients reported Long COVID symptoms (49 percent vs. 26 percent), and about four times as many hospitalized patients were unable to return to work (19 percent vs. 5 percent). In addition, in a U. S. Department of Veterans Affairs (VA) cohort of more than 150,000 individuals, Xie and colleagues (2022) and Xu and colleagues (2022) found that, compared with those who were not hospitalized, those who were hospitalized experienced approximately twice as great an excess burden of neurological outcomes and more than four times greater excess burden of cardiovascular outcomes at 12 months.

While severity of acute COVID-19 has been found consistently to be a strong risk factor for Long COVID and associated sequelae, individuals who experience mild SARS-CoV-2 infection can still develop Long COVID. Baseline demographic factors, including female gender, older age, obesity, and baseline disability, have also been identified as risk factors for functional disability (Asadi-Pooya et al., 2021; Damanti et al., 2022; Fernández-de-las-Peñas et al., 2022). Additionally, neurological complications, psychological morbidity (e.g., depression, anxiety, posttraumatic stress disorder), and psychosocial stressors (e.g., financial insecurity, food insecurity, death of close contact, new disability) have been found to confer risk for poor functional outcomes (Claflin et al., 2021; Frontera et al., 2021, 2022; McAuley et al., 2023; Sahanic et al., 2023; Sonnweber et al., 2022).

Recovery Trajectories

With respect to recovery trajectories, only a few studies have examined the functional disability burden of Long COVID longitudinally. Such studies have found that approximately half of patients hospitalized for severe COVID-19 may recover, whereas others may remain with persistent functional impairment at 12 months and beyond (Huang et al., 2021). One study found that among those reporting difficulty managing occupational or school responsibilities at 4 months, half continued to report difficulty at 2 years follow-up (Wahlgren et al., 2023). Another study found that approximately 47 percent of participants (n = 825) had at least one new impairment in ADLs or instrumental ADLs (IADLs) at 6 months following acute infection—a decrease from the reported 55 percent of patients reporting such impairments at 1 month (Admon et al., 2023). Approximately 26 percent of participants reported three or more new ADL or IADL impairments at 6 months (Admon et al., 2023).

Overall, these findings suggest that functional recovery is limited for patients hospitalized for COVID-19 (Admon et al., 2023; Wahlgren et al., 2023). Among those who do not recover by 6 months following acute infection, recovery appears to plateau between 6 and 12 months (Fernandez-de-las-Penas et al., 2023; Sahanic et al., 2023; Schlemmer et al., 2023; Steinbeis et al., 2022; Zhang et al., 2024). In the above-referenced study of 1,359 patients from China, the proportion with any post-COVID symptom at 3 years (54 percent) was nearly identical to that at 2 years (55 percent) (Zhang et al., 2024). Factors associated with not recovering included female sex, middle/older ages, two or more comorbidities, and more severe initial infection (Ahmad et al., 2023; Banic et al., 2022; Evans et al., 2021; Hodgson et al., 2021; Qin et al., 2023; Sahanic et al., 2023).

Given the relatively brief time since the onset of the pandemic, the long-term trajectories for recovery remain unclear. Extrapolating from other research areas and critical illnesses (e.g., post-intensive care syndrome [PICS]; acute respiratory distress syndrome), the likelihood of long-term functional recovery may be limited in a subset of individuals. Studies of PICS and acute respiratory distress syndrome have found that many affected individuals experience persistent functional disability up to 5 years later (Herridge et al., 2011; Hodgson et al., 2021). Research is needed to answer questions about variations in functional status or long-term effects in people hospitalized for COVID-19 based on different viral variants and vaccination status. However, studies have shown that even for the milder Omicron variant, rates of COVID-19 hospitalization have remained high, and vaccination and patients' immune status have been the greatest predictors of poor health outcomes (Nevejan et al., 2022).

LONG-TERM FUNCTIONAL OUTCOMES IN PATIENTS RECEIVING INTENSIVE CARE FOR COVID-19

PICS, a term used to describe new or worsening health impairments across physical, mental, cognitive, or social domains of health in survivors of critical illnesses that required hospitalization in an ICU, is a useful rubric for understanding the long-term functional outcomes in individuals with COVID-19 who were treated in ICUs (Needham et al., 2012). However, most of the studies examining long-term outcomes in COVID-19 survivors treated in the ICU are small case series or single-center inception cohort studies (Erber et al., 2021; Fischer et al., 2022; Gonzalez et al., 2022; Núñez-Seisdedos et al., 2022; Sassi et al., 2022). Since most people who survive the discharge from the ICU spend a significant time after discharge in hospital wards, disentangling post-ICU from posthospital effects is challenging (Admon et al., 2023; Iwashyna et al., 2021). Other methodological challenges to interpreting the literature on long-term outcomes after ICU treatment for COVID-19 include (1) a high degree of patient heterogeneity in many of the studies; (2) the absence of pre-ICU functional status in most studies; (3) variation in mortality in the months following hospital discharge, which can impact the estimates of impairments, particularly when the follow-up time is long; and (4) loss to follow-up (whether due to severe symptoms or impairments or to functional recovery), which can contribute to the study population's not being representative of the population of interest (Murphy et al., 2018).

Compared with COVID-19 survivors who were hospitalized but not treated in the ICU, COVID-19 ICU survivors have been shown to have higher rates of cardiovascular outcomes (Xie et al., 2022), neuromuscular weakness (Núñez-Seisdedos et al., 2022), abnormalities in pulmonary function (Erber et al., 2021; Schlemmer et al., 2023), mood disorders (Portacci et al., 2022), posttraumatic stress symptoms (Neville et al., 2022), and dysphagia (Sassi et al., 2022). In the above-cited VA cohort of more than 150,000 individuals with COVID-19, approximately twice as many ICU patients experienced cardiovascular outcomes compared with patients hospitalized but not admitted to the ICU (Xie et al., 2022). In a small cohort of 70 adult survivors, ICU-acquired neuromuscular weakness and gait dependence at hospital discharge were present in 31 percent and 54 percent, respectively (Núñez-Seisdedos et al., 2022). In a Spanish cohort of 97 adults treated for COVID-19 in the ICU, Gonzalez and colleagues found that about 60 percent of survivors reported either cognitive concerns, severe dyspnea, or fatigue at 12 months after hospital discharge, and that a high proportion of these survivors were also diagnosed with new medical conditions during the follow-up period (Gonzalez et al., 2022). In a French cohort of 41 adult COVID-19 ICU survivors who underwent a neurological consultation 4 months following ICU discharge, ICU-acquired weakness was present in 16 percent, depression or anxiety in 26 percent, and posttraumatic stress symptoms in 7 percent (Jaquet et al., 2022). In a Dutch cohort of 96 adult survivors of severe COVID-19, 30 percent met criteria for objective cognitive impairment 6 months after ICU discharge based on abnormalities in two or more neuropsychological tests, and 20 percent reported subjective cognitive concerns; there was no strong correlation between the subjective concerns and the objective cognitive impairment (Duindam et al., 2022). In a U.S. cohort of 132 ICU COVID-19 survivors from two academic institutions who were assessed at 6 months after hospital discharge, levels of anxiety, depression, fatigue, sleep disturbance, social activity participation, pain interference, and cognitive function were not significantly different from those found in the general U.S. population, but physical function was worse among the ICU survivors than in the average U.S. adult population (Neville et al., 2022). This study found that about 24 percent of the COVID-19 ICU survivors reported very low health status, as reflected by a health utility score ≤0.2 (Neville et al., 2022). In a large sample of more than 2,590 critically ill adult COVID-19 survivors who were eligible for follow-up at 180 days after hospital discharge, 1 in 3 reported at least moderate disability that persisted at 6 months after hospital discharge, and 37.9 percent reported moderate, severe, or complete disability (Higgins et al., 2023).

Risk Factors

Few risk factors have been elucidated by the studies examining health impairments in ICU-hospitalized COVID-19 survivors. Demographic factors such as older age and more comorbidities have been associated with a higher risk of neuromuscular weakness (Núñez-Seisdedos et al., 2022). Older age, the need for invasive mechanical ventilation, and/or longer stays in the hospital or ICU are factors associated with lower quality life or a higher risk of disability in the months after hospital discharge (Jaquet et al., 2022). Rapid resolution of both lung injury and multiorgan dysfunction have been found to be associated with better functional status 1 year after hospital discharge. Individuals who had low health status at 6 months after discharge were more likely to require supplemental oxygen, to have been rehospitalized, and to need informal caregivers (Neville et al., 2022). Risk factors for persistent postintubation dysphagia at hospital discharge include older age, greater severity of illness upon ICU admission, presence of neurological comorbidities, type 2 diabetes mellitus, and severe swallowing impairment shortly after extubation (Sassi et al., 2022). In one study, women were more likely than men to report subjective cognitive concerns, and type 2 diabetes was associated with objective cognitive impairment (Duindam et al., 2022).

Recovery Trajectories

Few studies have examined recovery trajectories in COVID-19 survivors beyond 1 year after ICU treatment. Information on the long-term outcomes in populations with acute respiratory distress syndrome from before COVID-19 indicates that physical, mental, and cognitive impairments improve steadily during the first year following hospital discharge but can persist for up to 5 years. Recent data from a cohort of 428 critically ill COVID-19 survivors through 1 year suggest that many of the health impairments peak in prevalence around 3 months after hospital discharge but persist in a minority of patients even at 1 year after discharge (Taniguchi et al., 2023). In a Danish cohort of about 200 ICU survivors, the prevalence of cognitive impairment decreased from 26 percent at 6 months after ICU admission to 17 percent at 12 months after admission. The prevalence of frailty and fatigue was similar at both time points (Weihe et al., 2022).

LONG-TERM FUNCTIONAL OUTCOMES IN CHILDREN AND ADOLESCENTS WITH COVID-19

Limited data are available on long-term outcomes in children and adolescents with Long COVID. Even though most children and adolescents experience a mild acute COVID-19 illness, Long COVID can occur in children with or without hospitalization (Fink et al., 2021; Jamaica Balderas et al., 2023; see Chapter 3). Some youth with persistent symptoms experience difficulties that affect their quality of life (Fink et al., 2021) and result in more school absences (Kikkenborg Berg et al., 2022). Risk factors for the development of Long COVID include acute-phase hospitalization, preexisting comorbidity, re-infection, and infection with pre-Omicron variants (Morello et al., 2023; Osmanov et al., 2022; Pazukhina et al., 2022; Pinto Pereira et al., 2023). Common symptoms of Long COVID in children and adolescents include tiredness, sleep difficulties, shortness of breath, and headaches (Pinto Pereira et al., 2023).

One study in a pediatric Long COVID clinic found that 60 percent of children with a mean age of 12 years reported functional impairment, which was assessed by self-report anywhere between 1 and 7 months after SARS-CoV-2 infection (Ashkenazi-Hoffnung et al., 2021). In this study, only 12 percent of the children were hospitalized during the acute phase of illness (Ashkenazi-Hoffnung et al., 2021). A more recent cohort study investigated symptom trajectory at 3, 6, 12, and 18 months after SARS-CoV-2 infection (Morello et al., 2023). In this study, 23 percent of children with a median age of 7.5 years met the definition of Long COVID, defined as symptoms persisting for at least 3 months after initial infection, symptoms having a negative impact on daily life, and other possible diagnoses being excluded (Morello et al., 2023). Of those with Long COVID, 48 percent remained symptomatic at 6 months, 13 percent at 12 months, and 5 percent (1 in 20) at 18 months after infection (Morello et al., 2023). A study conducted in the UK that included 20,202 11-to-17-year-olds found that at the

12-month follow-up, 24 percent of those who were reinfected compared to 10 percent of those who had no later infection experienced 5-plus symptoms (Pinto Pereira et al., 2023). A Canadian cohort study at 14 pediatric emergency departments studied long-term effects of COVID-19 in younger children (ages 0.9 to 5.0 years, median age 2.0 years). They found that in this population of young children, out of over 5,000 participants, only 10 children at the 6-month follow-up and 8 children at the 12-month follow-up had Long COVID-related symptoms (Dun-Dery et al., 2023).

Importantly, severity of symptoms and functional impairment from Long COVID symptoms *were not correlated* with traditional clinical testing (e.g., lung ultrasound, standard systolic and diastolic function on echocardiogram) (Ashkenazi-Hoffnung et al., 2021; Grager et al., 2023; Sabatino et al., 2022). However, one study found persistent subclinical changes in systolic cardiac impairment approximately 5 months after acute SARS-CoV-2 infection that was worse in children who were infected in the second wave versus the first wave of infections (Sabatino et al., 2022). This subtle impairment in myocardial function (with findings still within the "normal" range) was worse in children who recovered during the second compared with the first wave (i.e., those who had the alpha variant rather than the original strain), although functional impact and cardiopulmonary symptoms were not assessed in this cohort (Sabatino et al., 2022).

At this time, there is a dearth of prospective and cross-sectional studies on the prevalence, risk factors, and time course and pattern of Long COVID in children and adolescents. It is also important to note that in pediatrics, because of typical development, the baseline for comparison is constantly changing. Additionally, the duration of symptoms (e.g., 1 or 3 months) can feel very different to and have a greater impact on children and adolescents compared with adults. Overall, more research is needed to identify the long-term functional implications of Long COVID in pediatric populations, to whom information from adult studies may not be directly applicable.

LONG-TERM FUNCTIONAL OUTCOMES IN OTHER SELECTED POPULATIONS WITH COVID-19

Functional impacts from Long COVID vary among individuals, and there is no standardized approach for evaluation and treatment. Some populations that may disproportionally experience greater severity and prevalence of COVID-19 and of long-term symptoms after infection include but are not limited to racial and ethnic minorities, women (pregnant and nonpregnant), and individuals with disabilities (CDC, 2022). These differences in severity and prevalence could be due to a wide range of social or biopsychological factors, such as poor access to health care, repeat infections from workplaces, and higher rates of comorbidities (Jolley et al.,

2022; Mora et al., 2023). Although racial and ethnic minority populations experience greater severity of disease and complications from COVID-19, more data are needed on how race/ethnicity and other social factors impact the risk of long-term functional impairment after infection (Jolley et al., 2022; Khullar et al., 2023). Importantly, the same marginalized populations that are disproportionally impacted by higher rates of infection and severity of illness from COVID-19—racial and ethnic minorities, women, children, and individuals with disabilities—have also been shown to be at risk for less access to rehabilitation care (Katz et al., 2023). The combination of increased risk for and/or severity of COVID-19 and poor access to rehabilitation care may well translate into inequities in the severity and duration of Long COVID.

Data gathered by the U.S. Centers for Disease Control and Prevention (CDC) using household survey methods suggest that LGBTQIA persons may have higher rates of Long COVID, and may have distinct health issues in addition to experiencing challenges in accessing care during the pandemic (Jarrett et al., 2021; NCHS, 2023). Pregnant women can have more severe COVID-19 and may experience fatigue related to both pregnancy and Long COVID (Lassi et al., 2021). Considerations required for this at-risk population include diagnostic testing without radiation exposure; exercise prescriptions that may be limited by large girth, back pain, or preeclampsia; and return to work with appropriate accommodations. Individuals with versus those without disabilities have a higher fatality rate from COVID-19, a finding suggesting that impaired cognitive and physical function may be associated with COVID-19 mortality (Katz et al., 2023). Even before the COVID-19 pandemic, persons with disabilities already had reduced access to health care, resources, and social services (Lebrasseur et al., 2021). Stereotypes and biases toward these individuals can further lead to their disparate treatment (Fuentes et al., 2021). When appropriate, clinicians need to advocate for persons with disabilities to obtain appropriate therapy, accommodations (per the Americans with Disabilities Act and the Rehabilitations Act), home health aides, and/or medical equipment. Additionally, one study among farmworkers in California showed that a significant proportion experienced Long COVID and associated persistent symptoms, limiting their ability to continue working (Mora et al., 2023). Finally, though not a population of interest to SSA, it is worth mentioning that nursing home residents tend to experience modest declines in cognition after COVID-19 infection and may need more help with activities of daily living than their peers who were not infected. One study of nursing home residents aged 80 years or older found that most residents experienced improved functional status and cognition within one year after their illness (Harris, 2024).

Overall, research is limited on functional impacts and impairments from Long COVID affecting specific populations. A comprehensive approach to addressing the varying and unique needs of these populations is critical for the achievement of health equity.

EFFECTS OF REHABILITATION ON FUNCTIONAL TRAJECTORIES IN INDIVIDUALS WITH LONG COVID

Rehabilitation can be helpful in improving functional outcomes, as has been demonstrated in a variety of health conditions. In the rehabilitation literature, measuring function involves a variety of components, including cardiovascular and pulmonary fitness, muscle strength, coordination, cognitive function, and quality of life. The specific benefits of rehabilitation in individuals with Long COVID may vary depending on the individual's symptoms and severity of disease, but small studies consistently show improvements in physical function, fatigue, dyspnea, and quality of life (Calvo-Paniagua et al., 2022; de la Plaza San Frutos et al., 2023; Gloeckl et al., 2021; Nopp et al., 2022; Ostrowska et al., 2023; Parker et al., 2023; Spielmanns et al., 2023).

A recent systematic review and meta-analysis by Pouliopoulou and colleagues (2023) analyzed 14 randomized clinical trials involving 1,244 patients with Long COVID. The authors found improvements in functional exercise capacity, yet there was significant uncertainty regarding the probability of experiencing exercise-induced adverse events during rehabilitation. Additionally, studies have shown that the benefits of rehabilitation for people with Long COVID are greater for those who are younger and who have had Long COVID for a shorter period of time (Nopp et al., 2022; Ostrowska et al., 2023). However, people who have had Long COVID for a longer period of time may still benefit from an individualized, targeted rehabilitation program that monitors for any post-exertional symptom exacerbation. It is important to note that these studies are relatively small, and more research is needed to confirm their findings. Given the multidisciplinary nature of human function, the variables measured in studies of rehabilitation of persons with Long COVID may not provide a comprehensive understanding of their true functional capacity. Furthermore, the variables used to look at function in these studies need to be interpreted cautiously and alongside other variables that capture the multidisciplinary nature of functional capacity and quality of life.

At the beginning of the pandemic, health care systems recognized the urgent need for specialized rehabilitation programs to aid individuals in their recovery from COVID-19. Several types of rehabilitation programs have been used for recovering individuals (Table 4-1). The early reliance on evidence from post–intensive care syndrome rehabilitation was a pragmatic approach, given the similarities in the clinical trajectories of severe COVID-19 cases and patients with other critical illnesses. These established

TABLE 4-1 Types of Rehabilitation Programs Used in Long COVID Recovery

Type of therapy	Description
Physical therapy	Addresses physical symptoms and uses personalized exercise programs
Occupational therapy	Addresses challenges in activities of daily living and can develop strategies and accommodations to manage these tasks
Speech and language pathology	Addresses speech, swallowing, and cognitive impairments
Pulmonary rehabilitation	Aims to improve respiratory function and endurance
Neurocognitive rehabilitation	Manages and improves cognitive function
Pacing	Program that instructs in a phased pacing protocol to decrease post-exertional symptom exacerbation
Cardiac rehabilitation	Monitored multi-phase program to improve cardiovascular health
Autonomic conditioning therapy	Adapted program to manage autonomic dysregulation
Multidisciplinary rehabilitation programs	Comprehensive rehabilitation program involving a team of professions working together

NOTE: Many professionals from different backgrounds can provide the forms of rehabilitation listed.
SOURCE: Carda et al., 2020b.

strategies targeted respiratory, muscular, and neurological impairments that arise from prolonged hospitalization. Moreover, insights gleaned from past pandemics informed the design of those rehabilitation programs, aiding in the anticipation of potential long-term sequelae that Long COVID survivors might face (Carda et al., 2020a,b). Rehabilitation programs have evolved over time as more data have become available on the unique effects of COVID-19 on various populations.

Recommendations on the safe provision of rehabilitation for persons with Long COVID have been published (DeMars et al., 2023). The World Health Organization has created a Living Guideline for the Clinical Management of COVID-19 with up-to-date recommendations for clinical management, which includes a section on rehabilitation for patients with COVID-19 (WHO, 2023). Regardless of disease severity, individuals with COVID-19 can present with persistent symptoms and functional decline. The guideline provides suggestions across the continuum of care for persons with COVID-19 from the ICU to the outpatient setting for persons with persistent symptoms. Additionally, authors from the National Institute for Occupational Safety and Health published best practices for handling return to work in Long COVID patients (Howard et al., 2024). The guidelines suggest that returning to work too early may result in health deterioration, and a gradual return to work plan may be advised, especially in cases involving post-exertional malaise. They also address the importance of communication among affected workers and their employers and health care providers, as well as the potential role of workplace accommodations in facilitating return to work.

Research on the long-term effects of COVID-19 and the most effective rehabilitation approaches is incomplete, and understanding of the impacts of Long COVID rehabilitation is limited. Because some patients report post-exertional symptom exacerbation following physical exertion or have a phenotype of Long COVID consistent with myalgic encephalomyelitis/chronic fatigue syndrome (ME/CFS) (see Chapter 5), clearer guidelines are needed on safe rehabilitation for these individuals (Appelman et al., 2024). There is no one-size-fits-all approach to rehabilitation, and each individual will need a program tailored to their complex needs.

ASSESSING GLOBAL FUNCTIONING

Table 4-2 provides an overview of selected assessments that can be used to quantify the functional impacts of Long COVID. The assessments in the table can contribute to an overall picture of individuals' functioning, but given the heterogeneity of Long COVID, there are no gold standard tests specific for this population. The assessments are divided into domains of functioning, including full-body functioning, work-related functioning, pain, fatigue, and cognitive functioning. The assessments in the table include both performance-based and self-report measures and are just examples of ones that might be reported in the medical record. Performance-based measures assess the individual's ability to perform specific tasks, such as walking or climbing stairs, while self-report measures ask the individual to rate their symptoms and how those symptoms affect their daily life. Of note, these selected assessments are commonly used to assess disability based on specific complaints; however, the three newer, more unique symptoms described earlier in Chapter 3 (chronic fatigue and post-exertional malaise, post–COVID-19 cognitive impairment, and autonomic dysfunction) may not be adequately captured with these assessments. There also may be wide day-to-day variability in performance on these tests, which may make using the tests to assess disability challenging. More research is needed to develop and validate additional disability and functioning assessments for Long COVID.

TABLE 4-2 Global Functioning Associated with Long COVID

Domain	Selected Assessments
Full-body functioning, walking, standing (physical)	*Performance-based measures:* • Bruininks-Oseretsky Test of Motor Proficiency, 2nd edition (BOT-2)* (Bruininks and Bruininks, 2005) [pediatric population] • Bruininks Motor Ability Test (BMAT)* (Bruininks and Bruininks, 2012) [adult version of BOT-2] • Functional capacity evaluation (Chen, 2007; Fore et al., 2015; Genovese and Galper, 2009; Jahn et al., 2004; Kuijer et al., 2012; Soer et al., 2008) • Exercise testing to include aerobic capacity and neuromuscular performance (Liguori and American College of Sports Medicine, 2021) • 6-minute walk test • 10-meter walk test (Physiopedia, n.d.) • Functional Gait Assessment • Sensory Organization Test (Shirley Ryan AbilityLab, 2013e) • 30-second, 5x, or 10x sit-to-stand test (Shirley Ryan AbilityLab, 2013a) • Romberg (Shirley Ryan AbilityLab, 2013d) *Self-reported measures:* • Composite Autonomic Symptom Score-31 (COMPASS-31) (Sletten et al., 2012) • Lower Extremity Functional Scale (LEFS) (Shirley Ryan AbilityLab, 2013b) • Foot and Ankle Ability Measures (FAAM) (Shirley Ryan AbilityLab, 2015) • The Activities-Specific Balance Confidence (ABC) Scale (Powell and Myers, 1995) • Patient-Reported Outcomes Measurement Information System (PROMIS)—Physical Function (HealthMeasures, 2020)
Work-related functioning, activities of daily living (ADLs), and instrumental activities of daily living (IADLs)	*Performance-based measures:* • ADL Profile (head injury and stroke) (Dutil et al., 1990) • ADL-Focused Occupations-Based Neurobehavioral Evaluation (Gardarsdottir and Kaplan, 2002) • Assessment of Motor and Processing Skills [adult and pediatric populations] (Fisher and James, 2012; Shirley Ryan AbilityLab, 2019) • Bay Area Functional Performance Evaluation (Houston et al., 1989) • Executive Function Performance Test (Baum et al., 2008) • Functional Independence Measure (Ottenbacher et al., 1996) • Katz ADL Scale (elderly and chronically ill) (Katz, 1983; Katz and Akpom, 1976) • Kohlman Evaluation of Living Skills (IADLs—psychiatric geriatric) (Burnett et al., 2009; Kohlman-Thomson, 1992) *Observation and interview-based measures:* • Performance Assessment of Self-Care Skills (Chisholm et al., 2014)

TABLE 4-2 Continued

Domain	Selected Assessments
	Self-reported measures: • Work Disability Functional Assessment Battery (WD-FAB) Physical Function (Meterko et al., 2015; Meterko et al., 2019) • Work Ability (Illmaren, 2007; Tuomi et al., 1998) • Sheehan Disability Scale (Sheehan, 1983) • Barthel Index (Quinn et al., 2011) • Frenchay Activities Index (IADLs) (Schuling et al., 1993) • The Lawton IADL Scale (Graf, 2008) • Manual Ability Measure (neurological and musculoskeletal conditions) (Chen and Bode, 2010) *Caregiver-reported measures:* • Cleveland Scale of Activities of Daily Living (dementia) (Patterson and Mack, 2001)
Pain	*Self-reported measures:* • Visual Analog Scale (VAS) for Pain (Bijur et al., 2001) • Numeric Rating Scale (NRS) for Pain (Shirley Ryan AbilityLab, 2013c) • PROMIS—Pain Interference Instruments (HealthMeasures, 2021) • Functional Disability Inventory (Claar and Walker, 2006; Walker and Greene, 1991) [pediatric population]
Fatigue	*Performance-based measures:* • Polysomnography • Exercise testing to include aerobic capacity and neuromuscular performance (Liguori and American College of Sports Medicine, 2021) *Self-reported measures:* • Brief Fatigue Inventory [BFI] • Fatigue Severity Scale [FSS] • Fatigue Symptom Inventory • Multidimensional Assessment of Fatigue • Fatigue Impact Scale (modified) • Multidimensional Fatigue Symptom Inventory • Multidimensional Fatigue Symptom Inventory Short Form • Profile of Mood States-Brief • PedsQL Multidimensional Fatigue Scale [pediatric and young adult population] • Multi-Dimensional Fatigue Scale • Profile of Fatigue • Functional Assessment Chronic Illness • Therapy Checklist Individual Strength • Patient-Reported Outcomes Measurement Information System – Fatigue • Pittsburgh Sleep Quality Assessment (Buysse et al., 1989) • VAS to Evaluate Fatigue Severity • PROMIS—Fatigue (Shirley Ryan AbilityLab, 2018)

continued

TABLE 4-2 Continued

Domain	Selected Assessments

Cognitive dysfunction	*Attention and Working Memory*
	• Weschler Adult Intelligence Scale-IV (WAIS-IV) Digit Span
	• Continuous Performance Test-3 (CPT-3)
	• Digit Vigilance Test
	• Paced Auditory Serial Addition Test (PASAT)
	
	Processing Speed
	• Trail Making Test-Part A
	• Symbol Digit Modalities Test
	• WAIS-IV Coding
	
	Executive Functioning
	• Trail Making Test-Part B
	• Wisconsin Card Sorting Test-64 (WCST-64)
	• Stroop Color and Word Test
	• Delis-Kaplan Executive Function System (DKEFS) Tower Test
	• Frontal Systems Behavior Scale (FrSBe) (self-reported)
	• Behavior Rating Inventory of Executive Functioning (BRIEF) (self-reported)
	• PROMIS Short Form v2.0—Cognitive Function (self-reported)
	
	Language
	• Controlled Oral Word Association Test (COWAT) or DKEFS Verbal Fluency
	• Multilingual Naming Test or Boston Naming Test
	
	Memory
	• Verbal:
	  ○ California Verbal Learning Test-II (CVLT-II)
	  ○ Hopkins Verbal Learning Test-Revised (HVLT-R)
	  ○ Rey Auditory Verbal Learning Test (RAVLT)
	• Nonverbal:
	  ○ Brief Visual Memory Test Revised (BVMT-R)
	
	Visuospatial Ability
	• Judgment of Line Orientation
	• Rey-Osterrieth Complex Figure Test
	
	Estimated Premorbid Ability
	• Wide Range Achievement Test-4 (WRAT-4) Reading subtest
	• Test of Premorbid Functioning (TOPF)

NOTES: *Multi-dimensional assessment: Balance, coordination, dexterity, functional mobility, gait, strength, upper-extremity, function, vestibular.

SOURCES: Hodgson et al., 2021; Raj et al., 2018.

SUMMARY AND CONCLUSIONS

For many individuals, the effects of SARS-CoV-2 infection persist well beyond resolution of the acute infection and can result in significant disability. Functional disability associated with Long COVID has been characterized as inability to return to work, poor quality of life, diminished ability to perform ADLs, decreased physical and cognitive function, and overall disability. Severity of acute COVID-19 is a major risk factor for poor functional outcomes. By the committee's best estimate, people hospitalized for COVID-19 are two to three times more likely to have higher rates of Long COVID and more severe disease and to experience longer disease duration compared with nonhospitalized people. In addition, those whose severe COVID-19 required life support treatments in the ICU may be twice as likely to experience the aforementioned outcomes compared with those hospitalized without such intensive treatment. However, even people with mild initial illness can experience long-term functional impairments. In fact, those with mild initial illness make up the great majority of the population with long-term functional impairments simply because there are many times more people with mild than with severe initial infection. Increased number and severity of long-term symptoms correlates with decreased quality of life, physical functioning, and ability to work or perform in school. Other risk factors for poor functional outcomes include female sex, lack of vaccination against SARS-CoV-2, baseline disability or comorbidities, and smoking.

Data on recovery trajectories are rapidly evolving, and recovery is heterogenous. Initial data suggest that people with persistent Long COVID symptoms generally improve over time, although preliminary studies suggest that recovery can plateau between 6 and 12 months after acute infection. More information on recovery trajectories at 1 year or longer may become available in the next few years.

Long COVID in children and adolescents is a poorly understood condition. While most children recover from COVID-19 with no long-term problems, some may experience persistent symptoms that can affect their quality of life and result in more school absences. Risk factors for Long COVID in children include acute-phase hospitalization, preexisting comorbidity, being infected with pre-Omicron variants, and older age. More research is needed to identify the long-term functional implications of Long COVID for children, as information from adult studies may not be directly applicable to the pediatric population.

Rehabilitation can improve functional outcomes in people with Long COVID, regardless of the severity of disease or duration of symptoms, although the benefits are greater for people who are younger and who have had Long COVID for a shorter period of time. It is important to choose the right type of rehabilitation for the individual. Access to rehabilitation can be difficult, and there are often long waitlists.

REFERENCES

Admon, A. J., T. J. Iwashyna, L. A. Kamphuis, S. J. Gundel, S. K. Sahetya, I. D. Peltan, S. Y. Chang, J. H. Han, K. C. Vranas, K. P. Mayer, A. A. Hope, S. E. Jolley, E. Caldwell, M. L. Monahan, K. Hauschildt, S. M. Brown, N. R. Aggarwal, B. T. Thompson, C. L. Hough, and National Heart, Lung, and Blood Institute PETAL Network. 2023. Assessment of symptom, disability, and financial trajectories in patients hospitalized for COVID-19 at 6 months. *JAMA Network Open* 6(2):e2255795.

Ahmad, I., A. Edin, C. Granvik, L. Kumm Persson, S. Tevell, E. Månsson, A. Magnuson, I. Marklund, I. L. Persson, A. Kauppi, C. Ahlm, M. N. E. Forsell, J. Sundh, A. Lange, S. Cajander, and J. Normark. 2023. High prevalence of persistent symptoms and reduced health-related quality of life 6 months after COVID-19. *Frontiers in Public Health* 11:1104267.

Angulo, F. J., L. Finelli, and D. L. Swerdlow. 2021. Estimation of U.S. SARS-CoV-2 infections, symptomatic infections, hospitalizations, and deaths using seroprevalence surveys. *JAMA Network Open* 4(1):e2033706.

Appelman, B., B. T. Charlton, R. P. Goulding, T. J. Kerkhoff, E. A. Breedveld, W. Noort, C. Offringa, F. W. Bloemers, M. van Weeghel, B. V. Schomakers, P. Coelho, J. J. Posthuma, E. Aronica, W. Joost Wiersinga, M. van Vugt, and R. C. I. Wüst. 2024. Muscle abnormalities worsen after post-exertional malaise in long COVID. *Nature Communications* 15(1):17.

Asadi-Pooya, A. A., A. Akbari, A. Emami, M. Lotfi, M. Rostamihosseinkhani, H. Nemati, Z. Barzegar, M. Kabiri, Z. Zeraatpisheh, M. Farjoud-Kouhanjani, A. Jafari, F. Sasannia, S. Ashrafi, M. Nazeri, S. Nasiri, and M. Shahisavandi. 2021. Risk factors associated with long COVID syndrome: A retrospective study. *Iranian Journal of Medical Sciences* 46(6):428–436.

Ashkenazi-Hoffnung, L., E. Shmueli, S. Ehrlich, A. Ziv, O. Bar-On, E. Birk, A. Lowenthal, and D. Prais. 2021. Long COVID in children: Observations from a designated pediatric clinic. *Journal of Pediatric Infectious Diseases* 40(12):e509–e511.

Ayoubkhani, D., M. L. Bosworth, S. King, K. B. Pouwels, M. Glickman, V. Nafilyan, F. Zaccardi, K. Khunti, N. A. Alwan, and A. S. Walker. 2022. Risk of long COVID in people infected with severe acute respiratory syndrome coronavirus 2 after 2 doses of a coronavirus disease 2019 vaccine: Community-based, matched cohort study. *Open Forum Infectious Diseases* 9(9):ofac464.

Bahmer, T., C. Borzikowsky, W. Lieb, A. Horn, L. Krist, J. Fricke, C. Scheibenbogen, K. F. Rabe, W. Maetzler, C. Maetzler, M. Laudien, D. Frank, S. Ballhausen, A. Hermes, O. Muljukov, K. G. Haeusler, N. E. E. Mokhtari, M. Witzenrath, J. J. Vehreschild, D. Krefting, D. Pape, F. A. Montellano, M. Kohls, C. Morbach, S. Stork, J. P. Reese, T. Keil, P. Heuschmann, M. Krawczak, and S. Schreiber. 2022. Severity, predictors and clinical correlates of post-COVID syndrome (PCS) in Germany: A prospective, multi-centre, population-based cohort study. *eClinicalMedicine* 51:101549.

Banic, M., M. J. Makek, M. Samarzija, D. Mursic, Z. Boras, V. Trkes, D. Baricevic, M. Korsic, L. Basara, T. J. Gluncic, and A. V. Dugac. 2022. Risk factors and severity of functional impairment in long COVID: A single-center experience in Croatia. *Croatian Medical Journal* 63(1):27–35.

Baum, C. M., L. T. Connor, T. Morrison, M. Hahn, A. W. Dromerick, and D. F. Edwards. 2008. Reliability, validity, and clinical utility of the Executive Function Performance Test: A measure of executive function in a sample of people with stroke. *American Journal of Occupational Therapy* 62(4):446–455.

Becker, C., K. Beck, S. Zumbrunn, V. Memma, N. Herzog, B. Bissmann, S. Gross, N. Loretz, J. Mueller, S. A. Amacher, C. Bohren, R. Schaefert, S. Bassetti, C. Fux, B. Mueller, P. Schuetz, and S. Hunziker. 2021a. Long COVID 1 year after hospitalisation for COVID-19: A prospective bicentric cohort study. *Swiss Medical Weekly* 151:w30091.

Becker, J. H., J. J. Lin, M. Doernberg, K. Stone, A. Navis, J. R. Festa, and J. P. Wisnivesky. 2021b. Assessment of cognitive function in patients after COVID-19 infection. *JAMA Network Open* 4(10):e2130645.

Bellan, M., D. Apostolo, A. Albè, M. Crevola, N. Errica, G. Ratano, S. Tonello, R. Minisini, D. D'Onghia, A. Baricich, F. Patrucco, P. Zeppegno, C. Gramaglia, P. E. Balbo, G. Cappellano, S. Casella, A. Chiocchetti, E. Clivati, M. Giordano, M. Manfredi, G. Patti, D. J. Pinato, C. Puricelli, D. Raineri, R. Rolla, P. P. Sainaghi, and M. Pirisi. 2022. Determinants of long COVID among adults hospitalized for SARS-CoV-2 infection: A prospective cohort study. *Frontiers in Immunology* 13:1038227.

Bijur, P. E., W. Silver, and E. J. Gallagher. 2001. Reliability of the visual analog scale for measurement of acute pain. *Academic Emergency Medicine* 8(12):1153–1157.

Björsell, T., J. Sundh, A. Lange, C. Ahlm, M. N. E. Forsell, S. Tevell, A. Blomberg, A. Edin, J. Normark, and S. Cajander. 2023. Risk factors for impaired respiratory function post COVID-19: A prospective cohort study of nonhospitalized and hospitalized patients. *Journal of Internal Medicine* 293(5):600–614.

Bowe, B., Y. Xie, and Z. Al-Aly. 2023. Postacute sequelae of COVID-19 at 2 years. *Nature Medicine* 29:2347–2357.

Bruininks, B. D., and R. H. Bruininks. 2005. *Bruininks-Oseretsky Test of Motor Proficiency— Second edition.* https://www.pearsonassessments.com/store/usassessments/en/Store/ Professional-Assessments/Motor-Sensory/Bruininks-Oseretsky-Test-of-Motor-Proficiency- %7C-Second-Edition/p/100000648.html (accessed February 16, 2024).

Bruininks, B. D., and R. H. Bruininks. 2012. *Bruininks Motor Ability Test.* https://www.pearsonassessments.com/store/usassessments/en/Store/Professional-Assessments/Cognition- %26-Neuro/Bruininks-Motor-Ability-Test/p/100000324.html (accessed February 16, 2024).

Burnett, J., C. B. Dyer, and A. D. Naik. 2009. Convergent validation of the Kohlman Evaluation of Living Skills as a screening tool of older adults' ability to live safely and independently in the community. *Archives of Physical Medicine and Rehabilitation* 90(11):1948–1952.

Buysse, D. J., C. F. Reynolds, 3rd, T. H. Monk, S. R. Berman, and D. J. Kupfer. 1989. The Pittsburgh Sleep Quality Index: A new instrument for psychiatric practice and research. *Psychiatry Research* 28(2):193–213.

Calvo-Paniagua, J., M. J. Diaz-Arribas, J. A. Valera-Calero, M. I. Gallardo-Vidal, C. Fernandez-de-las-Penas, I. Lopez-De-Uralde-Villanueva, T. del Corral, and G. Plaza-Manzano. 2022. A tele-health primary care rehabilitation program improves self-perceived exertion in COVID-19 survivors experiencing post-COVID fatigue and dyspnea: A quasi-experimental study. *PLoS ONE* 17:e0271802.

Carda, S., M. Invernizzi, G. Bavikatte, D. Bensmaïl, F. Bianchi, T. Deltombe, N. Draulans, A. Esquenazi, G. E. Francisco, and R. Gross. 2020a. COVID-19 pandemic: What should physical and rehabilitation medicine specialists do? A clinician's perspective. *European Journal of Physical and Rehabilitation Medicine* 56(4):515–524.

Carda, S., M. Invernizzi, G. Bavikatte, D. Bensmaïl, F. Bianchi, T. Deltombe, N. Draulans, A. Esquenazi, G. E. Francisco, and R. Gross. 2020b. The role of physical and rehabilitation medicine in the COVID-19 pandemic: The clinician's view. *Annals of Physical and Rehabilitation Medicine* 63(6):554.

Cazé, A. B., T. Cerqueira-Silva, A. P. Bomfim, G. L. de Souza, A. C. Azevedo, M. Q. Brasil, N. R. Santos, R. Khouri, J. Dan, A. C. Bandeira, L. P. Cavalcanti, M. Barral-Netto, A. Barral, C. G. Barbosa, and V. S. Boaventura. 2023. Prevalence and risk factors for long COVID after mild disease: A cohort study with a symptomatic control group. *Journal of Global Health* 13:06015.

CDC (U.S. Centers for Disease Control and Prevention). 2022. *What is health equity?* https://www.cdc.gov/healthequity/whatis/index.html (accessed February 14, 2024).

Chatys-Bogacka, Z., I. Mazurkiewicz, J. Slowik, M. Bociaga-Jasik, A. Dzieza-Grudnik, A. Slowik, M. Wnuk, and L. Drabik. 2022. Brain fog and quality of life at work in non-hospitalized patients after COVID-19. *International Journal of Environmental Research and Public Health* 19(19):12816.

Chen, J. J. 2007. Functional capacity evaluation & disability. *Iowa Orthopedic Journal* 27:121-127.

Chen, C. C., and R. K. Bode. 2010. Psychometric validation of the Manual Ability Measure-36 (MAM-36) in patients with neurologic and musculoskeletal disorders. *Archives of Physical Medicine and Rehabilitation* 91(3):414–420.

Chisholm, D., P. Toto, K. Raina, M. Holm, and J. Rogers. 2014. Evaluating capacity to live independently and safely in the community: Performance assessment of self-care skills. *British Journal of Occupational Therapy* 77(2):59–63.

Claar, R. L., and L. S. Walker. 2006. Functional assessment of pediatric pain patients: Psychometric properties of the Functional Disability Inventory. *Pain* 121(1-2):77–84.

Claflin, E. S., A. K. Daunter, A. Bowman, J. Startup, E. Reed, C. Krishnan, and A. L. Kratz. 2021. Hospitalized patients with COVID-19 and neurological complications experience more frequent decline in functioning and greater rehabilitation needs. *American Journal of Physical Medicine & Rehabilitation* 100(8):725–729.

Coelho, D. H., E. R. Reiter, S. G. Budd, Y. Shin, Z. A. Kons, and R. M. Costanzo. 2021. Quality of life and safety impact of COVID-19 associated smell and taste disturbances. *American Journal of Otolaryngology* 42(4):103001.

D'Ettorre, G., E. Gentilini Cacciola, L. Santinelli, G. De Girolamo, O. Spagnolello, A. Russo, L. Tarsitani, M. Ciccozzi, C. M. Mastroianni, G. D'Ettorre, and G. Ceccarelli. 2022. COVID-19 sequelae in working age patients: A systematic review. *Journal of Medical Virology* 94(3):858–868.

Daher, A., P. Balfanz, C. Cornelissen, A. Müller, I. Bergs, N. Marx, D. Müller-Wieland, B. Hartmann, M. Dreher, and T. Müller. 2020. Follow up of patients with severe coronavirus disease 2019 (COVID-19): Pulmonary and extrapulmonary disease sequelae. *Respiratory Medicine* 174:106197.

Damanti, S., M. Cilla, M. Cilona, A. Fici, A. Merolla, G. Pacioni, R. De Lorenzo, S. Martinenghi, G. Vitali, C. Magnaghi, A. Fumagalli, M. Gennaro Mazza, F. Benedetti, M. Tresoldi, and P. Rovere Querini. 2022. Prevalence of long COVID-19 symptoms after hospital discharge in frail and robust patients. *Frontiers in Medicine* 9:834887.

de la Plaza San Frutos, M., V. Abuin Porras, M. Blanco Morales, M. G. Arrabe, C. Estrada Barranco, and M. Rubio Alonso. 2023. Telemedicine in pulmonary rehabilitation— Benefits of a telerehabilitation program in post-COVID-19 patients: A controlled quasi-experimental study. *Therapeutic Advances in Respiratory Disease* 17:17534666231167354.

DeMars, J., D. A. Brown, I. Angelidis, F. Jones, F. McGuire, K. K. O'Brien, D. Oller, S. Pemberton, R. Tarrant, M. Verduzco-Gutierrez, and D. P. Gross. 2023. What is safe long COVID rehabilitation? *Journal of Occupational Rehabilitation* 33(2):227–230.

Dennis, A., M. Wamil, J. Alberts, J. Oben, D. J. Cuthbertson, D. Wootton, M. Crooks, M. Gabbay, M. Brady, L. Hishmeh, E. Attree, M. Heightman, R. Banerjee, and A. Banerjee. 2021. Multiorgan impairment in low-risk individuals with post-COVID-19 syndrome: A prospective, community-based study. *BMJ Open* 11(3):e048391.

Dennis, A., D. J. Cuthbertson, D. Wootton, M. Crooks, M. Gabbay, N. Eichert, S. Mouchti, M. Pansini, A. Roca-Fernandez, H. Thomaides-Brears, M. Kelly, M. Robson, L. Hishmeh, E. Attree, M. Heightman, R. Banerjee, and A. Banerjee. 2023. Multi-organ impairment and long COVID: A 1-year prospective, longitudinal cohort study. *Journal of the Royal Society of Medicine* 116(3):97–112.

Duindam, H. B., R. P. C. Kessels, B. van den Borst, P. Pickkers, and W. F. Abdo. 2022. Long-term cognitive performance and its relation to anti-inflammatory therapy in a cohort of survivors of severe COVID-19. *Brain Behavior & Immunity—Health* 25:100513.

Dun-Dery, F., J. Xie, K. Winston, B. Burstein, J. Gravel, J. Emsley, V. Sabhaney, R. Zemek, S. Berthelot, D. Beer, A. Kam, G. Freire, A. Mater, R. Porter, N. Poonai, A. Moffatt, A. Dixon, M. I. Salvadori, and S. B. Freedman, for the Pediatric Emergency Research Canada (PERC) COVID Study Group. 2023. Post–COVID-19 condition in children 6 and 12 months after infection. *JAMA Network Open* 6(12):e2349613.

Dutil, E., A. Forget, M. Vanier, and C. Gaudreault. 1990. Development of the ADL profile: An evaluation for adults with severe head injury. *Occupational Therapy in Healthcare* 7(1):7–22.

Erber, J., J. R. Wiessner, G. S. Zimmermann, P. Barthel, E. Burian, F. Lohofer, E. Martens, H. Mijocevic, S. Rasch, R. M. Schmid, C. D. Spinner, R. Braren, J. Schneider, and T. Lahmer. 2021. Longitudinal assessment of health and quality of life of COVID-19 patients requiring intensive care—An observational study. *Journal of Clinical Medicine* 10(23):5469.

Evans, R. A., H. McAuley, E. M. Harrison, A. Shikotra, A. Singapuri, M. Sereno, O. Elneima, A. B. Docherty, N. I. Lone, O. C. Leavy, L. Daines, J. K. Baillie, J. S. Brown, T. Chalder, A. De Soyza, N. Diar Bakerly, N. Easom, J. R. Geddes, N. J. Greening, N. Hart, L. G. Heaney, S. Heller, L. Howard, J. R. Hurst, J. Jacob, R. G. Jenkins, C. Jolley, S. Kerr, O. M. Kon, K. Lewis, J. M. Lord, G. P. McCann, S. Neubauer, P. J. M. Openshaw, D. Parekh, P. Pfeffer, N. M. Rahman, B. Raman, M. Richardson, M. Rowland, M. G. Semple, A. M. Shah, S. J. Singh, A. Sheikh, D. Thomas, M. Toshner, J. D. Chalmers, L. P. Ho, A. Horsley, M. Marks, K. Poinasamy, L. V. Wain, and C. E. Brightling, on behalf of the PHOSP-COVID Collaborative Group. 2021. Physical, cognitive, and mental health impacts of COVID-19 after hospitalisation (PHOSP-COVID): A UK multicentre, prospective cohort study. *The Lancet Respiratory Medicine* 9(11):1275–1287.

Fernández-de-las-Peñas, C., J. D. Martín-Guerrero, Ó. J. Pellicer-Valero, E. Navarro-Pardo, V. Gómez-Mayordomo, M. L. Cuadrado, J. A. Arias-Navalón, M. Cigarán-Méndez, V. Hernández-Barrera, and L. Arendt-Nielsen. 2022. Female sex is a risk factor associated with long-term post-COVID related-symptoms but not with COVID-19 symptoms: The LONG-COVID-EXP-CM multicenter study. *Journal of Clinical Medicine* 11(2):413.

Fernández-de-las-Peñas, C., I. Cancela-Cilleruelo, J. Rodriguez-Jimenez, J. A. Arias-Navalón, J. D. Martín-Guerrero, Ó. J. Pellicer-Valero, L. Arendt-Nielsen, and M. Cigarán-Méndez. 2023. Trajectory of post-COVID brain fog, memory loss, and concentration loss in previously hospitalized COVID-19 survivors: The LONG-COVID-EXP multicenter study. *Frontiers in Human Neuroscience* 17:1259660.

Fink, T. T., H. H. S. Marques, B. Gualano, L. Lindoso, V. Bain, C. Astley, F. Martins, D. Matheus, O. M. Matsuo, P. Suguita, V. Trindade, C. S. Y. Paula, S. C. L. Farhat, P. Palmeira, G. N. Leal, L. Suzuki, V. Odone Filho, M. Carneiro-Sampaio, A. J. S. Duarte, L. Antonangelo, L. R. Batisttella, G. V. Polanczyk, R. M. R. Pereira, C. R. R. Carvalho, C. A. Buchpiguel, A. C. L. Xavier, M. Seelaender, C. A. Silva, M. F. B. Pereira, A. M. E. Sallum, A. V. M. Brentani, J. S. Neto Á, A. Ihara, A. R. Santos, A. P. M. Canton, A. Watanabe, A. C. D. Santos, A. C. Pastorino, B. Franco, B. Caruzo, C. Ceneviva, C. Martins, D. Prado, D. M. Abellan, F. B. Benatti, F. Smaria, F. T. Gonçalves, F. D. Penteado, G. S. F. Castro, G. S. Gonçalves, H. Roschel, I. R. Disi, I. G. Marques, I. A. Castro, I. M. Buscatti, J. Z. Faiad, J. Fiamoncini, J. C. Rodrigues, J. D. A. Carneiro, J. A. Paz, J. C. Ferreira, J. C. O. Ferreira, K. R. Silva, K. L. M. Bastos, K. Kozu, L. M. Cristofani, L. V. B. Souza, L. M. A. Campos, L. Silva Filho, M. T. Sapienza, M. S. Lima, M. P. Garanito, M. F. A. Santos, M. B. Dorna, N. E. Aikawa, N. Litvinov, N. K. Sakita, P. V. V. Gaiolla, P. Pasqualucci, R. K. Toma, S. Correa-Silva, S. M. Sieczkowska, M. Imamura, S. Forsait, V. A. Santos, and Y. Zheng. 2021. Persistent symptoms and decreased health-related quality of life after symptomatic pediatric COVID-19: A prospective study in a Latin American tertiary hospital. *Clinics (São Paulo)* 76:e3511.

Fisher, A. G., and K. B. James. 2012. *Assessment of Motor and Process Skills*. Fort Collins, CO: Three Star Press.

Fischer, D., S. B. Snider, M. E. Barra, W. R. Sanders, O. Rapalino, P. Schaefer, A. S. Foulkes, Y. G. Bodien, and B. L. Edlow. 2022. Disorders of consciousness associated with COVID 19: A prospective multimodal study of recovery and brain connectivity. *Neurology* 98(3):e315–e325.

Ford, N. D., D. Slaughter, D. Edwards, A. Dalton, C. Perrine, A. Vahratian, and S. Saydah. 2023. Long COVID and significant activity limitation among adults, by age—United States, June 1–13, 2022, to June 7–19, 2023. *MMWR Morbidity and Mortality Weekly Report* 72:866–870.

Fore, L., Y. Perez, R. Neblett, S. Asih, T. G. Mayer, and R. J. Gatchel. 2015. Improved functional capacity evaluation performance predicts successful return to work one year after completing a functional restoration rehabilitation program. *PM&R* 7(4):365–375.

Fortunato, F., D. Martinelli, G. Iannelli, M. Milazzo, U. Farina, G. Di Matteo, R. De Nittis, L. Ascatigno, M. Cassano, P. L. Lopalco, and R. Prato. 2022. Self-reported olfactory and gustatory dysfunctions in COVID-19 patients: A 1-year follow-up study in Foggia district, Italy. *BMC Infectious Diseases* 22(1):77.

Frontera, J. A., D. Yang, A. Lewis, P. Patel, C. Medicherla, V. Arena, T. Fang, A. Andino, T. Snyder, M. Madhavan, D. Gratch, B. Fuchs, A. Dessy, M. Canizares, R. Jauregui, B. Thomas, K. Bauman, A. Olivera, D. Bhagat, M. Sonson, G. Park, R. Stainman, B. Sunwoo, D. Talmasov, M. Tamimi, Y. Zhu, J. Rosenthal, L. Dygert, M. Ristic, H. Ishii, E. Valdes, M. Omari, L. Gurin, J. Huang, B. M. Czeisler, D. E. Kahn, T. Zhou, J. Lin, A. S. Lord, K. Melmed, S. Meropol, A. B. Troxel, E. Petkova, T. Wisniewski, L. Balcer, C. Morrison, S. Yaghi, and S. Galetta. 2021. A prospective study of long-term outcomes among hospitalized COVID-19 patients with and without neurological complications. *Journal of the Neurological Sciences* 426:117486.

Frontera, J. A., S. Sabadia, D. Yang, A. de Havenon, S. Yaghi, A. Lewis, A. S. Lord, K. Melmed, S. Thawani, L. J. Balcer, T. Wisniewski, and S. L. Galetta. 2022. Life stressors significantly impact long-term outcomes and post-acute symptoms 12-months after COVID-19 hospitalization. *Journal of the Neurological Sciences* 443:120487.

Fuentes, M., A. J. Houtrow, and M. V. Gutierrez. 2021. Ableism and quality of life during the coronavirus pandemic. *Journal of Hospital Medicine* 16(5):316–318.

Gardarsdottir, S., and S. Kaplan. 2002. Validity of the Arnadóttir OT-ADL Neurobehavioral Evaluation (A-ONE): Performance in activities of daily living and neurobehavioral impairments of persons with left and right hemisphere damage. *American Journal of Occupational Therapy* 56(5):499–508.

Genovese, E., and J. S. Galper. 2009. *Guide to the evaluation of functional ability: How to request, interpret, and apply functional capacity evaluations.* Chicago, IL: American Medical Association.

Ghossein-Doha, C., M. Wintjens, E. Janssen, D. Klein, S. C. M. Heemskerk, F. W. Asselbergs, E. Birnie, G. J. Bonsel, B. C. T. van Bussel, J. W. L. Cals, H. Ten Cate, J. Haagsma, B. Hemmen, I. C. C. van der Horst, B. Kietselaer, F. A. Klok, M. D. de Kruif, M. Linschoten, S. van Santen, K. Vernooy, L. H. Willems, R. Westerborg, M. Warle, and S. M. J. van Kuijk. 2022. Prevalence, pathophysiology, prediction and health-related quality of life of long COVID: Study protocol of the longitudinal multiple cohort CORona Follow Up (CORFU) study. *BMJ Open* 12(11):e065142.

Gloeckl, R., D. Leitl, I. Jarosch, T. Schneeberger, C. Nell, N. Stenzel, C. F. Vogelmeier, K. Kenn, and A. R. Koczulla. 2021. Benefits of pulmonary rehabilitation in COVID-19—A prospective observational cohort study. *ERJ Open Research* 7(2):00108–2021.

Golla, R., S. Vuyyuru, B. Kante, P. Kumar, D. M. Thomas, G. Makharia, S. Kedia, and V. Ahuja. 2023. Long-term gastrointestinal sequelae following COVID-19: A prospective follow-up cohort study. *Clinical Gastroenterology & Hepatology* 21(3):789–796.e1.

Gonzalez, J., M. Zuil, I. D. Benitez, D. de Gonzalo-Calvo, M. Aguilar, S. Santisteve, R. Vaca, O. Minguez, F. Seck, G. Torres, J. de Batlle, S. Gomez, S. Barril, A. Moncusi-Moix, A. Monge, C. Gort-Paniello, R. Ferrer, A. Ceccato, L. Fernandez, A. Motos, J. Riera, R. Menendez, D. Garcia-Gasulla, O. Penuelas, G. Labarca, J. Caballero, C. Barbera, A. Torres, and F. Barbe. 2022. One year overview and follow-up in a post-COVID consultation of critically ill patients. *Frontiers in Medicine* 9:897990.

Graf, C. 2008. The Lawton Instrumental Activities of Daily Living Scale. *American Journal of Nursing* 108(4):52–63.

Grager, S., R. Pfirschke, M. Lorenz, D. Vilser, M. Kramer, H. J. Mentzel, and K. Glutig. 2023. Lung ultrasound in children and adolescents with long-term effects of COVID-19: Initial results. *Frontiers in Pediatrics* 11:1112881.

Graham, E. L., J. R. Clark, Z. S. Orban, P. H. Lim, A. L. Szymanski, C. Taylor, R. M. DiBiase, D. T. Jia, R. Balabanov, S. U. Ho, A. Batra, E. M. Liotta, and I. J. Koralnik. 2021. Persistent neurologic symptoms and cognitive dysfunction in non-hospitalized COVID-19 "long haulers." *Annals of Clinical and Translational Neurology* 8(5):1073–1085.

Gutiérrez-Canales, L. G., C. Muñoz-Corona, I. Barrera-Chávez, C. Viloria-Álvarez, A. E. Macías, and E. Guaní-Guerra. 2022. Quality of life and persistence of symptoms in outpatients after recovery from COVID-19. *Medicina (Kaunas)* 58(12):1795.

Han, J. H., K. N. Womack, M. W. Tenforde, D. C. Files, K. W. Gibbs, N. I. Shapiro, M. E. Prekker, H. L. Erickson, J. S. Steingrub, N. Qadir, A. Khan, C. L. Hough, N. J. Johnson, E. W. Ely, T. W. Rice, J. D. Casey, C. J. Lindsell, M. N. Gong, V. Srinivasan, N. M. Lewis, M. M. Patel, and W. H. Self. 2022. Associations between persistent symptoms after mild COVID-19 and long-term health status, quality of life, and psychological distress. *Influenza and Other Respiratory Viruses* 16(4):680–689.

Harris, E. 2024. Long COVID in nursing home residents manifests as functional decline. *JAMA* 331(1):15.

Hartung, T. J., C. Neumann, T. Bahmer, I. Chaplinskaya-Sobol, M. Endres, J. Geritz, K. G. Haeusler, P. U. Heuschmann, H. Hildesheim, A. Hinz, S. Hopff, A. Horn, M. Krawczak, L. Krist, J. Kudelka, W. Lieb, C. Maetzler, A. Mehnert-Theuerkauf, F. A. Montellano, C. Morbach, S. Schmidt, S. Schreiber, F. Steigerwald, S. Störk, W. Maetzler, and C. Finke. 2022. Fatigue and cognitive impairment after COVID-19: A prospective multicentre study. *EClinicalMedicine* 53:101651.

Hastie, C. E., D. J. Lowe, A. McAuley, A. J. Winter, N. L. Mills, C. Black, J. T. Scott, C. A. O'Donnell, D. N. Blane, S. Browne, T. R. Ibbotson, and J. P. Pell. 2022. Outcomes among confirmed cases and a matched comparison group in the Long-COVID in Scotland study. *Nature Communications* 13(1):5663.

HealthMeasures. 2020. *PROMIS Physical Function.* https://www.healthmeasures.net/images/PROMIS/manuals/PROMIS_Physical_Function_Scoring_Manual.pdf (accessed February 20, 2024).

HealthMeasures. 2021. *Pain interference: A brief guide to the PROMIS Pain Interference instruments.* http://www.healthmeasures.net/images/PROMIS/manuals/PROMIS_Pain_Interference_Scoring_Manual.pdf (accessed February 20, 2024).

Herridge, M. S., C. M. Tansey, A. Matté, G. Tomlinson, N. Diaz-Granados, A. Cooper, C. B. Guest, C. D. Mazer, S. Mehta, T. E. Stewart, P. Kudlow, D. Cook, A. S. Slutsky, and A. M. Cheung. 2011. Functional disability 5 years after acute respiratory distress syndrome. *New England Journal of Medicine* 364(14):1293–1304.

Higgins, A. M., L. R. Berry, E. Lorenzi, S. Murthy, Z. McQuilten, P. R. Mouncey, F. Al-Beidh, D. Annane, Y. M. Arabi, A. Beane, W. van Bentum-Puijk, Z. Bhimani, M. J. M. Bonten, C. A. Bradbury, F. M. Brunkhorst, A. Burrell, A. Buzgau, M. Buxton, W. N. Charles, M. Cove, M. A. Detry, L. J. Estcourt, E. O. Fagbodun, M. Fitzgerald, T. D. Girard, E. C. Goligher, H. Goossens, R. Haniffa, T. Hills, C. M. Horvat, D. T. Huang, N. Ichihara, F. Lamontagne, J. C. Marshall, D. F. McAuley, A. McGlothlin, S. P. McGuinness, B. J. McVerry, M. D. Neal, A. D. Nichol, R. L. Parke, J. C. Parker, K. Parry-Billings, S. E. C. Peters, L. F. Reyes, K. M. Rowan, H. Saito, M. S. Santos, C. T. Saunders, A. Serpa-Neto, C. W. Seymour, M. Shankar-Hari, L. M. Stronach, A. F. Turgeon, A. M. Turner, F. L. van de Veerdonk, R. Zarychanski, C. Green, R. J. Lewis, D. C. Angus, C. J. McArthur, S. Berry, L. P. G. Derde, A. C. Gordon, S. A. Webb, P. R. Lawler, and Writing Committee for the RE-MAP Investigators. 2023. Long-term (180-day) outcomes in critically ill patients with COVID-19 in the REMAP-CAP randomized clinical trial. *JAMA* 329(1):39–51.

Hodgson, C. L., A. M. Higgins, M. J. Bailey, A. M. Mather, L. Beach, R. Bellomo, B. Bissett, I. J. Boden, S. Bradley, A. Burrell, D. J. Cooper, B. J. Fulcher, K. J. Haines, J. Hopkins, A. Y. M. Jones, S. Lane, D. Lawrence, L. Van Der Lee, J. Liacos, N. J. Linke, L. M. Gomes, M. Nickels, G. Ntoumenopoulos, P. S. Myles, S. Patman, M. Paton, G. Pound, S. Rai, A. Rix, T. C. Rollinson, J. Sivasuthan, C. J. Tipping, P. Thomas, T. Trapani, A. A. Udy, C. Whitehead, I. T. Hodgson, S. Anderson, A. S. Neto, N. Burgess, K. Hearn, D. Brewster, A. Waanders, S. Simpson, Y. De Silva, J. Lang, S. Burleigh, E. Killer, M. Wang, L. O'Connor, L. Thomas, L. Dennis, J. Caruana, W. Al-Bassam, M. Shealy, M. Chapman, S. O'Connor, J. Sheehan, E. Alexander, A. Sukkar, L. Davis, F. Bass, N. Hammond, A. O'Connor, E. Yarad, R. T. H. Buhr, N. Reddy, W. Chaseling, K. Ip, O. Tronstad, A. Mahoney, C. Fanning, H. Esterman, A. Kozary, B. Scott, and D. Urquhart. 2021. The impact of COVID-19 critical illness on new disability, functional outcomes and return to work at 6 months: A prospective cohort study. *Critical Care* 25(1):382.

Hossain, M. A., K. M. A. Hossain, K. Saunders, Z. Uddin, L. M. Walton, V. Raigangar, M. Sakel, R. Shafin, M. S. Hossain, M. F. Kabir, R. Faruqui, M. S. Rana, M. S. Ahmed, S. K. Chakrovorty, M. A. Hossain, and I. K. Jahid. 2021. Prevalence of long COVID symptoms in Bangladesh: A prospective inception cohort study of COVID-19 survivors. *BMJ Global Health* 6(12):e006838.

Houston, D., S. L. Williams, J. Bloomer, and W. C. Mann. 1989. The Bay Area Functional Performance Evaluation: Development and standardization. *American Journal of Occupational Therapy* 43(3):170–183.

Howard, J., M. Cloeren, and G. Vanichkachorn. 2024. Long COVID and occupational medicine practice. *Journal of Occupational and Environmental Medicine* 66(1):1–5.

Huang, L., Q. Yao, X. Gu, Q. Wang, L. Ren, Y. Wang, P. Hu, L. Guo, M. Liu, J. Xu, X. Zhang, Y. Qu, Y. Fan, X. Li, C. Li, T. Yu, J. Xia, M. Wei, L. Chen, Y. Li, F. Xiao, D. Liu, J. Wang, X. Wang, and B. Cao. 2021. 1-year outcomes in hospital survivors with COVID-19: A longitudinal cohort study. *The Lancet* 398(10302):747–758.

Illmaren, J. 2007. The Work Ability Index (WAI). *Occupational Medicine* 57(2):160.

Iwashyna, T. J., L. A. Kamphuis, S. J. Gundel, A. A. Hope, S. Jolley, A. J. Admon, E. Caldwell, M. L. Monahan, K. Hauschildt, B. T. Thompson, C. L. Hough, and NHLBI Prevention and Early Treatment of Acute Lung Injury (PETAL) Network. 2021. Continuing cardiopulmonary symptoms, disability, and financial toxicity 1 month after hospitalization for third-wave COVID-19: Early results from a US nationwide cohort. *Journal of Hospital Medicine* 16(9):531–537.

Jahn, W. T., L. N. Cupon, and J. H. Steinbaugh. 2004. Functional and work capacity evaluation issues. *Journal of Chiropractic Medicine* 3(1):1–5.

Jamaica Balderas, L., A. Navarro Fernández, S. A. Dragustinovis Garza, M. I. Orellana Jerves, W. E. Solís Figueroa, S. G. Koretzky, H. Márquez González, M. Klünder Klünder, J. G. Espinosa, J. Nieto Zermeño, M. Villa Guillén, R. E. Rosales Uribe, and V. Olivar López. 2023. Long COVID in children and adolescents: COVID-19 follow-up results in third-level pediatric hospital. *Frontiers in Pediatrics* 11:1016394.

Jaquet, P., C. Legouy, L. Le Fevre, A. Grinea, F. Sinnah, G. Franchineau, J. Patrier, M. Marzouk, P. H. Wicky, P. Alexis Geoffroy, F. Arnoult, S. Vledouts, E. de Montmollin, L. Bouadma, J. F. Timsit, T. Sharshar, and R. Sonneville. 2022. Neurologic outcomes of survivors of COVID-19-associated acute respiratory distress syndrome requiring intubation. *Critical Care Medicine* 50(8):e674–e682.

Jarrett, B. A., S. M. Peitzmeier, A. Restar, T. Adamson, S. Howell, S. Baral, and S. W. Beckham. 2021. Gender-affirming care, mental health, and economic stability in the time of COVID-19: A multi-national, cross-sectional study of transgender and nonbinary people. *PLoS ONE* 16(7):e0254215.

Jassat, W., C. Mudara, C. Vika, R. Welch, T. Arendse, M. Dryden, L. Blumberg, N. Mayet, S. Tempia, A. Parker, J. Nel, R. Perumal, M. J. Groome, F. Conradie, N. Ndjeka, L. Sigfrid, L. Merson, and C. Cohen. 2023. A cohort study of post-COVID-19 condition across the Beta, Delta, and Omicron waves in South Africa: 6-month follow-up of hospitalized and nonhospitalized participants. *International Journal of Infectious Disease* 128:102–111.

Jolley, S., A. Nordon-Craft, M. P. Wilson, K. Ridgeway, M. R. Rauzi, J. Capin, L. M. Heery, J. Stevens-Lapsley, and K. M. Erlandson. 2022. Disparities in the allocation of inpatient physical and occupational therapy services for patients with COVID-19. *Journal of Hospital Medicine* 17(2):88–95.

Katz, S. 1983. Assessing self-maintenance: Activities of daily living, mobility, and instrumental activities of daily living. *Journal of the American Geriatric Society* 31(12):721–727.

Katz, S., and C. A. Akpom. 1976. 12. Index of ADL. *Medical Care* 14(5 Suppl):116–118.

Katz, N. B., T. L. Hunter, L. E. Flores, and J. K. Silver. 2023. Addressing rehabilitation health care disparities during the coronavirus disease-2019 pandemic and beyond. *Physical Medicine and Rehabilitation Clinics of North America* 34(3):657–675.

Kenny, G., K. McCann, C. O'Brien, S. Savinelli, W. Tinago, O. Yousif, J. S. Lambert, C. O'Broin, E. R. Feeney, E. De Barra, P. Doran, and P. W. G. Mallon. 2022. Identification of distinct long COVID clinical phenotypes through cluster analysis of self-reported symptoms. *Open Forum Infectious Diseases* 9(4):ofac060.

Kersten, J., A. Wolf, L. Hoyo, E. Hüll, M. Tadic, S. Andreß, S. d'Almeida, D. Scharnbeck, E. Roder, P. Beschoner, W. Rottbauer, and D. Buckert. 2022. Symptom burden correlates to impairment of diffusion capacity and exercise intolerance in long COVID patients. *Scientific Reports* 12(1):8801.

Khullar, D., Y. Zhang, C. Zang, Z. Xu, F. Wang, M. G. Weiner, T. W. Carton, R. L. Rothman, J. P. Block, and R. Kaushal. 2023. Racial/ethnic disparities in post-acute sequelae of SARS-CoV-2 infection in New York: An EHR-based cohort study from the recover program. *Journal of General Internal Medicine* 38(5):1127–1136.

Kikkenborg Berg, S., S. Dam Nielsen, U. Nygaard, H. Bundgaard, P. Palm, C. Rotvig, and A. Vinggaard Christensen. 2022. Long COVID symptoms in SARS-CoV-2-positive adolescents and matched controls (LongCOVIDKidsDK): A national, cross-sectional study. *The Lancet Child & Adolescent Health* 6(4):240–248.

Kim, S. G., H. C. Kwon, T. K. Kang, M. Y. Kwak, S. Lee, K. Lee, and K. Ko. 2022a. COVID-19 sequelae and their implications on social services. *Journal of Korean Medical Science* 37(48):e342.

Kim, Y., H. Bitna, S. W. Kim, H. H. Chang, K. T. Kwon, S. Bae, and S. Hwang. 2022b. Post-acute COVID-19 syndrome in patients after 12 months from COVID-19 infection in Korea. *BMC Infectious Diseases* 22(1):93.

Kohlman-Thomson, L. 1992. *Kohlman Evaluation of Living Skills*. Rockville, MD: American Occupational Therapy Association.

Krysa, J. A., M. Buell, K. Pohar Manhas, K. Kovacs Burns, M. J. Santana, S. Horlick, K. Russell, E. Papathanassoglou, and C. Ho. 2023. Understanding the experience of long COVID symptoms in hospitalized and non-hospitalized individuals: A random, cross-sectional survey study. *Healthcare (Basel)* 11(9):1309.

Kuijer, P. P. F. M., V. Gouttebarge, S. Brouwer, M. F. Reneman, and M. H. W. Frings-Dresen. 2012. Are performance-based measures predictive of work participation in patients with musculoskeletal disorders? A systematic review. *International Archives of Occupational and Environmental Health* 85(2):109–123.

Lassi, Z. S., A. Ana, J. K. Das, R. A. Salam, Z. A. Padhani, O. Irfan, and Z. A. Bhutta. 2021. A systematic review and meta-analysis of data on pregnant women with confirmed COVID-19: Clinical presentation, and pregnancy and perinatal outcomes based on COVID-19 severity. *Journal of Global Health* 11:05018.

Lebrasseur, A., N. Fortin-Bedard, J. Lettre, E. L. Bussieres, K. Best, N. Boucher, M. Hotton, S. Beaulieu-Bonneau, C. Mercier, M. E. Lamontagne, and F. Routhier. 2021. Impact of COVID-19 on people with physical disabilities: A rapid review. *Disability and Health Journal* 14(1):101014.

Lenoir, A., A. Christe, L. Ebner, C. Beigelman-Aubry, P. O. Bridevaux, M. Brutsche, C. Clarenbach, B. Erkosar, C. Garzoni, T. Geiser, S. A. Guler, D. Heg, F. Lador, M. Mancinetti, S. R. Ott, L. Piquilloud, M. Prella, Y. A. Que, C. von Garnier, and M. Funke-Chambour. 2023. Pulmonary recovery 12 months after non-severe and severe COVID-19: The prospective Swiss COVID-19 lung study. *Respiration* 102(2):120–133.

Liguori, G., and American College of Sports Medicine. 2021. *ACSM's guidelines for exercise testing and prescription, 11th ed.* Philadelphia, PA: Lippincott Williams & Wilkins.

Mahajan, S., C. Caraballo, S. X. Li, Y. Dong, L. Chen, S. K. Huston, R. Srinivasan, C. A. Redlich, A. I. Ko, J. S. Faust, H. P. Forman, and H. M. Krumholz. 2021. SARS-CoV-2 infection hospitalization rate and infection fatality rate among the non-congregate population in Connecticut. *American Journal of Medicine* 134(6):812–816.e2.

Mateu, L., C. Tebe, C. Loste, J. R. Santos, G. Lladós, C. López, S. España-Cueto, R. Toledo, M. Font, A. Chamorro, F. Muñoz-López, M. Nevot, N. Vallejo, A. Teis, J. Puig, C. R. Fumaz, J. A. Muñoz-Moreno, A. Prats, C. Estany-Quera, R. Coll-Fernández, C. Herrero, P. Casares, A. Garcia, B. Clotet, R. Paredes, and M. Massanella. 2023. Determinants of the onset and prognosis of the post-COVID-19 condition: A 2-year prospective observational cohort study. *The Lancet Regional Health—Europe* 33:100724.

McAuley, H. J. C., R. A. Evans, C. E. Bolton, C. E. Brightling, J. D. Chalmers, A. B. Docherty, O. Elneima, P. L. Greenhaff, A. Gupta, V. C. Harris, E. M. Harrison, L. P. Ho, A. Horsley, L. Houchen-Wolloff, C. J. Jolley, O. C. Leavy, N. I. Lone, W. D. Man, M. Marks, D. Parekh, K. Poinasamy, J. K. Quint, B. Raman, M. Richardson, R. M. Saunders, M. Sereno, A. Shikotra, A. Singapuri, S. J. Singh, M. Steiner, A. L. Tan, L. V. Wain, C. Welch, J. Whitney, M. D. Witham, J. Lord, and N. J. Greening. 2023. Prevalence of physical frailty, including risk factors, up to 1 year after hospitalisation for COVID-19 in the UK: A multicentre, longitudinal cohort study. *EClinicalMedicine* 57:101896.

Menachemi, N., B. E. Dixon, K. K. Wools-Kaloustian, C. T. Yiannoutsos, and P. K. Halverson. 2021. How many SARS-CoV-2-infected people require hospitalization? Using random sample testing to better inform preparedness efforts. *Journal of Public Health Management and Practice* 27(3):246–250.

Menges, D., T. Ballouz, A. Anagnostopoulos, H. E. Aschmann, A. Domenghino, J. S. Fehr, and M. A. Puhan. 2021. Burden of post-COVID-19 syndrome and implications for healthcare service planning: A population-based cohort study. *PLoS ONE* 16(7):e0254523.

Meterko, M., E. E. Marfeo, C. M. McDonough, A. M. Jette, P. Ni, K. Bogusz, E. K. Rasch, D. E. Brandt, and L. Chan. 2015. Work Disability Functional Assessment Battery: Feasibility and psychometric properties. *Archives of Physical Medicine and Rehabilitation* 96(6):1028–1035.

Meterko, M., M. Marino, P. Ni, E. Marfeo, C. M. McDonough, A. Jette, K. Peterik, E. Rasch, D. E. Brandt, and L. Chan. 2019. Psychometric evaluation of the improved Work-Disability Functional Assessment Battery. *Archives of Physical Medicine and Rehabilitation* 100(8):1442–1449.

Miller, M. J., L. R. Feldstein, J. Holbrook, I. D. Plumb, E. K. Accorsi, Q. C. Zhang, Q. Cheng, J. Y. Ko, V. Wanga, S. Konkle, L. V. Dimitrov, J. Bertolli, and S. Saydah. 2023. Post-COVID conditions and healthcare utilization among adults with and without disabilities–2021 Porter Novelli Fallstyles survey. *Disability and Health Journal* 16(2):101436.

Miskowiak, K. W., J. K. Pedersen, D. V. Gunnarsson, T. K. Roikjer, D. Podlekareva, H. Hansen, C. H. Dall, and S. Johnsen. 2023. Cognitive impairments among patients in a long-COVID clinic: Prevalence, pattern and relation to illness severity, work function and quality of life. *Journal of Affective Disorders* 324:162–169.

Mohamed Hussein, A. A., M. Saad, H. E. Zayan, M. Abdelsayed, M. Moustafa, A. R. Ezzat, R. Helmy, H. Abd-Elaal, K. Aly, S. Abdelrheem, and I. Sayed. 2021. Post-COVID-19 functional status: Relation to age, smoking, hospitalization, and previous comorbidities. *Annals of Thoracic Medicine* 16(3):260–265.

Mora, A. M., K. Kogut, N. K. Sandhu, D. Ridgway, C. M. Patty, M. Renteria, N. Morga, M. T. Rodriguez, M. Romero, J. M. Valdovinos, A. Torres-Nguyen, O. Guzman, M. Martinez, R. L. Doty, A. Padilla, E. Flores, P. M. Brown, and B. Eskenazi. 2023. SARS-CoV-2 infection and long COVID among California farmworkers. *The Journal of Rural Health* 40(2):292–302.

Morello, R., F. Mariani, L. Mastrantoni, C. De Rose, G. Zampino, D. Munblit, L. Sigfrid, P. Valentini, and D. Buonsenso. 2023. Risk factors for post-COVID-19 condition (long COVID) in children: A prospective cohort study. *EClinicalMedicine* 59:101961.

Muccioli, L., G. Sighinolfi, M. Mitolo, L. Ferri, M. Jane Rochat, U. Pensato, L. Taruffi, C. Testa, M. Masullo, P. Cortelli, R. Lodi, R. Liguori, C. Tonon, and F. Bisulli. 2023. Cognitive and functional connectivity impairment in post-COVID-19 olfactory dysfunction. *NeuroImage: Clinical* 38:103410.

Murphy, T. E., T. M. Gill, L. S. Leo-Summers, E. A. Gahbauer, M. A. Pisani, and L. E. Ferrante. 2018. The competing risk of death in longitudinal geriatric outcomes. *Journal of the American Geriatrics Society* 67(2):357–362.

NCHS (National Center for Health Statistics). 2023. *U.S. Census Bureau, household pulse survey, 2022-2023. Long COVID.* https://www.cdc.gov/nchs/covid19/pulse/long-covid.htm (accessed February 14, 2024).

Needham, D. M., J. Davidson, H. Cohen, R. O. Hopkins, C. Weinert, H. Wunsch, C. Zawistowski, A. Bemis-Dougherty, S. C. Berney, O. J. Bienvenu, S. L. Brady, M. B. Brodsky, L. Denehy, D. Elliott, C. Flatley, A. L. Harabin, C. Jones, D. Louis, W. Meltzer, S. R. Muldoon, J. B. Palmer, C. Perme, M. Robinson, D. M. Schmidt, E. Scruth, G. R. Spill, C. P. Storey, M. Render, J. Votto, and M. A. Harvey. 2012. Improving long-term outcomes after discharge from intensive care unit: Report from a stakeholders' conference. *Critical Care Medicine* 40(2):502–509.

Nevejan, L., S. Ombelet, L. Laenen, E. Keyaerts, T. Demuyser, L. Seyler, O. Soetens, E. Van Nedervelde, R. Naesens, D. Geysels, W. Verstrepen, L. Cattoir, S. Martens, C. Michel, E. Mathieu, M. Reynders, A. Evenepoel, J. Hellemans, M. Vanhee, K. Magerman, J. Maes, V. Matheeussen, H. Boogaerts, K. Lagrou, L. Cuypers, and E. André. 2022. Severity of COVID-19 among hospitalized patients: Omicron remains a severe threat for immuno-compromised hosts. *Viruses* 14(12):2736.

Neville, T. H., R. D. Hays, C. H. Tseng, C. A. Gonzalez, L. Chen, A. Hong, M. Yamamoto, L. Santoso, A. Kung, K. Schwab, S. Y. Chang, N. Qadir, T. Wang, and N. S. Wenger. 2022. Survival after severe COVID-19: Long-term outcomes of patients admitted to an intensive care unit. *Journal of Intensive Care Medicine* 37(8):1019–1028.

Niedziela, J. T., J. Głowacki, M. Ochman, R. Pudlo, M. Adamczyk-Sowa, A. Nowowiejska-Wiewióra, Z. Kułaczkowska, B. Sobala-Szczygieł, K. Myrda, M. Wiewióra, I. Jaworska, K. Czapla, A. Grzanka, M. Gąsior, and J. Jaroszewicz. 2022. Post-COVID-19 complications in hospitalized and nonhospitalized patients: The Silesian database of COVID-19 complications (SILCOV-19). *Polish Archives of Internal Medicine* 132(6):16233.

Nopp, S., F. Moik, F. A. Klok, D. Gattinger, M. Petrovic, K. Vonbank, A. R. Koczulla, C. Ay, and R. H. Zwick. 2022. Outpatient pulmonary rehabilitation in patients with long COVID improves exercise capacity, functional status, dyspnea, fatigue, and quality of life. *Respiration* 101(6):593–601.

Núñez-Seisdedos, M. N., I. Lázaro-Navas, L. López-González, and L. López-Aguilera. 2022. Intensive care unit-acquired weakness and hospital functional mobility outcomes following invasive mechanical ventilation in patients with COVID-19: A single-centre prospective cohort study. *Journal of Intensive Care Medicine* 37(8):1005–1014.

O'Kelly, B., L. Vidal, G. Avramovic, J. Broughan, S. P. Connolly, A. G. Cotter, W. Cullen, S. Glaspy, T. McHugh, J. Woo, and J. S. Lambert. 2022. Assessing the impact of COVID-19 at 1-year using the SF-12 questionnaire: Data from the anticipate longitudinal cohort study. *International Journal of Infectious Diseases* 118:236–243.

Osmanov, I. M., E. Spiridonova, P. Bobkova, A. Gamirova, A. Shikhaleva, M. Andreeva, O. Blyuss, Y. El-Taravi, A. DunnGalvin, P. Comberiati, D. G. Peroni, C. Apfelbacher, J. Genuneit, L. Mazankova, A. Miroshina, E. Chistyakova, E. Samitova, S. Borzakova, E. Bondarenko, A. A. Korsunskiy, I. Konova, S. W. Hanson, G. Carson, L. Sigfrid, J. T. Scott, M. Greenhawt, E. A. Whittaker, E. Garralda, O. V. Swann, D. Buonsenso, D. E. Nicholls, F. Simpson, C. Jones, M. G. Semple, J. O. Warner, T. Vos, P. Olliaro, D. Munblit, and the Sechenov StopCOVID Research Team. 2022. Risk factors for post-COVID-19 condition in previously hospitalised children using the ISARIC Global follow-up protocol: A prospective cohort study. *European Respiratory Journal* 59(2):2101341.

Ostrowska, M., A. Rzepka-Cholasinska, L. Pietrzykowski, P. Michalski, A. Kosobucka-Ozdoba, M. Jasiewicz, M. Kasprzak, J. Krys, and A. Kubica. 2023. Effects of multidisciplinary rehabilitation program in patients with long COVID-19: Post-COVID-19 rehabilitation (PCR SIRIO 8) study. *Journal of Clinical Medicine* 12(2):420.

Ottenbacher, K. J., Y. Hsu, C. V. Granger, and R. C. Fiedler. 1996. The reliability of the functional independence measure: A quantitative review. *Archives of Physical Medicine and Rehabilitation* 77(12):1226–1232.

Parker, M., H. B. Sawant, T. Flannery, R. Tarrant, J. Shardha, R. Bannister, D. Ross, S. Halpin, D. C. Greenwood, and M. Sivan. 2023. Effect of using a structured pacing protocol on post-exertional symptom exacerbation and health status in a longitudinal cohort with the post-COVID-19 syndrome. *Journal of Medical Virology* 95(1):e28373.

Patterson, M. B., and J. L. Mack. 2001. Cleveland Scale for Activities of Daily Living (CSADL): Its reliability and validity. *Journal of Clinical Geropsychology* 7(1):15–28.

Pazukhina, E., M. Andreeva, E. Spiridonova, P. Bobkova, A. Shikhaleva, Y. El-Taravi, M. Rumyantsev, A. Gamirova, A. Bairashevskaia, P. Petrova, D. Baimukhambetova, M. Pikuza, E. Abdeeva, Y. Filippova, S. Deunezhewa, N. Nekliudov, P. Bugaeva, N. Bulanov, S. Avdeev, V. Kapustina, A. Guekht, A. DunnGalvin, P. Comberiati, D. G. Peroni, C. Apfelbacher, J. Genuneit, L. F. Reyes, C. L. H. Brackel, V. Fomin, A. A. Svistunov, P. Timashev, L. Mazankova, A. Miroshina, E. Samitova, S. Borzakova, E. Bondarenko, A. A. Korsunskiy, G. Carson, L. Sigfrid, J. T. Scott, M. Greenhawt, D. Buonsenso, M. G. Semple, J. O. Warner, P. Olliaro, D. M. Needham, P. Glybochko, D. Butnaru, I. M. Osmanov, D. Munblit, and the Sechenov StopCOVID Research Team. 2022. Prevalence and risk factors of post-COVID-19 condition in adults and children at 6 and 12 months after hospital discharge: A prospective, cohort study in Moscow (StopCOVID). *BMC Medicine* 20(1):244.

Perez Giraldo, G. S., S. T. Ali, A. K. Kang, T. R. Patel, S. Budhiraja, J. I. Gaelen, G. K. Lank, J. R. Clark, S. Mukherjee, T. Singer, A. Venkatesh, Z. S. Orban, P. H. Lim, M. Jimenez, J. Miller, C. Taylor, A. L. Szymanski, J. Scarpelli, E. L. Graham, R. D. Balabanov, B. E. Barcelo, J. G. Cahan, K. Ruckman, A. G. Shepard, M. W. Slutzky, K. LaFaver, P. U. Kumthekar, N. K. Shetty, K. S. Carroll, S. U. Ho, R. V. Lukas, A. Batra, E. M. Liotta, and I. J. Koralnik. 2023. Neurologic manifestations of long COVID differ based on acute COVID-19 severity. *Annals of Neurology* 94(1):146–159.

Perlis, R. H., K. Lunz Trujillo, A. Safarpour, M. Santillana, K. Ognyanova, J. Druckman, and D. Lazer. 2023. Association of post-COVID-19 condition symptoms and employment status. *JAMA Network Open* 6(2):e2256152.

Physiopedia. n.d. *10 Metre Walk Test.* https://www.physio-pedia.com/10_Metre_Walk_Test (accessed February 14, 2024).

Pinto Pereira, S. M., M. D. Nugawela, K. McOwat, E. Dalrymple, L. Xu, S. N. Ladhani, R. Simmons, T. Chalder, O. Swann, T. Ford, I. Heyman, T. Segal, M. Semple, N. Rojas, R. Shafran, T. Stephenson, and the CLoCk Consortium. 2023. Symptom profiles of children and young people 12 months after SARS-CoV-2 testing: A national matched cohort study (The CLoCk Study). *Children* 10(7):1227.

Portacci, A., V. N. Quaranta, I. Iorillo, E. Buonamico, F. Diaferia, S. Quaranta, C. Locorotondo, S. Dragonieri, and G. E. Carpagnano. 2022. The impact of healthcare setting on post-COVID mood disorders: A single-centre perspective from Southern Italy Respiratory Intensive Care Unit. *Respiratory Medicine* 203:107006.

Pouliopoulou, D. V., J. C. Macdermid, E. Saunders, S. Peters, L. Brunton, E. Miller, K. L. Quinn, T. V. Pereira, and P. Bobos. 2023. Rehabilitation interventions for physical capacity and quality of life in adults with post-COVID-19 condition: A systematic review and meta-analysis. *JAMA Network Open* 6(9):e2333838.

Powell, L. E., and A. M. Myers. 1995. The Activities-specific Balance Confidence (ABC) scale. *Journals of Gerontology. Series A, Biological Sciences and Medical Sciences* 50A(1):M28–34.

Public Health Agency of Canada. 2023. *COVID-19: Longer-term symptoms among Canadian adults—Highlights.* https://health-infobase.canada.ca/COVID-19/post-COVID-condition/ (accessed February 14, 2024).

Qin, E. S., L. S. Gold, N. Singh, K. D. Wysham, C. L. Hough, P. B. Patel, A. E. Bunnell, and J. S. Andrews. 2023. Physical function and fatigue recovery at 6 months after hospitalization for COVID-19. *PM&R* 15(3):314–324.

Quinn, T. J., P. Langhorne, and D. J. Stott. 2011. Barthel Index for stroke trials: Development, properties, and application. *Stroke* 42(4):1146–1151.

Raj, V., M. Opie, and A. C. Arnold. 2018. Cognitive and psychological issues in postural tachycardia syndrome. *Autonomic Neuroscience* 215:46–55.

Rass, V., R. Beer, A. J. Schiefecker, A. Lindner, M. Kofler, B. A. Ianosi, P. Mahlknecht, B. Heim, M. Peball, F. Carbone, V. Limmert, P. Kindl, L. Putnina, E. Fava, S. Sahanic, T. Sonnweber, W. N. Löscher, J. V. Wanschitz, L. Zamarian, A. Djamshidian, I. Tancevski, G. Weiss, R. Bellmann Weiler, S. Kiechl, K. Seppi, J. Loeffler Ragg, B. Pfausler, and R. Helbok. 2022. Neurological outcomes 1 year after COVID-19 diagnosis: A prospective longitudinal cohort study. *European Journal of Neurology* 29(6):1685–1696.

Rea, M., P. Pawelek, and D. Ayoubkhani. *Prevalence of ongoing symptoms following coronavirus (COVID-19) infection in the UK: 30 March 2023.* Office for National Statistics. https://www.ons.gov.uk/peoplepopulationandcommunity/healthandsocialcare/conditionsanddiseases/bulletins/prevalenceofongoingsymptomsfollowingcoronaviruscovid19infectionintheuk/30march2023 (accessed February 20, 2024).

Sabatino, J., C. Di Chiara, A. Di Candia, D. Sirico, D. Donà, J. Fumanelli, A. Basso, P. Pogacnik, E. Cuppini, L. R. Romano, B. Castaldi, E. Reffo, A. Cerutti, R. Biffanti, S. Cozzani, C. Giaquinto, and G. Di Salvo. 2022. Mid- and long-term atrio-ventricular functional changes in children after recovery from COVID-19. *Journal of Clinical Medicine* 12(1):186.

Sahanic, S., P. Tymoszuk, A. K. Luger, K. Hufner, A. Boehm, A. P. C. Schwabl, S. Koppelstatter, K. Kurz, M. Asshoff, B. Mosheimer-Feistritzer, M. Coen, B. Pfeifer, V. Rass, A. Egger, G. Hormann, B. Sperner-Unterweger, R. Helbok, E. Woll, G. Weiss, G. Widmann, I. Tancevski, T. Sonnweber, and J. Loffler-Ragg. 2023. COVID-19 and its continuing burden after 12 months: A longitudinal observational prospective multicentre trial. *ERJ Open Research* 9(2):00317–02022.

Sassi, F. C., A. P. Ritto, M. S. de Lima, C. N. Valente Junior, P. F. G. Cardoso, B. Zilberstein, P. H. N. Saldiva, and C. R. F. de Andrade. 2022. Characteristics of postintubation dysphagia in ICU patients in the context of the COVID-19 outbreak: A report of 920 cases from a Brazilian reference center. *PLoS ONE* 17(6):e0270107.

Schlemmer, F., S. Valentin, L. Boyer, A. Guillaumot, F. Chabot, C. Dupin, P. Le Guen, G. Lorillon, A. Bergeron, D. Basille, J. Delomez, C. Andrejak, V. Bonnefoy, H. Goussault, J.-B. Assié, P. Choinier, A.-M. Ruppert, J. Cadranel, M. C. Mennitti, M. Roumila, C. Colin, S. Günther, O. Sanchez, T. Gille, L. Sésé, Y. Uzunhan, M. Faure, M. Patout, C. Morelot-Panzini, P. Laveneziana, M. Zysman, E. Blanchard, C. Raherison-Semjen, V. Giraud, E. Giroux-Leprieur, S. Habib, N. Roche, A. T. Dinh-Xuan, I. Sifaoui, P.-Y. Brillet, C. Jung, E. Boutin, R. Layese, F. Canoui-Poitrine, and B. Maitre. 2023. Respiratory recovery trajectories after severe-to-critical COVID-19: A 1-year prospective multicentre study. *European Respiratory Journal* 61(4):2201532.

Schuling, J., R. de Haan, M. Limburg, and K. H. Groenier. 1993. The Frenchay Activities Index. Assessment of functional status in stroke patients. *Stroke* 24(8):1173–1177.

Seeßle, J., T. Waterboer, T. Hippchen, J. Simon, M. Kirchner, A. Lim, B. Müller, and U. Merle. 2022. Persistent symptoms in adult patients 1 year after coronavirus disease 2019 (COVID-19): A prospective cohort study. *Clinical Infectious Disease* 74(7):1191–1198.

Sheehan, D. V. 1983. The Sheehan Disability Scale. In *The Anxiety Disease and How to Overcome It*. New York: Charles Scribner and Sons. P. 151.

Shirakawa, C., R. Tachikawa, R. Yamamoto, C. Miyakoshi, K. Iwata, K. Endo, Y. Shimada, Y. Shima, A. Matsunashi, M. Osaki, R. Hirabayashi, Y. Sato, K. Nagata, A. Nakagawa, and K. Tomii. 2023. Longitudinal changes in mental health outcomes after COVID-19 hospitalization: A prospective study. *Respiratory Investigation* 61(3):321–331.

Shirley Ryan AbilityLab. 2013a. *30 Second Sit to Stand Test*. https://www.sralab.org/rehabilitation-measures/30-second-sit-stand-test (accessed February 14, 2024).

Shirley Ryan AbilityLab. 2013b. *Lower Extremity Functional Scale*. https://www.sralab.org/rehabilitation-measures/lower-extremity-functional-scale (accessed February 14, 2024).

Shirley Ryan AbilityLab. 2013c. *Numeric pain rating scale*. https://www.sralab.org/rehabilitation-measures/numeric-pain-rating-scale (accessed February 14, 2024).

Shirley Ryan AbilityLab. 2013d. *Romberg test*. https://www.sralab.org/rehabilitation-measures/romberg-test (accessed February 14, 2024).

Shirley Ryan AbilityLab. 2013e. *Sensory Organization Test*. https://www.sralab.org/rehabilitation-measures/sensory-organization-test (accessed February 14, 2024).

Shirley Ryan AbilityLab. 2015. *Foot and Ankle Ability Measures*. https://www.sralab.org/rehabilitation-measures/foot-and-ankle-ability-measures (accessed February 14, 2024).

Shirley Ryan AbilityLab. 2018. *PROMIS fatigue*. https://www.sralab.org/rehabilitation-measures/promis-fatigue (accessed February 14, 2024).

Shirley Ryan AbilityLab. 2019. *Assessment of Motor and Process Skills*. https://www.sralab.org/rehabilitation-measures/assessment-motor-and-process-skills (accessed February 14, 2024).

Sletten, D. M., G. A. Suarez, P. A. Low, J. Mandrekar, and W. Singer. 2012. COMPASS 31: A refined and abbreviated composite autonomic symptom score. *Mayo Clinic Proceedings* 87(12):1196–1201.

Soer, R., C. P. van der Schans, J. W. Groothoff, J. H. Geertzen, and M. F. Reneman. 2008. Towards consensus in operational definitions in functional capacity evaluation: A Delphi survey. *Journal of Occupational Rehabilitation* 18(4):389–400.

Sonnweber, T., P. Tymoszuk, S. Sahanic, A. Boehm, A. Pizzini, A. Luger, C. Schwabl, M. Nairz, P. Grubwieser, K. Kurz, S. Koppelstätter, M. Aichner, B. Puchner, A. Egger, G. Hoermann, E. Wöll, G. Weiss, G. Widmann, I. Tancevski, and J. Löffler-Ragg. 2022. Investigating phenotypes of pulmonary COVID-19 recovery: A longitudinal observational prospective multicenter trial. *Elife* 11:e72500.

Spielmanns, M., C. E. Schaer, A. M. Pekacka-Egli, S. Spielmanns, O. Ibish, G. Gafina, A. Stiube, and M. Hermann. 2023. Pulmonary rehabilitation outcomes of post-acute COVID-19 patients during different waves of the pandemic. *International Journal of Environmental Research and Public Health* 20(10):5907.

Stavem, K., G. Einvik, and C. Lundqvist. 2022. Cognitive impairment 13 months after hospitalization for COVID-19. *Open Forum Infectious Diseases* 9(7):ofac355.

Steinbeis, F., C. Thibeault, F. Doellinger, R. M. Ring, M. Mittermaier, C. Ruwwe-Glosenkamp, F. Alius, P. Knape, H. J. Meyer, L. J. Lippert, E. T. Helbig, D. Grund, B. Temmesfeld-Wollbruck, N. Suttorp, L. E. Sander, F. Kurth, T. Penzkofer, M. Witzenrath, and T. Zoller. 2022. Severity of respiratory failure and computed chest tomography in acute COVID-19 correlates with pulmonary function and respiratory symptoms after infection with SARS-CoV-2: An observational longitudinal study over 12 months. *Respiratory Medicine* 191:106709.

Taboada, M., N. Rodríguez, M. Diaz-Vieito, M. J. Domínguez, A. Casal, V. Riveiro, A. Cariñena, E. Moreno, A. Pose, L. Valdés, J. Alvarez, and T. Seoane-Pillado. 2022. Quality of life and persistent symptoms after hospitalization for COVID-19. A prospective observational study comparing ICU with non-ICU patients. *Revista Española de Anestesiologia Reanimación (England Edition)* 69(6):326–335.

Tanguay, P., S. Decary, S. Lemaire-Paquette, G. Leonard, A. Piche, M. F. Dubois, D. Kairy, G. Bravo, H. Corriveau, N. Marquis, M. Tousignant, M. Chasse, and L. P. Carvalho. 2023. Trajectories of health-related quality of life and their predictors in adult COVID-19 survivors: A longitudinal analysis of the Biobanque québécoise de la COVID-19 (BQC-19). *Quality of Life Research* 32(9):2707–2717.

Taniguchi, L. U., M. J. R. Aliberti, M. B. Dias, W. Jacob-Filho, and T. J. Avelino-Silva. 2023. Twelve months and counting: Following clinical outcomes in critical COVID-19 survivors. *Annals of the American Thoracic Society* 20(2):289–295.

Thaweethai, T., S. E. Jolley, E. W. Karlson, E. B. Levitan, B. Levy, G. A. McComsey, L. McCorkell, G. N. Nadkarni, S. Parthasarathy, U. Singh, T. A. Walker, C. A. Selvaggi, D. J. Shinnick, C. C. M. Schulte, R. Atchley-Challenner, L. I. Horwitz, and A. S. Foulkes, RECOVER Consortium Authors, for the RECOVER Consortium. 2023. Development of a definition of postacute sequelae of SARS-CoV-2 infection. *JAMA* 329(22):1934–1946.

Thronicke, A., M. Hinse, S. Weinert, A. Jakubowski, G. Grieb, and H. Matthes. 2022. Factors associated with self-reported post/long-COVID-a real-world data study. *International Journal of Environmental Research and Public Health* 19(23):16124.

Tuomi, K., J. Ilmarinen, A. Jahkola, L. Katajarinne, and A. Tulkki. 1998. *Work Ability Index*. 2nd revised ed. Helsinki, Finland: Finnish Institute of Occupational Health.

Valdes, E., B. Fuchs, C. Morrison, L. Charvet, A. Lewis, S. Thawani, L. Balcer, S. L. Galetta, T. Wisniewski, and J. A. Frontera. 2022. Demographic and social determinants of cognitive dysfunction following hospitalization for COVID-19. *Journal of the Neurological Sciences* 438:120146.

Wahlgren, C., G. Forsberg, A. Divanoglou, Å. Östholm Balkhed, K. Niward, S. Berg, and R. Levi. 2023. Two-year follow-up of patients with post-COVID-19 condition in Sweden: A prospective cohort study. *The Lancet Regional Health—Europe* 28:100595.

Walker, L. S., and J. W. Greene. 1991. The Functional Disability Inventory: Measuring a neglected dimension of child health status. *Journal of Pediatric Psychology* 16(1):39–58.

Weber, B., H. Siddiqi, G. Zhou, J. Vieira, A. Kim, H. Rutherford, X. Mitre, M. Feeley, K. Oganezova, A. S. Varshney, A. S. Bhatt, V. Nauffal, D. S. Atri, R. Blankstein, E. W. Karlson, M. Di Carli, L. R. Baden, D. L. Bhatt, and A. E. Woolley. 2022. Relationship between myocardial injury during index hospitalization for SARS-CoV-2 infection and longer-term outcomes. *Journal of the American Heart Association* 11(1):e022010.

Weihe, S., C. B. Mortensen, N. Haase, L. P. K. Andersen, T. Mohr, H. Siegel, M. Ibsen, V. R. L. Jorgensen, D. L. Buck, H. B. S. Pedersen, H. P. Pedersen, S. Iversen, N. Ribergaard, B. S. Rasmussen, R. Winding, U. S. Espelund, H. Bundgaard, C. G. Solling, S. Christensen, R. S. Garcia, A. C. Brochner, J. Michelsen, G. Michagin, L. Kirkegaard, A. Perner, O. Mathiesen, and L. M. Poulsen. 2022. Long-term cognitive and functional status in Danish ICU patients with COVID-19. *Acta Anaesthesiolgica Scandinavica* 66(8):978–986.

WHO (World Health Organization). 2023. *Clinical management of COVID-19: Living guideline: Version 7.* Geneva, Switzerland: WHO. 18 August 2023. https://www.who.int/publications/i/item/WHO-2019-nCoV-clinical-2023.2 (accessed February 20, 2024).

Xie, Y., E. Xu, B. Bowe, and Z. Al-Aly. 2022. Long-term cardiovascular outcomes of COVID-19. *Nature Medicine* 28(3):583–590.

Xu, E., Y. Xie, and Z. Al-Aly. 2022. Long-term neurologic outcomes of COVID-19. *Nature Medicine* 28(11):2406–2415.

Zhang, Y., H. Hu, V. Fokaidis, V, C. Lewis, J. Xu, C. Zang, Z. Xu, F. Wang, M. Koropsak, J. Bian, J. Hall, R. L. Rothman, E. A. Shenkman, W. Q. Wei, M. G. Weiner, T. W. Carton, and R. Kaushal. 2023. Identifying environmental risk factors for post-acute sequelae of SARS-CoV-2 infection: An EHR-based cohort study from the RECOVER program. *Environmental Advances* 11:100352.

Zhang, H., C. Huang, X. Gu, Y. Wang, X. Li, M. Liu, Q. Wang, J. Xu, Y. Wang, H. Dai, D. Zhang, and B. Cao. 2024. 3-year outcomes of discharged survivors of COVID-19 following the SARS-CoV-2 Omicron (B.1.1.529) wave in 2022 in China: A longitudinal cohort study. *The Lancet Respiratory Medicine* 12(1):55–66.

5

Chronic Conditions Similar
to Long COVID

While Long COVID has recently garnered significant attention because of its wide-ranging effects on a considerable portion of the global population, infection-associated chronic conditions (IACCs) are not a new phenomenon. Additionally, Long COVID shares many features with other complex multisystem chronic conditions, including myalgic encephalomyelitis/chronic fatigue syndrome (ME/CFS) and fibromyalgia (FM). This chapter focuses on Long COVID's similarities with those two conditions, which are requested in the committee's statement of task. The committee also reviewed Long COVID's similarities with other conditions, including postural orthostatic tachycardia syndrome (POTS), posttreatment Lyme disease, and hypermobile Ehlers-Danlos syndrome, and data on those similarities are included where available; however, the research here is limited. A discussion of autonomic dysfunction, including POTS, is provided in Chapter 3.

SARS-CoV-2 is the viral trigger for Long COVID. It is also hypothesized to be one potential viral trigger for ME/CFS and FM. Other mechanistic links have been suggested among these conditions, including abnormalities involving the immune system, central and autonomic nervous systems, cardiopulmonary system, gut microbiome, and energy metabolism. Additionally, given their common symptoms, treatments for ME/CFS and FM can help inform treatment for Long COVID. Beginning with a review of ME/CFS and FM and their shared symptoms with Long COVID, this chapter explores the parallels among those disorders, including a review of the common potential mechanisms of action, testing procedures, prognosis and progression, and management and treatment.

183

CASE DEFINITIONS AND EPIDEMIOLOGY

Myalgic Encephalomyelitis/Chronic Fatigue Syndrome

ME/CFS is a severe systemic illness with symptoms based predominantly on neurological, immunological, and endocrinological dysfunction (Carruthers et al., 2011). The Institute of Medicine's (IOM's) diagnostic criteria for adults and children with ME/CFS are the most widely used (IOM, 2015). According to the IOM, ME/CFS is diagnosed when a patient meets the following criteria: a new-onset substantial activity impairment lasting at least 6 months, post-exertional malaise, and unrefreshing sleep, in addition to cognitive impairment or orthostatic intolerance. In addition to the IOM criteria, there exist more than 20 clinical case definitions for ME/CFS (Brurberg et al., 2014), presenting a challenge in standardization and comparison across research studies.

It is estimated that 17–24 million people globally have ME/CFS (Lim et al., 2020a). Prevalence estimates for the United States range from 0.2 percent to 1.3 percent (Lim et al., 2020a; Vahratian et al., 2023). ME/CFS is more prevalent among women than men (Wessely, 1995), and peak ages of onset are during adolescence and ages 30–50 years (Bakken et al., 2014). Data on ME/CFS in children and adolescents are sparse; however, pediatric populations are generally considered to have a better recovery prognosis than adults (Moore et al., 2021; Rowe et al., 2017).

Diagnosis of ME/CFS is difficult due to limited knowledge about the pathomechanism of ME/CFS and lack of a consensus biomarker. In addition to being an obstacle to accurate diagnosis, poor knowledge of ME/CFS is detrimental to efficient patient care. In an early publication, estimates of misdiagnosis are reported to be as high as 84–91 percent as a result of physician misinformation (Solomon and Reeves, 2004), while other authors have reported that 71 percent of patients needed to see four or more physicians to receive a diagnosis (Tidmore et al., 2015).

The percentage of patients with Long COVID that meet criteria for ME/CFS varies in the literature. An overview of the literature shows that on average, 40–70 percent of Long COVID patients meet the criteria for ME/CFS (Bonilla et al., 2023; Jason and Islam, 2022; Kedor et al., 2022; Mancini et al., 2021; Twomey et al., 2022). In contrast, González-Hermosillo and colleagues (2021) found that only 13 percent of Long COVID patients met the criteria for ME/CFS, and AlMuhaissen and colleagues (2023) found an overlap of 8.1 percent. These differences could be due to the varied case definitions for both Long COVID and ME/CFS.

Fibromyalgia

FM is characterized by chronic and widespread musculoskeletal pain, accompanied by fatigue and sleep disturbances (Bhargava and Hurley, 2023;

Häuser et al., 2015; Sarzi-Puttini et al., 2020). Patients with FM present with a range of other clinical symptoms, including cognitive dysfunction, anxiety or mood disturbances, and variable gastrointestinal symptoms (Fialho et al., 2023). Pain and stiffness are usually found in the muscles of the neck, shoulders, back, hips, arms, and legs. In addition to fatigue and sleep disturbances, other signs and symptoms include headaches, and fatigue (Bhargava and Hurley, 2023). FM impacts approximately 2 percent of the U.S. adult population (CDC, 2022). The rates of FM increase with age between 20 and 55, with dominance in middle-aged and older women, although the condition can occur in anyone, including children (Brill et al., 2012; Lindell et al., 2000).

Diagnoses of FM may involve dynamic evoked pain assessments with neuroimaging (Boquete et al., 2022; de la Coba et al., 2022; Mosch et al., 2023). Several of the features leading to diagnosis of FM are also present in other rheumatologic diseases, such as connective tissue disorders, ankylosing spondylitis, and spondylarthritis. Other researchers have investigated the differentiation of FM from other chronic pain disorders or ME/CFS. The distinct symptoms of FM are persistent deep aching within the body, poor balance, environmental sensitivity, tenderness to touch, and pain after exercise (Bennett et al., 2022). Studies show that up to 39 percent of people with Long COVID also meet the 2011 criteria for FM (Plaut, 2023; Ursini et al., 2021).

SHARED SYMPTOMS AND FUNCTIONAL IMPLICATIONS

Shared Symptoms

Systemic postinfectious syndromes share several symptom profiles, including post-exertional malaise, chronic fatigue, impaired concentration and memory, pain, and sleep disturbances (Jason et al., 2023). Interestingly, the IOM (2015) core criteria for ME/CFS noted above are also core symptoms of Long COVID, as described in Chapter 3 of this report. One key difference is that for an ME/CFS diagnosis, symptoms must be present for at least 6 months, whereas for Long COVID, the timeframe varies in the literature from 2 to 6 months. A systematic review comparing clinical presentation and symptoms for ME/CFS and Long COVID found that only 3 of 21 Long COVID studies assessed patients who had had symptoms for at least 6 months (Wong and Weitzer, 2021). The authors compared the 21 selected studies with ME/CFS case definitions and found that of 29 ME/CFS symptoms, 25 were reported in at least one Long COVID study. Fatigue, reduced daily activity, and post-exertional malaise were reported in multiple studies, with fatigue appearing in 12 of the 21 reviewed. Komaroff and Lipkin (2023) provide a helpful table summarizing the overlap in clinical presentation between Long COVID and ME/CFS, based on the work of Wong and Weitzer (2021). The committee adapted this table to include symptoms of FM (Table 5-1).

TABLE 5-1 Overlap in Common Symptoms among Long COVID, ME/CFS, and Fibromyalgia

	Long COVID	ME/CFS	Fibromyalgia
Common Symptoms			
Post-exertional malaise	✓	✓	
Chronic fatigue	✓	✓	✓
Orthostatic intolerance	✓	✓	
Cognitive impairment	✓	✓	✓
Pain/Lower threshold for pain	✓	✓	✓
Sleep disturbances	✓	✓	✓
Neurosensory, perceptual, and motor disturbances	✓	✓	
Muscle abnormalities	✓	✓	✓
Sensitivity to food, medications, and odors	✓	✓	
Altered smell/taste	✓		
Palpitations or cardiovascular conditions	✓	✓	
Breathlessness	✓	✓	
Gastrointestinal and genitourinary issues	✓	✓	✓
Loss of thermostatic stability	✓	✓	
Anxiety and depression	✓	✓	✓
Hair loss	✓		

NOTE: This is a list of common symptoms and is not intended to be a diagnostic tool. Not all people with Long COVID, ME/CFS, and fibromyalgia will have the checked symptoms. Additionally, the symptoms listed may present in individuals who do not have those conditions.
SOURCES: AMA, 2023; American College of Rheumatology, 2024; Bhargava and Hurley, 2023; Cabrera Martimbianco et al., 2021; Carruthers et al., 2011; Komaroff and Lipkin, 2023; Raveendran et al., 2021; Sukocheva et al., 2021; WHO, 2020; Wong and Weitzer, 2021.

Functional Implications

People with Long COVID, ME/CFS, and FM have decreased quality of life, including reduced physical and cognitive capacity, impairment in work performance, and reduced participation in society. In a study by Haider and colleagues (2023), individuals with Long COVID, ME/CFS, and FM reported a similar impact on physical and cognitive function; however, individuals with Long COVID versus those with the other two conditions reported lower pain and fatigue. Other studies suggest that the functional impairment in people with ME/CFS may be greater than in those with Long COVID (Komaroff and Lipkin, 2023). A comorbid diagnosis of Long COVID with ME/CFS and/or FM further exacerbated pain, fatigue, and psychological domains compared with Long COVID alone (Haider et al., 2023).

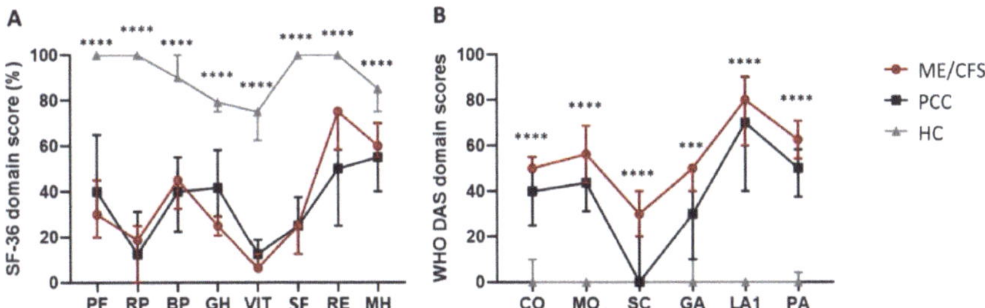

FIGURE 5-1 36-Item Short Form Survey (SF-36) and World Health Organization Disability Assessment Schedule (WHODAS) scores among ME/CFS, Long COVID, and control populations.
NOTES: (A) Line graph representing median and 95% confidence interval (CI) of SF-36v2 domains. (B) Line graph representing median and 95% CI of WHODAS 2.0 domains. Abbreviations: BP = bodily pain; CO = cognition; GA = getting along; GH = general health perceptions; HC = healthy control; LA1 = life activities 1; ME/CFS = myalgic encephalomyelitis/chronic fatigue syndrome; MH = general mental health; MO = mobility; PA = participation; PCC = post-COVID-19 condition; PF = physical functioning; RE = role limitations due to personal or emotional problems; RP = role limitations due to physical health problems; SC = self-care; SF = social functioning; SF-36v2 = 36-Item Short-Form Health Survey (version 2); VIT = vitality; WHODAS = 2.0 World Health Organization Disability Assessment Schedule (version 2). ***p<0.001 ****p<0.0001
SOURCE: Based on data published in Weigel et al., 2023.

Data currently under review show that ME/CFS and Long COVID cohorts do not differ significantly in any domain of quality of life using either the 36-Item Short Form Survey (SF-36) or the World Health Organization Disability Assessment Schedule (WHODAS) (Figure 5-1), the Hospital Anxiety and Depression Scale (HADS), or the Modified Fatigue Impact Scale (MFIS). For all three chronic conditions, symptoms are cyclic, with some relatively "good" days and frequent "bad" days. Some people with the conditions are able to perform their responsibilities at home and work, while others are bedridden and unable to work (Komaroff and Lipkin, 2023).

COMMON MECHANISMS OF ACTION

The COVID-19 pandemic has generated interest in virally associated fatigue syndromes, though not all fatigue syndromes result from viral pandemics. The Epstein-Barr virus (EBV) is the most common cause of infectious mononucleosis and has been the most researched source of post-viral fatigue. There is evidence indicating the onset of ME/CFS following viral infections such as EBV, Q fever, influenza, and other coronaviruses (Sasso et al., 2022). In 2003, 4 years following an outbreak of severe acute respiratory syndrome (SARS) caused by SARS-CoV-1, one study found that 40.3 percent of patients reported persistent chronic fatigue, 27.1 percent of whom qualified for a diagnosis of ME/CFS (Lam et al., 2009). Although SARS-CoV-2 infection has received attention as a potential infectious trigger for ME/CFS (Sasso et al., 2022), additional research is needed to confirm this hypothesis. Indeed, the underlying pathomechanism of ME/CFS also remains unknown because of the multitude of symptoms, including cognitive, endocrine, gastrointestinal, and cardiovascular dysfunction.

FM is a complex disease with uncertain etiology and pathophysiology; however, symptom worsening has been reported following infectious triggers, including SARS-CoV-2 (Attal et al., 2021; Clauw et al., 2020; Fialho et al., 2023). Approximately 30 percent of individuals with FM report physical or psychological triggers prior to disease onset (Fitzcharles et al., 2021). Viral infections linked with FM include hepatitis C virus, human immunodeficiency virus (HIV), parvovirus, and EBV (Buskila et al., 2008). Lyme disease also has overlapping features with FM, contributing to diagnostic confusion.

The significant overlap in clinical presentation between Long COVID and ME/CFS and FM raises the question of common mechanisms that could be involved in the pathogenesis of these conditions and offers the potential to use past clinical and biomedical research to accelerate the understanding of pathomechanisms specific to Long COVID. This section provides an overview of the potential overlapping pathomechanisms for which there is published evidence, summarized in Table 5-2. It should be noted that the discussion here focuses on biological mechanisms of action, given the available literature. As described in Chapter 1, the *International Classification of Functioning, Disability and Health* (ICF) framework developed by the World Health Organization provides a comprehensive perspective that includes not only biological conditions but also the impact of these conditions on an individual's functioning in various aspects of life. In addition to biological mechanisms, illness and disability are mediated by stress and stress response, behaviors and social forces, and environmental factors.

Immune Dysregulation

The underlying pathomechanism of Long COVID is not yet clear. However, varying degrees of immune dysregulation have been reported in Long COVID patients (Gottschalk et al., 2023). Similarly, immune dysregulation is commonly reported in ME/CFS and FM (Brenu et al., 2011; Hardcastle et al., 2015a; Klimas and Koneru, 2007; Klimas et al., 1990; Ojo-Amaize et al., 1994), with noted abnormalities in cytokines (Broderick et al., 2010; Corbitt et al., 2019; Fletcher et al., 2009), lymphocyte subsets (Curriu et al., 2013; Huth et al., 2014; Rivas et al., 2018), and cytotoxic function (Brenu et al., 2011; Hardcastle et al., 2015b; Huth et al., 2016; Klimas et al., 1990;

TABLE 5-2 Summary of Potential Biological Mechanisms of Long COVID, Myalgic Encephalomyelitis/Chronic Fatigue Syndrome (ME/CFS), and Fibromyalgia (FM)

Postinfectious onset		Long COVID	ME/CFS	FM
Immune dysregulation	Innate immune exhaustion	✓	✓	
	Cytokine dysregulation	✓	✓	
	Autoantibodies	✓	✓	✓
Neurological disturbances	Neuroinflammation	✓	✓	
	Reduced cerebral blood flow	✓	✓	
	Impaired functional connectivity	✓	✓	
	Abnormal brain metabolites	✓	✓	✓
	Changes in brain region volumes	✓	✓	
Cardiovascular disturbances	Orthostatic intolerance	✓	✓	
	Endothelial dysfunction	✓	✓	
	Coagulopathies	✓		
Gastrointestinal disturbances	Dysbiosis	✓	✓	✓
	Gut–immune–brain axis	✓	✓	
Metabolic and mitochondrial dysfunction	Mitochondrial dysfunction	✓	✓	
	Mitochondrial metabolite abnormalities	✓	✓	
	Down-regulation of the hypothalamic-pituitary-adrenal axis	✓	✓	✓

SOURCES: Augustin et al., 2021; Bakken et al., 2014; Bhargava and Hurley, 2023; Cao, 2020; Carruthers et al., 2011; Cervia et al., 2022; de Miranda et al., 2022; Demitrack et al., 1991; Farhadian et al., 2023; Garg et al., 2021b; Guasp et al., 2022; Jason et al., 2009; Komaroff and Lipkin, 2023; Lindell et al., 2000; NICE, 2020; Ram-Mohan et al., 2022; Raveendran et al., 2021; Srikanth et al., 2023; Su et al., 2022; Sukocheva et al., 2021; Tay et al., 2020; Urhan et al., 2022; Wessely, 1995; Yelin et al., 2022.

Ojo-Amaize et al., 1994; Whiteside and Friberg, 1998), with the caveat that many of those markers are not very specific, and proper measurement of some poses technical challenges. Dysregulation of innate immune responses has been reported in some patients with Long COVID, ME/CFS, and FM, as well as hypermobile Ehlers-Danlos syndrome (Bagga and Bouchard, 2014; Jukema et al., 2022; Mohandas et al., 2023; Wirth and Löhn, 2023).

Immune dysregulation tends to pair closely with cytokine dysregulation (Freidin et al., 2023; Prompetchara et al., 2020). Indeed, severe acute SARS-CoV-2 infection is associated with a well-described cytokine storm, characterized by elevated levels of proinflammatory cytokines (McGonagle et al., 2020; Prompetchara et al., 2020). In a similar fashion, multisystem inflammatory syndrome in children (MIS-C) can be seen 2–8 weeks after acute

SARS-CoV-2 infection, requiring anti-inflammatory agents for treatment (CDC, 2023; Consiglio et al., 2020; Gruber et al., 2023; Vella et al., 2021). Notably, aberrations in cytokines reported in ME/CFS and FM are equivocal (Corbitt et al., 2019). Finally, while autoantibodies have been reported in acute COVID-19, ME/CFS, and FM, the underlying autoimmunity primary pathomechanism does not currently meet the classification criteria for autoimmune diseases, although it does open a theoretical field of potential therapeutic options if proven to have a relevant role in the pathophysiology of those entities (Akbari et al., 2023; Arthur et al., 2021; Casciola-Rosen et al., 2022; Freitag et al., 2021; Hallmann et al., 2023; Malkova and Shoenfeld, 2023; Marshall-Gradisnik et al., 2015; Rodriguez-Perez et al., 2021; Vojdani et al., 2023; Wallukat et al., 2021).

Neurological Disturbances

Neurological and cognitive disturbances are reported in individuals with Long COVID, ME/CFS, and FM. Neuroinflammation has been suggested in Long COVID and ME/CFS (Tate et al., 2022). Supporting this hypothesis, microglial activation has been reported in Long COVID and ME/CFS (Fernández-Castañeda et al., 2022; Nakatomi et al., 2020; Tomo et al., 2022). Other neurological mechanisms include reduced cerebral blood flow (Barnden et al., 2016, 2019; Davis et al., 2023; Gay et al., 2015; Monje and Iwasaki, 2022; Shungu et al., 2012; Thapaliya et al., 2020, 2022; van Campen et al., 2022) and anatomical and/or connectivity changes (Douaud et al., 2022; Monje and Iwasaki, 2022; Morris and Maes, 2013); however, findings are inconsistent, and there is no overlap in anatomical brain region changes between the two disorders. Changes in brain metabolites have been reported in Long COVID, ME/CFS, and FM (Baraniuk et al., 2004; Deters et al., 2023; Martínez-Lavín and Miguel-Álvarez, 2023; Martini et al., 2022; Mueller et al., 2020; Puri et al., 2002; Russell et al., 1992). Overall, there are inconsistencies in research findings across various measures, and further comprehensive studies are required to elucidate the role of neurological disturbances in the pathomechanism of Long COVID.

Cardiovascular Damage

Cardiovascular disturbances, including endothelial dysfunction (Scherbakov et al., 2020; Xu et al., 2023b), coagulation issues (Nunes et al., 2023; Patell et al., 2020; Roberts et al., 2020), and orthostatic intolerance, are reported in Long COVID, ME/CFS, and FM (Gyöngyösi et al., 2023), and are quoted globally in the majority of chronic inflammatory diseases. Individuals with ME/CFS have reduced total blood volume, plasma volume, and red blood cell volume compared with control groups (Hurwitz et al., 2009).

Similarly, patients with ME/CFS and FM and some patients with Long COVID have impaired autonomic and cardiovascular responses to postural challenges that reduce autonomic flexibility and adaptability to situational demands.

Gastrointestinal Manifestations

Gastrointestinal manifestations are commonly reported in Long COVID and ME/CFS, and FM is associated with concurrent diagnosis of irritable bowel disorders. Changes resulting in gut dysbiosis, defined by an imbalance in the gut microbiome, are associated with recovery from COVID-19 (D'Amico et al., 2020; Tian et al., 2021). A pro-inflammatory gut microbiome has been documented in some patients with Long COVID and ME/CFS. This is hypothesized to allow microbial antigens (including endotoxins) to breach the gut-blood barrier, potentially contributing to inflammation at different systemic levels (Giloteaux et al., 2016; Guo et al., 2023; Haran et al., 2021; Liu et al., 2022; Nagy-Szakal et al., 2017; Xiong et al., 2023; Yeoh et al., 2021).

Metabolic

Energy insufficiency increased reactive oxygen species (ROS), and mitochondrial dysfunction are features that may be shared in patients with Long COVID, ME/CFS, and FM. Identified phenomena also include the down-regulation of the hypothalamic-pituitary-adrenal axis (Urhan et al., 2022; Demitrack et al., 1991). While mitochondrial dysfunction may correlate with severity of SARS-CoV-2 infection (Ganji and Reddy, 2021; Holder and Reddy, 2021), findings in Long COVID and ME/CFS are equivocal and require further investigation to confirm commonalities and differences (Domingo et al., 2021; Fukuda et al., 2016; Guarnieri et al., 2023; Holden et al., 2020; Missailidis et al., 2020; Sweetman et al., 2020). Studies have shown increased risk of diabetes mellitus, hyperlipidemia, and kidney disease in the post-acute phase of SARS-CoV-2 infection (Bowe et al., 2021; Xie and Al-Aly, 2022; Xu et al., 2023a). Although the evidence base is less well developed, similar metabolic abnormalities have also been reported in ME/CFS and FM.

Gene Structure and Expression

Variations in gene structure and gene expression have been reported in Long COVID, ME/CFS and FM. Thus far, published genome-wide association studies (GWAS) have involved small numbers of patients; predictably, given the sample sizes, no risk loci have been identified or validated for either ME/CFS or Long COVID (Lammi at al., 2023; Li et al, 2021; Pairo-Castineira et al, 2021; Thibord et al, 2022). However, in both ME/CFS and FM, a recent publication employing combinatorial analysis reported potentially significant associations involving genes involved in the response to infection, mitochondrial function, and autoimmunity (Das et al., 2022). Attempts to replicate this potentially important result in different and larger groups of patients are underway.

Studies of gene expression have primarily analyzed levels of microRNAs (miRNAs). Different studies involving different tissues have identified different miRNAs that distinguish people with ME/CFS and Long COVID from healthy control subjects. One would not expect the same miRNAs to be identified in every study. Instead, one would expect the miRNAs identified by different studies to act on genes involved in the same underlying physiological processes. Indeed, a recent published pathway analysis finds that the different miRNAs identified in these different studies, in fact, control the expression of genes involved in the same physiologic processes (Kaczmarek, 2023). Other epigenetic phenomena, like DNA methylation, that have been postulated as having impact in acute COVID infection may also have an impact in the pathophysiology of Long COVID or other post-viral syndromes, and research is ongoing (Balnis et al., 2022).

There currently is no specific diagnostic test for Long COVID, ME/CFS, or FM. Diagnosis can involve the following laboratory tests and self-report questionnaires, as well as elimination of other potential causes of the patient's symptoms.

Initial Laboratory Tests

Clinical criteria for ME/CFS can be used as a guide for laboratory testing in patients presenting with suspected Long COVID, which then can be used to exclude other diagnoses that are similar or that may copresent. The 2021 National Institute for Health and Care Excellence (NICE) guidelines for ME/CFS suggest testing for white blood cell count, erythrocyte sedimentation rate (ESR), C-reactive protein (CRP), presence of HIV, blood urea nitrogen (BUN), creatine and electrolytes, blood glucose, calcium and phosphorus, thyroid-stimulating hormone (TSH), alkaline phosphatase, and aspartate and alanine aminotransferases, as well as total protein, albumin, and globulin (NICE, 2021). Elevated ferritin levels have been reported in female participants meeting criteria for ME/CFS compared with female participants not meeting those criteria, while ferritin levels are often low in individuals with Long COVID with or without true anemia (Dignass et al., 2018; Lechuga et al., 2023; Ruscitti et al., 2023; Yamamoto et al., 2023). Additionally, iron deficiency and anemia of chronic disease are very common in people with fatigue-related illnesses. Emerging evidence requires further validation with objective analysis of study limitations (Dignass et al., 2018; Lechuga et al., 2023). Additional testing such as sleep studies and exercise testing (including VO_2max) may be needed to address specific symptoms, often performed in consultation with a specialist (CDC, 2021; Lim et al., 2020b).

Symptom Inventory Questionnaires

Jason and colleagues (2023) suggest that one of the challenges in diagnosing ME/CFS accurately and reliably is the use of ambiguous questions or psychometrically invalid questionnaires. The NICE guidelines recommend the use of a screening questionnaire during the initial consultation to capture the patient's symptoms, in addition to clinical assessment. Concurrent with laboratory-based testing, a symptom inventory questionnaire can be used to determine the severity and frequency of a symptom, as well as whether a symptom is preexisting (same vs. worsened), new since acute COVID-19 infection and stable/improving, or new since acute infection and worsening. Symptom inventory questionnaires are used to diagnose and research ME/CFS. For example, the DePaul Symptom Questionnaire (DSQ), consists of 54 questions assessing key symptoms of ME/CFS (such as fatigue; post-exertional malaise; sleep, pain, and cognitive disturbances; autonomic dysfunction; and immune dysregulation) (Bedree et al., 2019; Jason and Sunnquist, 2018). Indeed, the DSQ has since been used for research on Long COVID (Jason et al., 2021; Oliveira et al., 2023), although it does not incorporate all symptoms of Long COVID because of minimal differences in symptomology between ME/CFS and Long COVID (for example, hair loss). Other symptom inventory questionnaires used to evaluate health effects of these chronic conditions include the 31-question Composite Autonomic Symptom Score (COMPASS 31) for autonomic dysfunction and the Patient-Reported Outcomes Measurement Information System (PROMIS) for cognitive function (Larsen et al., 2022; Weerahandi et al., 2021).

Symptom inventory questionnaires for cognitive concerns are an integral part of a comprehensive cognitive assessment, as they capture the impact of cognitive symptoms on patients' daily functioning. While such symptom inventories have not been validated specifically for patients with Long COVID, measures such as the Patient's Assessment of Own Functioning Inventory (PAOFI), Cognitive Failures Questionnaire (CFQ), and Everyday Cognition scale (ECog) have excellent psychometric properties and are known as reliable tools for the detection of self-reported cognitive impairment in a variety of conditions and with diverse populations (Broadbent et al., 1982; Tomaszewski Farias et al., 2011).

PROGNOSIS AND PROGRESSION

ME/CFS is a chronic debilitating multisystem condition with poor prognosis for complete recovery. Recovery trajectories vary widely across studies, although most conclude that the prognosis is unfavorable. Studies have found that 0–8 percent of patients recover fully, while 17–64 percent experience some improvement (Ghali et al., 2022). There is a severity spectrum for ME/CFS, which is relative to the patient's premorbid activity level. Patients with mild ME/CFS report a reduction from preillness activity of approximately 50 percent, including reduced ability to maintain employment and interpersonal relationships (Pendergrast et al., 2016). A moderate case of ME/CFS is associated with a significant reduction in activity, restricted mobility, and inability to perform activities of daily living consistently. Generally, patients classified as having moderate ME/CFS are restricted to home (Pendergrast et al., 2016). A person with a severe case of ME/CFS is typically bedbound and will be dependent on mobility aids and a caregiver (Pendergrast et al., 2016). Approximately 25 percent of ME/CFS cases are considered severe (Pendergrast et al., 2016). Studies have identified a worse prognosis in ME/CFS patients with comorbid Long COVID or FM (Ghali et al., 2022; Komaroff and Lipkin, 2023).

Limited research on FM outcomes has suggested that patients rarely achieve remission, although some may experience improvement or waxing and waning of symptoms over time (Schaefer et al., 2016). In general, it can be said that FM is a chronic condition that does not significantly improve or worsen, although longitudinal data are sparse and heterogeneous. One study on established FM patients (median disease duration of 7.8 years at the beginning of the study) found that functional disability worsened over the 7-year study period, while pain, fatigue, sleep disturbances, anxiety, and depression remained unchanged (Wolfe et al., 1997). In another study conducted in the United States that followed patients for 10 years, two-thirds of patients indicated that their symptoms were a little to a lot better, 10 percent reported no change, and a quarter reported they were a little or a lot worse at the end of the study period (Kennedy and Felson, 1996). Another study in the United States followed FM patients for 2 years and found that patients reported high levels of burden at both time points, with few significant changes over time. Outcomes varied among patients and were better among those whose pain improved (Schaefer et al., 2016).

As discussed in Chapter 4 of this report, preliminary studies suggest that many people with persistent Long COVID symptoms improve over time, and recovery can plateau 6–12 months after acute infection. Disease severity, functional disability, and duration vary, with severity of acute COVID-19 being a major risk factor for poor functional outcomes, although such outcomes can be experienced even by those with mild initial illness.

Some studies have compared the prognosis and progression of Long COVID and ME/CFS. In general, it appears that Long COVID (especially Long COVID that does not meet criteria for ME/CFS) has a better prognosis than ME/CFS (Oliveira et al., 2023). Like ME/CFS, Long COVID appears to be a chronic illness, with few patients achieving full remission (Wong and Weitzer, 2021), though the chronicity and duration of full recovery for patients with Long COVID are currently unknown (Oliveira et al., 2023). Studies comparing Long COVID and ME/CFS have several limitations, however. First, Long COVID is a new disease, so that study participants are usually newly diagnosed, while ME/CFS study participants often have had the condition for a longer time and so are less likely to improve. Additionally, to qualify for a diagnosis of ME/CFS, symptoms need to be ongoing for 6 months or more, whereas the criteria for Long COVID vary in the literature from 2 to 6 months. Thus, the two conditions are difficult to compare. At this time, the committee did not identify any studies comparing the prognosis and progression of Long COVID and FM.

For all three conditions, comorbid medical illnesses tend to worsen the overall course of the condition as it progresses. Additionally, Long COVID may be a trigger for ME/CFS and FM, and it may exacerbate the symptoms of people already living with fatigue or chronic pain (Fialho et al., 2023).

TREATMENT AND MANAGEMENT

The CDC "Post-COVID Conditions: Information for Healthcare Providers" page suggests symptom management approaches for Long COVID that have been helpful for disorders such as ME/CFS, FM, posttreatment Lyme disease, dysautonomia, and mast cell activation syndrome (CDC, 2024). Indeed, the goal of treatment and management for Long COVID and similar infection-associated chronic conditions is to optimize function and quality of life. These conditions represent many potentially overlapping entities, with different biological causes, risk factors, and outcomes. Different treatment approaches are needed for different individuals depending on their symptoms. This section provides an overview of nonpharmacological management and pharmacological treatments in clinical trial.

Nonpharmacological Management and Treatments

Pacing

Pacing refers to a self-management strategy whereby individuals alternate activities with small, interspersed rest intervals. Successful pacing is believed to be a beneficial treatment for ME/CFS according to NICE, the CDC, and the National Institutes of Health (NIH). Pacing is accompanied by the concept of an energy envelope. In the case of ME/CFS, an energy envelope provides people with a strategy for managing their exertional tolerance, especially in activities of daily living. The size of the energy envelope is defined by the varying day-to-day tolerance and resources of patients; exceeding the energy envelope may result in worsening or exacerbation of symptoms. Pacing provides an approach to reduce the burden of fatigue and post-exertional malaise when accompanied by assistive devices and flexibility in approaching activities of daily living or employment/school (Friedberg et al., 2020; NICE, 2021; Smith et al., 2015). Wearable technologies may be used to provide just-in-time assessments of physiological exertion (Clague-Baker et al., 2023).

Environmental Control

Patients who report sensitivities to light, noise, or odors are often diagnosed with comorbid multiple chemical sensitivities. Therefore, it is pertinent to limit the impact of these sensory triggers by (1) removing perfume and chemicals from the environment and (2) using eye masks and ear plugs. Environmental control provides an effective technique for improving sleep hygiene and lessening the burden of sleep disturbances.

Mobility Support

Depending on the severity of illness, occupation therapy referrals for home adaption may be essential to incorporate the use of aids that can improve quality of life. Such aids may include (1) disability parking permits, (2) wheelchairs or motorized scooters and appropriate home modifications, and (3) shower chairs and handrails. Additionally, alternative forms of pain management accompanied by physical therapy (within the energy envelope of the patient) may support patient mobility.

Multidisciplinary Care and Rehabilitation

Multidisciplinary care comprises the primary physician, appropriate medical and surgical and allied health professionals, and the patient advocacy community. A systematic review of nonpharmacological treatments in post-viral syndromes (including Long COVID) suggested interventions using Pilates exercises, resistance exercise, telerehabilitation, neuromodulation, and music therapy (Chandan et al., 2023). According to the NICE guidelines, recommendations for health care planning include the following:

- Self-management advice
  - Self-management and monitoring of symptoms
  - Support groups and forums
  - Housing, employment, financial, and other supports

- Support from integrated coordinated primary care, community, rehabilitation, and mental health services
- Multidisciplinary assessment

Patients with neuromuscular weakness can benefit from physical rehabilitation. It has been hypothesized that standardized exercise testing for cardiorespiratory fitness after recovery from acute COVID-19 can be used to improve the understanding of Long COVID. However, the use of graded exercise therapy (GET) requires caution in the treatment of ME/CFS because of the potential for iatrogenic harm. There is widespread and valid concern that exercise programs, even graded, may result in deterioration of the patient's condition given the underlying pathology of disease and the potential to trigger post-exertional malaise and exacerbate symptoms following activity (Tuller and Vink, 2023). It is important at this time to highlight the lessons that can be learned from ME/CFS regarding this need for caution in the use of GET (Torjesen, 2020; Tuller and Vink, 2023; Twisk and Maes, 2009).

Psychosocial Support

Chronic conditions pose a significant burden with respect to psychological health. Protocols for cognitive-behavioral therapy (CBT) or mindfulness are not standardized for the treatment of Long COVID, ME/CFS, or FM (Friedberg, 2016; O'Dowd et al., 2006; Worm-Smeitink et al., 2016). CBT and mindfulness are the most widely studied psychological interventions for managing pain. Changes in different brain regions observed after CBT include grey matter volume, activation/deactivation, and intrinsic connectivity. CBT involves cognitive and emotional regulation, with the dorsolateral prefrontal cortex, orbitofrontal cortex, right ventrolateral prefrontal cortex, posterior cingulate cortex, and amygdala being key regions. After CBT, the brain shows stronger top-down pain control, cognitive reassessment, and altered perception of stimulus signals (Arroyo-Fernández et al., 2022). Research is currently ongoing on the effectiveness of CBT (NCT05676047, NCT05597722, NCT05731570) or forms of cognitive rehabilitation in Long COVID, including behavioral amygdala-insula retraining (NCT05851846), sound mindfulness strategies (NCT05848401), mind–body reprocessing therapy (NCT05703074 & NCT05422924), behavioral and coping coaching (NCT05752331 & NCT05453201), and mindfulness (NCT05566379 & NCT05422924).

Diet Modulation

Symptoms akin to food intolerances and irritable bowel syndrome are reported in people with Long COVID, ME/CFS, and FM (Weigel et al., 2022).

The NICE guidelines encourage referral for dietic assessment and creation of a management plan by a dietitian (NICE, 2020, 2021). Lifestyle interventions and dietary supplementation in Long COVID are to be investigated (NCT05836402 & NCT05705648).

Endothelial Modulation

Both Long COVID and ME/CFS have demonstrated and been characterized by endothelial dysfunction (Haffke et al., 2022; McLaughlin et al., 2023; Varga et al., 2020). Enhanced external counterpulsation (EECP) is a Food and Drug Administration (FDA)–approved, noninvasive treatment for refractory angina and ischemic heart failure that has been effective for symptoms associated with heart disease such as chest pain, shortness of breath, and fatigue. A handful of studies have been published showing the benefit of EECP in Long COVID (Dayrit et al., 2021; Sathyamoorthy et al., 2022; Wu et al., 2023). ClinicalTrials.gov also reports an EECP study under way (NCT05668039).

Pharmacological Treatments

Currently, no standardized FDA-approved treatments are available for Long COVID, ME/CFS, or FM (Jason et al., 2023). Recently updated NICE guidelines for ME/CFS highlight that agents currently prescribed to treat cognitive impairment, fatigue, and sleep disturbances are of low quality and efficacy. Those treatments include, for cognitive disturbances and fatigue, modafinil, amantadine, and methylphenidate (Garg et al., 2021a; Pliszka, 2022; Randall et al., 2005), and for sleep disturbances, trazadone, low-dose tricyclic antidepressants, and cyclobenzaprine (Calandre et al., 2011; Clemons et al., 2011; Morillas-Arques et al., 2010). Treatment of chronic pain in ME/CFS follows the guidelines for the treatment of FM, and includes duloxetine, pregabalin, amitriptyline. ClinicalTrials.gov lists clinical trials evaluating the efficacy of various treatments for Long COVID, ME/CFS, and FM aimed at addressing the underlying disease and disease-associated manifestations. As of December 2023, the database included a total of 18 completed and ongoing clinical trials in Phase III or IV for ME/CFS, 124 for FM, and 30 for Long COVID. The limited overlap in treatment trials among the three conditions is discussed in this section.

Rintatolimod, also known as ampligen, has received attention as a potential treatment for ME/CFS and Long COVID because of its immuno-modulatory and antiviral activities as a toll-like receptor 3 (TLR-3) agonist (Mitchell, 2016; Strayer et al., 2020). Trials have shown that it increases exercise tolerance and decreases drug dependence in patients with ME/CFS (Mitchell, 2016; Strayer et al., 2020). Given concerns about toxicity, however, rintatolimod is approved only in Argentina for the treatment of severe ME/CFS.

It is included within the AMP-511 Expanded Access Program in the United States, but of note was rejected for approval by the FDA in 2009 for an indication of ME/CFS. The reason it was not approved, according to the FDA, was that the two randomized controlled trials "did not provide credible evidence of efficacy," and there were "clinical, statistical, clinical pharmacology, nonclinical, product quality, and facilities inspections deficiencies" (Castro-Marrero et al., 2017). Given the overlap with ME/CFS, including similar potential mechanisms of action, the efficacy of rintatolimod is under investigation in people with Long COVID (NCT05592418).

Metformin, an insulin response enhancer, is being investigated for use in Long COVID, ME/CFS, and FM (NCT06147050, NCT06128967, NCT05900466). Bramante and colleagues found that the incidence of Long COVID was reduced by 42 percent with metformin treatment (Bramante et al., 2022). Previous research has suggested the potential benefit of metformin in improving bioenergetic profiles in patients with FM (Alcocer-Gómez et al., 2015).

Immunomodulation is a treatment trial target for Long COVID, ME/CFS, and FM, and given their shared potential mechanism of action. Intravenous administration of immunoglobin shows efficacy in some autoimmune conditions and is used at a higher dose for anti-inflammatory effects (which also leads to increased side effect potential). It has been investigated for use in ME/CFS; however, it is no longer recommended for ME/CFS under the NICE guidelines published in 2021 because of inconsistent findings (NICE, 2021).

In general, pharmacological treatments for Long COVID, ME/CFS, and FM are not yet effective, and management of these conditions involves primarily the symptom management and functional improvement techniques described in the previous section.

SUMMARY AND CONCLUSIONS

Long COVID shares many features with other complex multisystem conditions. This review focused on similarities with ME/CFS and FM. Other less researched similar conditions include, but are not limited to, POTS, posttreatment Lyme disease, and hypermobile Ehlers-Danlos syndrome. More research is needed to understand infection-associated chronic illnesses.

The mechanism of action for these conditions remains unclear, and further investigation is needed. Current theories for potential shared mechanisms of action supported by published literature include immune dysregulation (including dysregulation of innate immune responses, cytokine dysregulation, or mast cell activation); neurological disturbances (neuroinflammation has been suggested in ME/CFS and Long COVID); cardiovascular damage (endothelial dysfunction, coagulation issues, and orthostatic intolerance have been reported in some patients with Long COVID, ME/CFS, and FM); gastrointestinal symptoms (due to gut microbiome dysbiosis); metabolic issues (energy insufficiency, reactive oxygen species production, and mitochondrial dysfunction are shared features in Long COVID, ME/CFS, and FM); and genetic variations.

There is currently no specific laboratory-based diagnostic test for Long COVID or ME/CFS. Rather, diagnosis is a process of exclusion and consideration of other potential causes of the patient's symptoms. Secondary testing should be at the discretion of the attending physician. The NICE guidelines recommend the use of a screening questionnaire during the initial consultation to capture the patient's symptoms, in addition to clinical assessment. Concurrent with laboratory-based testing, a symptom inventory questionnaire can be used to determine the severity and frequency of a symptom, as well as to determine whether a symptom is preexisting (same vs. worsened), new since acute SARS-CoV-2 infection and stable/improving, or new since acute infection and worsening. Symptom inventory questionnaires are used to diagnose and research ME/CFS.

Studies have compared the prognosis and progression of Long COVID and ME/CFS. It appears that in general, Long COVID (especially for Long COVID that does not meet ME/CFS criteria) has a better prognosis than ME/CFS, with some manifestations of Long COVID being similar to those of ME/CFS. Like ME/CFS, Long COVID appears to be a chronic illness, with few patients achieving full remission. Studies comparing Long COVID and ME/CFS have several limitations, however. First, Long COVID is a new disease, so that Long COVID study participants are usually newly diagnosed, while ME/CFS study participants often have had the condition for a longer time and so are less likely to improve. Additionally, to qualify for a diagnosis of ME/CFS, symptoms need to be ongoing for 6 months or more, whereas the criteria for Long COVID vary in the literature from 2 to 6 months. Thus, the two conditions are difficult to compare. The full recovery duration for Long COVID patients remains uncertain, but early diagnosis and treatment may help prevent progression to chronic conditions such as ME/CFS and FM.

Currently there are no FDA approved drugs or evidence-based treatments for Long COVID, ME/CFS, or FM. The primary approach to managing the three conditions involves the use of techniques, such as pacing and rehabilitation, to manage symptoms and improve functional ability. However, this approach is complicated by multisystem clinical presentation, and treatment approaches may need to be tailored to the individual. Numerous randomized controlled trials are currently under way to determine the efficacy of a number of identified pharmacological agents; however, limited data have been published, and these trials have yet to be finalized. Moreover, the use of some pharmacological agents is not supported by current research because of the limited understanding of the pathomechanism of Long COVID.

REFERENCES

Akbari, A., A. Hadizadeh, M. Islampanah, E. Salavati Nik, S. L. Atkin, and A. Sahebkar. 2023. COVID-19, G protein-coupled receptor, and renin-angiotensin system autoantibodies: Systematic review and meta-analysis. *Autoimmunity Reviews* 22(9):103402.

Alcocer-Gómez, E., J. Garrido-Maraver, P. Bullón, F. Marín-Aguilar, D. Cotán, A. M. Carrión, J. M. Alvarez-Suarez, F. Giampieri, J. A. Sánchez-Alcazar, M. Battino, and M. D. Cordero. 2015. Metformin and caloric restriction induce an AMPK-dependent restoration of mitochondrial dysfunction in fibroblasts from fibromyalgia patients. *Biochimica et Biophysica Acta* 1852(7):1257–1267.

AlMuhaissen, S., A. Abu Libdeh, Y. ElKhatib, R. Alshayeb, A. Jaara, and S. K. Bardaweel. 2023. Myalgic encephalomyelitis/chronic fatigue syndrome (ME/CFS) and COVID-19: Is there a connection? *Current Medical Research and Opinion* 39(8):1119–1126.

AMA (American Medical Association). 2023. *Long COVID and the brain: Neurological symptoms may persist.* https://www.ama-assn.org/delivering-care/public-health/long-covid-and-brain-neurological-symptoms-may-persist (accessed February 26, 2024).

American College of Rheumatology. 2024. *Fibromyalgia.* https://rheumatology.org/patients/fibromyalgia (accessed February 26, 2024).

Arroyo-Fernández, R., J. Avendaño-Coy, R. Velasco-Velasco, R. Palomo-Carrión, E. Bravo-Esteban, and A. Ferri-Morales. 2022. Effectiveness of transcranial direct current stimulation combined with exercising in people with fibromyalgia: A randomized sham-controlled clinical trial. *Archives of Physical Medicine and Rehabilitation* 103(8):1524–1532.

Arthur, J. M., J. C. Forrest, K. W. Boehme, J. L. Kennedy, S. Owens, C. Herzog, J. Liu, and T. O. Harville. 2021. Development of ACE2 autoantibodies after SARS-CoV-2 infection. *PLoS ONE* 16(9):e0257016.

Attal, N., V. Martinez, and D. Bouhassira. 2021. Potential for increased prevalence of neuropathic pain after the COVID-19 pandemic. *Pain Reports* 6(1):e884.

Augustin, M., P. Schommers, M. Stecher, F. Dewald, L. Gieselmann, H. Gruell, C. Horn, K. Vanshylla, V. D. Cristanziano, L. Osebold, M. Roventa, T. Riaz, N. Tschernoster, J. Altmueller, L. Rose, S. Salomon, V. Priesner, J. C. Luers, C. Albus, S. Rosenkranz, B. Gathof, G. Fatkenheuer, M. Hallek, F. Klein, I. Suarez, and C. Lehmann. 2021. Post-COVID syndrome in non-hospitalised patients with COVID-19: A longitudinal prospective cohort study. *The Lancet Regional Health—Europe* 6:100122.

Bagga, S., and M. J. Bouchard. 2014. Cell cycle regulation during viral infection. *Cell Cycle Control* 1170:165–227.

Bakken, I. J., K. Tveito, N. Gunnes, S. Ghaderi, C. Stoltenberg, L. Trogstad, S. E. Håberg, and P. Magnus. 2014. Two age peaks in the incidence of chronic fatigue syndrome/myalgic encephalomyelitis: A population-based registry study from Norway 2008-2012. *BMC Medicine* 12:167.

Balnis, J., A. Madrid, K. J. Hogan, L. A. Drake, A. Adhikari, R. Vancavage, H. A. Singer, R. S. Alisch, and A. Jaitovich. 2022. Persistent blood DNA methylation changes one year after SARS-COV-2 infection. *Clinical Epigenetics* 14(1):94.

Baraniuk, J. N., G. Whalen, J. Cunningham, and D. J. Clauw. 2004. Cerebrospinal fluid levels of opioid peptides in fibromyalgia and chronic low back pain. *BMC Musculoskeletal Disorders* 5(1):48.

Barnden, L. R., R. Kwiatek, B. Crouch, R. Burnet, and P. Del Fante. 2016. Autonomic correlations with MRI are abnormal in the brainstem vasomotor centre in chronic fatigue syndrome. *NeuroImage: Clinical* 11:530–537.

Barnden, L. R., Z. Y. Shan, D. R. Staines, S. Marshall-Gradisnik, K. Finegan, T. Ireland, and S. Bhuta. 2019. Intra-brainstem connectivity is impaired in chronic fatigue syndrome. *NeuroImage: Clinical* 24:102045.

Bedree, H., M. Sunnquist, and L. A. Jason. 2019. The DePaul Symptom Questionnaire-2: A validation study. *Fatigue: Biomedicine, Health & Behavior* 7(3):166–179.

Bennett, R. M., K.D. Jones, J. H. Aebischer, A. W. St John, and R. Friend. 2022. Which symptoms best distinguish fibromyalgia patients from those with other chronic pain disorders? *Journal of Evaluation in Clinical Practice* 28(2):225–234.

Bhargava, J., and J. A. Hurley. 2023. Fibromyalgia. In *Statpearls*. Treasure Island (FL): StatPearls Publishing.

Bonilla, H., T. C. Quach, A. Tiwari, A. E. Bonilla, M. Miglis, P. C. Yang, L. E. Eggert, H. Sharifi, A. Horomanski, A. Subramanian, L. Smirnoff, N. Simpson, H. Halawi, O. Sum-Ping, A. Kalinowski, Z. M. Patel, R. W. Shafer, and L. N. Geng. 2023. Myalgic encephalomyelitis/chronic fatigue syndrome is common in post-acute sequelae of SARS-CoV-2 infection (PASC) Results from a post-COVID-19 multidisciplinary clinic. *Frontiers in Neurology* 14:1090747.

Boquete, L., M.-J. Vicente, J.-M. Miguel-Jiménez, E.-M. Sánchez-Morla, M. Ortiz, M. Satue, and E. Garcia-Martin. 2022. Objective diagnosis of fibromyalgia using neuroretinal evaluation and artificial intelligence. *International Journal of Clinical and Health Psychology* 22(2):100294.

Bowe, B., Y. Xie, E. Xu, and Z. Al-Aly. 2021. Kidney outcomes in long COVID. *Journal of the American Society of Nephrology* 32(11):2851–2862.

Bramante, C. T., J. B. Buse, D. Liebovitz, J. Nicklas, M. A. Puskarich, K. Cohen, H. Belani, B. Anderson, J. D. Huling, C. Tignanelli, J. Thompson, M. Pullen, L. Siegel, J. Proper, D. J. Odde, N. Klatt, N. Sherwood, S. Lindberg, E. L. Wirtz, A. Karger, K. Beckman, S. Erickson, S. Fenno, K. Hartman, M. Rose, B. Patel, G. Griffiths, N. Bhat, T. A. Murray, and D. R. Boulware. 2022. Outpatient treatment of COVID-19 with metformin, ivermectin, and fluvoxamine and the development of long COVID over 10-month follow-up. *medRxiv* [Preprint]. 2022 Dec 23:2022.12.21.22283753. https://doi.org/10.1101/2022.12.21.22283753.

Brenu, E. W., M. L. van Driel, D. R. Staines, K. J. Ashton, S. B. Ramos, J. Keane, N. G. Klimas, and S. M. Marshall-Gradisnik. 2011. Immunological abnormalities as potential biomarkers in chronic fatigue syndrome/myalgic encephalomyelitis. *Journal of Translational Medicine* 9(1):81.

Broadbent, D. E., P. F. Cooper, P. Fitzgerald, and K. R. Parkes. 1982. The Cognitive Failures Questionnaire (CFQ) and its correlates. *British Journal of Clinical Psychology* 21(1):1–16.

Broderick, G., J. Fuite, A. Kreitz, S. D. Vernon, N. Klimas, and M. A. Fletcher. 2010. A formal analysis of cytokine networks in chronic fatigue syndrome. *Brain, Behavior, and Immunity* 24(7):1209–1217.

Brurberg, K. G., M. S. Fønhus, L. Larun, S. Flottorp, and K. Malterud. 2014. Case definitions for chronic fatigue syndrome/myalgic encephalomyelitis (CFS/ME): A systematic review. *BMJ Open* 4(2):e003973.

Buskila, D., F. Atzeni, and P. Sarzi-Puttini. 2008. Etiology of fibromyalgia: The possible role of infection and vaccination. *Autoimmunity Reviews* 8(1):41–43.

Cabrera Martimbianco, A. L., R. L. Pacheco, Â. M. Bagattini, and R. Riera. 2021. Frequency, signs and symptoms, and criteria adopted for long COVID-19: A systematic review. *International Journal of Clinical Practice* 75(10):e14357.

Calandre, E. P., P. Morillas-Arques, R. Molina-Barea, C. M. Rodriguez-Lopez, and F. Rico-Villademoros. 2011. Trazodone plus pregabalin combination in the treatment of fibromyalgia: A two-phase, 24-week, open-label uncontrolled study. *BMC Musculoskeletal Disorders* 12:95.

Cao, X. 2020. COVID-19: Immunopathology and its implications for therapy. *Nature Reviews Immunology* 20(5):269–270.

Carruthers, B. M., M. I. van de Sande, K. L. D. Meirleir, N. G. Klimas, G. Broderick, T. Mitchell, D. Staines, A. C. P. Powles, N. Speight, R. Vallings, L. Bateman, B. Baumgarten-Austrheim, D. S. Bell, N. Carlo-Stella, J. Chia, A. Darragh, D. Jo, D. Lewis, A. R. Light, S. Marshall-Gradisnik, I. Mena, J. A. Mikovits, K. Miwa, M. Murovska, M. L. Pall, and S. Stevens. 2011. Myalgic encephalomyelitis: International consensus criteria. *Journal of Internal Medicine* 270(4):327–338.

Casciola-Rosen, L., D. R. Thiemann, F. Andrade, M. I. Trejo Zambrano, J. E. Hooper, E. K. Leonard, J. B. Spangler, A. L. Cox, C. E. Machamer, L. Sauer, O. Laeyendecker, B. T. Garibaldi, S. C. Ray, C. A. Mecoli, L. Christopher-Stine, L. Gutierrez-Alamillo, Q. Yang, D. Hines, W. A. Clarke, R. Rothman, A. Pekosz, K. J. Fenstermacher, Z. Wang, S. L. Zeger, and A. Rosen. 2022. IgM anti-ACE2 autoantibodies in severe COVID-19 activate complement and perturb vascular endothelial function. *JCI Insight* 7(9):e158362.

Castro-Marrero, J., N. Sáez-Francàs, D. Santillo, and J. Alegre. 2017. Treatment and management of chronic fatigue syndrome/myalgic encephalomyelitis: All roads lead to Rome. *British Journal of Pharmacology* 174(5):345–369.

CDC (U.S. Centers for Disease Control and Prevention). 2021. *Myalgic encephalomyelitis/ chronic fatigue syndrome evaluation.* https://www.cdc.gov/me-cfs/healthcare-providers/ diagnosis/evaluation.html (accessed March 12, 2024).

CDC. 2022. *Fibromyalgia.* https://www.cdc.gov/arthritis/types/fibromyalgia.htm (accessed February 26, 2024).

CDC. 2023. *For parents: Multisystem inflammatory syndrome in children (MIS-C) associated with COVID-19.* https://www.cdc.gov/mis/mis-c.html#print (accessed February 26, 2024).

CDC. 2024. *Post-COVID Conditions: Information for healthcare providers.* https://www.cdc. gov/coronavirus/2019-ncov/hcp/clinical-care/post-covid-conditions.html (accessed February 26, 2024).

Cervia, C., Y. Zurbuchen, P. Taeschler, T. Ballouz, D. Menges, S. Hasler, S. Adamo, M. E. Raeber, E. Bachli, A. Rudiger, M. Stussi-Helbling, L. C. Huber, J. Nilsson, U. Held, M. A. Puhan, and O. Boyman. 2022. Immunoglobulin signature predicts risk of post-acute COVID-19 syndrome. *Nature Communications* 13(1):446.

Chandan, J. S., K. R. Brown, N. Simms-Williams, N. Z. Bashir, J. Camaradou, D. Heining, G. M. Turner, S. C. Rivera, R. Hotham, S. Minhas, K. Nirantharakumar, M. Sivan, K. Khunti, D. Raindi, S. Marwaha, S. E. Hughes, C. McMullan, T. Marshall, M. J. Calvert, S. Haroon, and O. L. Aiyegbusi. 2023. Non-pharmacological therapies for post-viral syndromes, including long COVID: A systematic review. *International Journal of Environmental Research and Public Health* 20(4):3477.

Clague-Baker, N., T. E. Davenport, M. Madi, K. Dickinson, K. Leslie, M.Bull, and N. Hilliard. 2023. An international survey of experiences and attitudes towards pacing using a heart rate monitor for people with myalgic encephalomyelitis/chronic fatigue syndrome. *Work* 74(4):1225–1234.

Clauw, D. J., W. Häuser, S. P. Cohen, and M.-A. Fitzcharles. 2020. Considering the potential for an increase in chronic pain after the COVID-19 pandemic. *Pain* 161(8):1694–1697.

Clemons, A., M. Vasiadi, D. Kempuraj, T. Kourelis, G. Vandoros, and T. C. Theoharides. 2011. Amitriptyline and prochlorperazine inhibit pro-inflammatory mediator release from human mast cells–Possible relevance to chronic fatigue syndrome. *Journal of Clinical Psychopharmacology* 31(3):385–387.

Consiglio, C. R., N. Cotugno, F. Sardh, C. Pou, D. Amodio, L. Rodriguez, Z. Tan, S. Zicari, A. Ruggiero, G. R. Pascucci, V. Santilli, T. Campbell, Y. Bryceson, D. Eriksson, J. Wang, A. Marchesi, T. Lakshmikanth, A. Campana, A. Villani, P. Rossi, CACTUS Study Team, N. Landegren, P. Palma, and P. Brodin. 2020. The immunology of multisystem inflammatory syndrome in children with COVID-19. *Cell* 183(4):968–981.

Corbitt, M., N. Eaton-Fitch, D. Staines, H. Cabanas, and S. Marshall-Gradisnik. 2019. A systematic review of cytokines in chronic fatigue syndrome/myalgic encephalomyelitis/ systemic exertion intolerance disease (CFS/ME/SEID). *BMC Neurology* 19(1):207.

Curriu, M., J. Carrillo, M. Massanella, J. Rigau, J. Alegre, J. Puig, A. M. Garcia-Quintana, J. Castro-Marrero, E. Negredo, B. Clotet, C. Cabrera, and J. Blanco. 2013. Screening NK-, B- and T-cell phenotype and function in patients suffering from chronic fatigue syndrome. *Journal of Translational Medicine* 11:68.

D'Amico, F., D. C. Baumgart, S. Danese, and L. Peyrin-Biroulet. 2020. Diarrhea during COVID-19 infection: Pathogenesis, epidemiology, prevention, and management. *Clinical Gastroenterology and Hepatology* 18(8):1663–1672.

Das, S., K. Taylor, J. Kozubek, J. Sardell, and S. Gardner. 2022. Genetic risk factors for ME/CFS identified using combinatorial analysis. *Journal of Translational Medicine* 20(1):598.

Davis, H. E., L. McCorkell, J. M. Vogel, and E. J. Topol. 2023. Long COVID: Major findings, mechanisms and recommendations. *Nature Reviews Microbiology* 21(3):133–146.

Dayrit, J. K., M. Verduzco-Gutierrez, A. Teal, and S. A. Shah. 2021. Enhanced external counterpulsation as a novel treatment for post-acute COVID-19 sequelae. *Cureus* 13(4):e14358.

de la Coba, P., C. I. Montoro, G. A. Reyes Del Paso, and C. M. Galvez-Sánchez. 2022. Algometry for the assessment of central sensitisation to pain in fibromyalgia patients: A systematic review. *Annals of Medicine* 54(1):1403–1422.

de Miranda, D. A. P., S. V. C. Gomes, P. S. Filgueiras, C. A. Corsini, N. B. F. Almeida, R. A. Silva, M. I. V. A. R. C. Medeiros, R. V. R. Vilela, G. R. Fernandes, and R. F. Q. Grenfell. 2022. Long COVID-19 syndrome: A 14-months longitudinal study during the two first epidemic peaks in southeast Brazil. *Transactions of the Royal Society of Tropical Medicine and Hygiene* 116(11):1007–1014.

Demitrack, M. A., J. K. Dale, S. E. Straus, L. Laue, S. J. Listwak, M. J. Kruesi, G. P. Chrousos, and P. W. Gold. 1991. Evidence for impaired activation of the hypothalamic-pituitary-adrenal axis in patients with chronic fatigue syndrome. *Journal of Clinical Endocrinology and Metabolism* 73(6):1224–1234.

Deters, J. R., A. C. Fietsam, P. E. Gander, L. L. Boles Ponto, and T. Rudroff. 2023. Effect of post-COVID-19 on brain volume and glucose metabolism: Influence of time since infection and fatigue status. *Brain Sciences* 13(4):675.

Dignass, A., K. Farrag, and J. Stein. 2018. Limitations of serum ferritin in diagnosing iron deficiency in inflammatory conditions. *International Journal of Chronic Diseases* 2018:1–11.

Domingo, J. C., B. Cordobilla, R. Ferrer, M. Giralt, J. Alegre-Martín, and J. Castro-Marrero. 2021. Are circulating fibroblast growth factor 21 and N-terminal prohormone of brain natriuretic peptide promising novel biomarkers in myalgic encephalomyelitis/chronic fatigue syndrome? *Antioxidants & Redox Signaling* 34(18):1420–1427.

Douaud, G., S. Lee, F. Alfaro-Almagro, C. Arthofer, C. Wang, P. McCarthy, F. Lange, J. L. R. Andersson, L. Griffanti, E. Duff, S. Jbabdi, B. Taschler, P. Keating, A. M. Winkler, R. Collins, P. M. Matthews, N. Allen, K. L. Miller, T. E. Nichols, and S. M. Smith. 2022. SARS-CoV-2 is associated with changes in brain structure in UK Biobank. *Nature* 604(7907):697–707.

Farhadian, S. F., H. D. Reisert, L. McAlpine, J. Chiarella, P. Kosana, J. Yoon, and S. Spudich. 2023. Self-reported neuropsychiatric post-COVID-19 condition and CSF markers of neuroinflammation. *JAMA Network Open* 6(11):e2342741.

Fernández-Castañeda, A., P. Lu, A. C. Geraghty, E. Song, M.-H. Lee, J. Wood, M. R. O'Dea, S. Dutton, K. Shamardani, K. Nwangwu, R. Mancusi, B. Yalçın, K. R. Taylor, L. Acosta-Alvarez, K. Malacon, M. B. Keough, L. Ni, P. J. Woo, D. Contreras-Esquivel, A. M. S. Toland, J. R. Gehlhausen, J. Klein, T. Takahashi, J. Silva, B. Israelow, C. Lucas, T. Mao, M. A. Peña-Hernández, A. Tabachnikova, R. J. Homer, L. Tabacof, J. Tosto-Mancuso, E. Breyman, A. Kontorovich, D. McCarthy, M. Quezado, H. Vogel, M. M. Hefti, D. P. Perl, S. Liddelow, R. Folkerth, D. Putrino, A. Nath, A. Iwasaki, and M. Monje. 2022. Mild respiratory COVID can cause multi-lineage neural cell and myelin dysregulation. *Cell* 185(14):2452–2468.e16.

Fialho, M. F. P., E. S. Brum, and S. M. Oliveira. 2023. Could the fibromyalgia syndrome be triggered or enhanced by COVID-19? *Inflammopharmacology* 31(2):633–651.

Fitzcharles, M.-A., S. P. Cohen, D. J. Clauw, G. Littlejohn, C. Usui, and W. Häuser. 2021. Nociplastic pain: Towards an understanding of prevalent pain conditions. *The Lancet* 397(10289):2098–2110.

Fletcher, M. A., X. R. Zeng, Z. Barnes, S. Levis, and N. G. Klimas. 2009. Plasma cytokines in women with chronic fatigue syndrome. *Journal of Translational Medicine* 7:96.

Freidin, M. B., N. Cheetham, E. L. Duncan, C. J. Steves, K. J. Doores, M. H. Malim, N. Rossi, J. M. Lord, P. W. Franks, A. Borsini, I. Granville Smith, M. Falchi, C. Pariante, and F. M. K. Williams. 2023. Long-COVID fatigue is not predicted by pre-pandemic plasma IL-6 levels in mild COVID-19. *Inflammation Research* 72(5):947–953.

Freitag, H., M. Szklarski, S. Lorenz, F. Sotzny, S. Bauer, A. Philippe, C. Kedor, P. Grabowski, T. Lange, G. Riemekasten, H. Heidecke, and C. Scheibenbogen. 2021. Autoantibodies to vasoregulative G-protein-coupled receptors correlate with symptom severity, autonomic dysfunction and disability in myalgic encephalomyelitis/chronic fatigue syndrome. *Journal of Clinical Medicine* 10(16):3675.

Friedberg, F. 2016. Cognitive-behavior therapy: Why is it so vilified in the chronic fatigue syndrome community? *Fatigue: Biomedicine, Health & Behavior* 4(3):127–131.

Friedberg, F., M. Sunnquist, and L. Nacul. 2020. Rethinking the standard of care for myalgic encephalomyelitis/chronic fatigue syndrome. *Journal of General Internal Medicine* 35(3):906–909.

Fukuda, S., J. Nojima, Y. Motoki, K. Yamaguti, Y. Nakatomi, N. Okawa, K. Fujiwara, Y. Watanabe, and H. Kuratsune. 2016. A potential biomarker for fatigue: Oxidative stress and anti-oxidative activity. *Biological Psychology* 118:88–93.

Ganji, R., and P. H. Reddy. 2021. Impact of COVID-19 on mitochondrial-based immunity in aging and age-related diseases. *Frontiers in Aging Neuroscience* 12:614650.

Garg, H., M. Douglas, G. D. Turkington, and D. Turkington. 2021a. Recovery from refractory chronic fatigue syndrome with CBT and modafinil. *BMJ Case Reports* 14(3):e240283.

Garg, P., U. Arora, A. Kumar, and N. Wig. 2021b. The "post-COVID" syndrome: How deep is the damage? *Journal of Medical Virology* 93(2):673–674.

Gay, C., A. O'Shea, M. Robinson, J. Craggs, and R. Staud. 2015. Default mode network connectivity in chronic fatigue syndrome patients. *Journal of Pain* 16(4):S54.

Ghali, A., C. Lacout, J.-O. Fortrat, K. Depres, M. Ghali, and C. Lavigne. 2022. Factors influencing the prognosis of patients with myalgic encephalomyelitis/chronic fatigue syndrome. *Diagnostics* 12(10):2540.

Giloteaux, L., J. K. Goodrich, W. A. Walters, S. M. Levine, R. E. Ley, and M. R. Hanson. 2016. Reduced diversity and altered composition of the gut microbiome in individuals with myalgic encephalomyelitis/chronic fatigue syndrome. *Microbiome* 4(1):30.

González-Hermosillo, J. A., J. P. Martínez-López, S. A. Carrillo-Lampón, D. Ruiz-Ojeda, S. Herrera-Ramírez, L. M. Amezcua-Guerra, and M. D. R. Martínez-Alvarado. 2021. Post-acute COVID-19 symptoms, a potential link with myalgic encephalomyelitis/chronic fatigue syndrome: A 6-month survey in a Mexican cohort. *Brain Sciences* 11(6):760.

Gottschalk, C. G., D. Peterson, J. Armstrong, K. Knox, and A. Roy. 2023. Potential molecular mechanisms of chronic fatigue in long haul COVID and other viral diseases. *Infectious Agents and Cancer* 18(1):7.

Gruber, C. N., R. S. Patel, R. Trachtman, L. Lepow, F. Amanat, F. Krammer, K. M. Wilson, K. Onel, D. Geanon, K. Tuballes, M. Patel, K. Mouskas, T. O'Donnell, E. Merritt, N. W. Simons, V. Barcessat, D. M. Del Valle, S. Udondem, G. Kang, C. Agashe, N. Karekar, J. Grabowska, K. Nie, J. Le Berichel, H. Xie, N. Beckmann, S. Gangadharan, G. Ofori-Amanfo, U. Laserson, A. Rahman, S. Kim-Schulze, A. W. Charney, S. Gnjatic, B. D. Gelb, M. Merad, and D. Bogunovic. 2023. Mapping systemic inflammation and antibody responses in multisystem inflammatory syndrome in children (MIS-C). *Cell* 186(15):3325.

Guarnieri, J. W., J. M. Dybas, H. Fazelinia, M. S. Kim, J. Frere, Y. Zhang, Y. Soto Albrecht, D. G. Murdock, A. Angelin, L. N. Singh, S. L. Weiss, S. M. Best, M. T. Lott, S. Zhang, H. Cope, V. Zaksas, A. Saravia-Butler, C. Meydan, J. Foox, C. Mozsary, Y. Bram, Y. Kidane, W. Priebe, M. R. Emmett, R. Meller, S. Demharter, V. Stentoft-Hansen, M. Salvatore, D. Galeano, F. J. Enguita, P. Grabham, N. S. Trovao, U. Singh, J. Haltom, M. T. Heise, N. J. Moorman, V. K. Baxter, E. A. Madden, S. A. Taft-Benz, E. J. Anderson, W. A. Sanders, R. J. Dickmander, S. B. Baylin, E. S. Wurtele, P. M. Moraes-Vieira, D. Taylor, C. E. Mason, J. C. Schisler, R. E. Schwartz, A. Beheshti, and D. C. Wallace. 2023. Core mitochondrial genes are down-regulated during SARS-CoV-2 infection of rodent and human hosts. *Science Translational Medicine* 15(708):eabq1533.

Guasp, M., G. Muñoz-Sánchez, E. Martínez-Hernández, D. Santana, Á. Carbayo, L. Naranjo, U. Bolós, M. Framil, A. Saiz, M. Balasa, R. Ruiz-García, R. Sánchez-Valle, and Barcelona Neuro-COVID Study Group. 2022. CSF biomarkers in COVID-19 associated encephalopathy and encephalitis predict long-term outcome. *Frontiers in Immunology* 13:866153.

Guo, C., X. Che, T. Briese, A. Ranjan, O. Allicock, R. A. Yates, A. Cheng, D. March, M. Hornig, A. L. Komaroff, S. Levine, L. Bateman, S. D. Vernon, N. G. Klimas, J. G. Montoya, D. L. Peterson, W. I. Lipkin, and B. L. Williams. 2023. Deficient butyrate-producing capacity in the gut microbiome is associated with bacterial network disturbances and fatigue symptoms in ME/CFS. *Cell Host Microbe* 31(2):288–304.e8.

Gyöngyösi, M., P. Alcaide, F. W. Asselbergs, B. J. J. M. Brundel, G. G. Camici, P. da Costa Martins, P. Ferdinandy, M. Fontana, H. Girao, M. Gnecchi, C. Gollmann-Tepeköylü, P. Kleinbongard, T. Krieg, R. Madonna, M. Paillard, A. Pantazis, C. Perrino, M. Pesce, G. G. Schiattarella, J. P. G. Sluijter, S. Steffens, C. Tschöpe, S. Van Linthout, and S. M. Davidson. 2023. Long COVID and the cardiovascular system- elucidating causes and cellular mechanisms in order to develop targeted diagnostic and therapeutic strategies: A joint scientific statement of the ESC working groups on cellular biology of the heart and myocardial and pericardial diseases. *Cardiovascular Research* 119(2):336–356.

Haffke, M., H. Freitag, G. Rudolf, M. Seifert, W. Doehner, N. Scherbakov, L. Hanitsch, K. Wittke, S. Bauer, F. Konietschke, F. Paul, J. Bellmann-Strobl, C. Kedor, C. Scheibenbogen, and F. Sotzny. 2022. Endothelial dysfunction and altered endothelial biomarkers in patients with post-COVID-19 syndrome and chronic fatigue syndrome (ME/CFS). *Journal of Translational Medicine* 20(1):138.

Haider, S., A. J. Janowski, J. B. Lesnak, K. Hayashi, D. L. Dailey, R. Chimenti, L. A. Frey-Law, K. A. Sluka, and G. Berardi. 2023. A comparison of pain, fatigue, and function between post-COVID-19 condition, fibromyalgia, and chronic fatigue syndrome: A survey study. *Pain* 164(2):385–401.

Hallmann, E., D. Sikora, B. Poniedziałek, K. Szymański, K. Kondratiuk, J. Żurawski, L. Brydak, and P. Rzymski. 2023. IgG autoantibodies against ACE2 in SARS-CoV-2 infected patients. *Journal of Medical Virology* 95(1):e28273.

Haran, J. P., E. Bradley, A. L. Zeamer, L. Cincotta, M. C. Salive, P. Dutta, S. Mutaawe, O. Anya, M. Meza-Segura, A. M. Moormann, D. V. Ward, B. A. McCormick, and V. Bucci. 2021. Inflammation-type dysbiosis of the oral microbiome associates with the duration of COVID-19 symptoms and long COVID. *JCI Insight* 6(19):e152346.

Hardcastle, S. L., E. W. Brenu, S. Johnston, T. Nguyen, T. Huth, S. Ramos, D. Staines, and S. Marshall-Gradisnik. 2015a. Longitudinal analysis of immune abnormalities in varying severities of chronic fatigue syndrome/myalgic encephalomyelitis patients. *Journal of Translational Medicine* 13:299.

Hardcastle, S. L., E. W. Brenu, S. Johnston, T. Nguyen, T. Huth, N. Wong, S. Ramos, D. Staines, and S. Marshall-Gradisnik. 2015b. Characterisation of cell functions and receptors in chronic fatigue syndrome/myalgic encephalomyelitis (CFS/ME). *BMC Immunology* 16:35.

Häuser, W., J. Ablin, M.-A. Fitzcharles, G. Littlejohn, J. V. Luciano, C. Usui, and B. Walitt. 2015. Fibromyalgia. *Nature Reviews. Disease Primers* 1:15022.

Holden, S., R. Maksoud, N. Eaton-Fitch, H. Cabanas, D. Staines, and S. Marshall-Gradisnik. 2020. A systematic review of mitochondrial abnormalities in myalgic encephalomyelitis/chronic fatigue syndrome/systemic exertion intolerance disease. *Journal of Translational Medicine* 18:290.

Holder, K., and P. H. Reddy. 2021. The COVID-19 effect on the immune system and mitochondrial dynamics in diabetes, obesity, and dementia. *Neuroscientist* 27(4):331–339.

Hurwitz, B. E., V. T. Coryell, M. Parker, P. Martin, A. Laperriere, N. G. Klimas, G. N. Sfakianakis, and M. S. Bilsker. 2009. Chronic fatigue syndrome: Illness severity, sedentary lifestyle, blood volume and evidence of diminished cardiac function. *Clinical Science (London, England: 1979)* 118(2):125–135.

Huth, T. K., E. W. Brenu, T. Nguyen, S. L. Hardcastle, S. Johnston, S. Ramos, D. Staines, and Marshall-Gradisnik. 2014. Characterization of natural killer cell phenotypes in chronic fatigue syndrome/myalgic encephalomyelitis. *Journal of Clinical & Cellular Immunology* 5:223.

Huth, T. K., E. W. Brenu, S. Ramos, T. Nguyen, S. Broadley, D. Staines, and S. Marshall-Gradisnik. 2016. Pilot study of natural killer cells in chronic fatigue syndrome/myalgic encephalomyelitis and multiple sclerosis. *Scandinavian Journal of Immunology* 83(1):44–51.

IOM (Institute of Medicine). 2015. *Beyond myalgic encephalomyelitis/chronic fatigue syndrome: Redefining an illness.* Washington, DC: The National Academies Press.

Jason, L. A., and M. F. Islam. 2022. A classification system for post-acute sequelae of SARS-CoV-2 infection. *Central Asian Journal of Medical Hypotheses and Ethics* 3(1):38–51.

Jason, L. A., and M. Sunnquist. 2018. The development of the DePaul Symptom Questionnaire: Original, expanded, brief, and pediatric versions. *Frontiers in Pediatrics* 6:330.

Jason, L. A., N. Porter, M. Brown, V. Anderson, A. Brown, J. Hunnell, and A. Lerch. 2009. CFS: A review of epidemiology and natural history studies. *Bulletin of the IACFS/ME* 17(3):88–106.

Jason, L. A., M. Islam, K. Conroy, J. Cotler, C. Torres, M. Johnson, and B. Mabie. 2021. COVID-19 symptoms over time: Comparing long-haulers to ME/CFS. *Fatigue: Biomedicine, Health & Behavior* 9(2):59–68.

Jason, L.A., B. H. Natelson, H. Bonilla, Z. A. Sherif, S. D. Vernon, M. Verduzco-Gutierrez, L. O'Brien, E. Taylor. 2023. What Long COVID investigators can learn from four decades of ME/CFS research. *Brain Behavior and Immunity Integrative*, Volume 4:100022.

Jukema, B. N., K. Smit, M. T. E. Hopman, C. C. W. G. Bongers, T. C. Pelgrim, M. H. Rijk, T. N. Platteel, R. P. Venekamp, D. L. M. Zwart, F. H. Rutten, and L. Koenderman. 2022. Neutrophil and eosinophil responses remain abnormal for several months in primary care patients with COVID-19 disease. *Frontiers in Allergy* 3:942699.

Kaczmarek, M. P. 2023. Heterogenous circulating mirna changes in ME/CFS converge on a unified cluster of target genes: A computational analysis. *PLoS ONE* 18(12):e0296060.

Kedor, C., H. Freitag, L. Meyer-Arndt, K. Wittke, L. G. Hanitsch, T. Zoller, F. Steinbeis, M. Haffke, G. Rudolf, B. Heidecker, T. Bobbert, J. Spranger, H. D. Volk, C. Skurk, F. Konietschke, F. Paul, U. Behrends, J. Bellmann-Strobl, and C. Scheibenbogen. 2022. A prospective observational study of post-COVID-19 chronic fatigue syndrome following the first pandemic wave in Germany and biomarkers associated with symptom severity. *Nature Communications* 13(1):5104.

Kennedy, M., and D. T. Felson. 1996. A prospective long-term study of fibromyalgia syndrome. *Arthritis & Rheumatism* 39(4):682–685.

Klimas, N. G., and A. O. B. Koneru. 2007. Chronic fatigue syndrome: Inflammation, immune function, and neuroendocrine interactions. *Current Rheumatology Reports* 9(6):482–487.

Klimas, N. G., F. R. Salvato, R. Morgan, and M. A. Fletcher. 1990. Immunologic abnormalities in chronic fatigue syndrome. *Journal of Clinical Microbiology* 28(6):1403–1410.

Komaroff, A. L., and W. I. Lipkin. 2023. ME/CFS and long COVID share similar symptoms and biological abnormalities: Road map to the literature. *Frontiers in Medicine (Lausanne)* 10:1187163.

Lam, M. H.-B., Y.-K. Wing, M. W.-M. Yu, C.-M. Leung, R. C. W. Ma, A. P. S. Kong, W. Y. So, S. Y.-Y. Fong, and S.-P. Lam. 2009. Mental morbidities and chronic fatigue in severe acute respiratory syndrome survivors: Long-term follow-up. *Archives of Internal Medicine* 169(22):2142–2147.

Lammi, V., T. Nakanishi, S. E. Jones, S. J. Andrews, J. Karjalainen, B. Cortés, H. E. O'Brien, B. E. Fulton-Howard, H. H. Haapaniemi, A. Schmidt, R. E. Mitchell, A. Mousas, M. Mangino, A. Huerta-Chagoya, N. Sinnott-Armstrong, E. T. Cirulli, M. Vaudel, A. S. F. Kwong, A. K. Maiti, M. Marttila, C. Batini, F. Minnai, A. R. Dearman, C. A. R. Warmerdam, C. B. Sequeros, T. W. Winkler, D. M. Jordan, L. Guare, E. Vergasova, E. Marouli, P. Striano, U. A. Zainulabid, A. Kumar, H. F. Ahmad, R. Edahiro, S. Azekawa, Long COVID Host Genetics Initiative, FinnGen, DBDS Genomic Consortium, GEN-COVID Multicenter Study, J. J. Grzymski, M. Ishii, Y. Okada, N. D. Beckmann, M. Kumari, R. Wagner, I. M. Heid, C. John, P. J. Short, P. Magnus, K. Banasik, F. Geller, L. H. Franke, A. Rakitko, E. L. Duncan, A. Renieri, K. K. Tsilidis, R. d. Cid, A. Niavarani, T. Tusié-Luna, S. S. Verma, G. D. Smith, N. J. Timpson, M. J. Daly, A. Ganna, E. C. Schulte, J. B. Richards, K. U. Ludwig, M. Hultström, H. Zeberg, and H. M. Ollila. 2023. Genome-wide association study of Long COVID. *medRxiv* [Preprint]. 2023.06.29.23292056. https://doi.org/10.1101/2023.06.29.23292056.

Larsen, N. W., L. E. Stiles, R. Shaik, L. Schneider, S. Muppidi, C. T. Tsui, L. N. Geng, H. Bonilla, and M. G. Miglis. 2022. Characterization of autonomic symptom burden in long COVID: A global survey of 2,314 adults. *Frontiers in Neurology* 13:1012668.

Lechuga, G. C., C. M. Morel, and S. G. De-Simone. 2023. Hematological alterations associated with long COVID-19. *Frontiers in Physiology* 14:1203472.

Li, Y., Y. Ke, X. Xia, Y. Wang, F. Cheng, X. Liu, X. Jin, B. Li, C. Xie, S. Liu, W. Chen, C. Yang, Y. Niu, R. Jia, Y. Chen, X. Liu, Z. Wang, F. Zheng, Y. Jin, Z. Li, N. Yang, P. Cao, H. Chen, J. Ping, F. He, C. Wang, and G. Zhou. 2021. Genome-wide association study of COVID-19 severity among the Chinese population. *Cell Discovery* 7:76.

Lim, E.-J., Y.-C. Ahn, E.-S. Jang, S.-W. Lee, S.-H. Lee, and C.-G. Son. 2020a. Systematic review and meta-analysis of the prevalence of chronic fatigue syndrome/myalgic encephalomyelitis (CFS/ME). *Journal of Translational Medicine* 18(1):100.

Lim, E.-J., E.-B. Kang, E.-S. Jang, and C.-G. Son. 2020b. The prospects of the two-day cardio-pulmonary exercise test (CPET) in ME/CFS patients: A meta-analysis. *Journal of Clinical Medicine* 9(12):4040.

Lindell, L., S. Bergman, I. F. Petersson, L. T. H. Jacobsson, and P. Herrström. 2000. Prevalence of fibromyalgia and chronic widespread pain. *Scandinavian Journal of Primary Health Care* 18(3):149–153.

Liu, Q., J. W. Y. Mak, Q. Su, Y. K. Yeoh, G. C. Lui, S. S. S. Ng, F. Zhang, A. Y. L. Li, W. Lu, D. S. Hui, P. K. Chan, F. K. L. Chan, and S. C. Ng. 2022. Gut microbiota dynamics in a prospective cohort of patients with post-acute COVID-19 syndrome. *Gut* 71(3):544–552.

Malkova, A. M., and Y. Shoenfeld. 2023. Autoimmune autonomic nervous system imbalance and conditions: Chronic fatigue syndrome, fibromyalgia, silicone breast implants, COVID and post-COVID syndrome, sick building syndrome, post-orthostatic tachycardia syndrome, autoimmune diseases and autoimmune/inflammatory syndrome induced by adjuvants. *Autoimmunity Reviews* 22(1):103230.

Mancini, D. M., D. L. Brunjes, A. Lala, M. G. Trivieri, J. P. Contreras, and B. H. Natelson. 2021. Use of cardiopulmonary stress testing for patients with unexplained dyspnea post-coronavirus disease. *JACC: Heart Failure* 9(12):927–937.

Marshall-Gradisnik, S., P. Smith, B. Nilius, and D. R. Staines. 2015. Examination of single nucleotide polymorphisms in acetylcholine receptors in chronic fatigue syndrome patients. *Immunology and Immunogenetics Insights* 7:III.S25105.

Martínez-Lavín, M., and A. Miguel-Álvarez. 2023. Hypothetical framework for post-COVID 19 condition based on a fibromyalgia pathogenetic model. *Clinical Rheumatology* 42(11):3167–3171.

Martini, A. L., G. Carli, L. Kiferle, P. Piersanti, P. Palumbo, S. Morbelli, M. L. Calcagni, D. Perani, and S. Sestini. 2022. Time-dependent recovery of brain hypometabolism in neuro-COVID-19 patients. *European Journal of Nuclear Medicine and Molecular Imaging* 50(1):90–102.

McGonagle, D., K. Sharif, A. O'Regan, and C. Bridgewood. 2020. The role of cytokines including interleukin-6 in COVID-19 induced pneumonia and macrophage activation syndrome-like disease. *Autoimmunity Reviews* 19(6):102537.

McLaughlin, M., N. E. M. Sanal-Hayes, L. D. Hayes, E. C. Berry, and N. F. Sculthorpe. 2023. People with long COVID and myalgic encephalomyelitis/chronic fatigue syndrome exhibit similarly impaired vascular function. *American Journal of Medicine* October 12:S0002-9343(23):00609-5. Advance online publication.

Missailidis, D., O. Sanislav, C. Y. Allan, S. J. Annesley, and P. R. Fisher. 2020. Cell-based blood biomarkers for myalgic encephalomyelitis/chronic fatigue syndrome. *International Journal of Molecular Sciences* 21(3):1142.

Mitchell, W. M. 2016. Efficacy of rintatolimod in the treatment of chronic fatigue syndrome/myalgic encephalomyelitis (CFS/ME). *Expert Review of Clinical Pharmacology* 9(6): 755–770.

Mohandas, S., P. Jagannathan, T. J. Henrich, Z. A. Sherif, C. Bime, E. Quinlan, M. A. Portman, M. Gennaro, J. Rehman, and RECOVER Mechanistic Pathways Task Force. 2023. Immune mechanisms underlying COVID-19 pathology and post-acute sequelae of SARS-CoV-2 infection (PASC). *eLife* 12:e86014.

Monje, M., and A. Iwasaki. 2022. The neurobiology of long COVID. *Neuron* 110(21): 3484–3496.

Moore, Y., T. Serafimova, N. Anderson, H. King, A. Richards, A. Brigden, P. Sinai, J. Higgins, C. Ascough, P. Clery, and E. M. Crawley. 2021. Recovery from chronic fatigue syndrome: A systematic review-heterogeneity of definition limits study comparison. *Archives of Disease in Childhood* 106(11):1087–1094.

Morillas-Arques, P., C. M. Rodriguez-Lopez, R. Molina-Barea, F. Rico-Villademoros, and E. P. Calandre. 2010. Trazodone for the treatment of fibromyalgia: An open-label, 12-week study. *BMC Musculoskeletal Disorders* 11:204.

Morris, G., and M. Maes. 2013. A neuro-immune model of myalgic encephalomyelitis/chronic fatigue syndrome. *Metabolic Brain Disease* 28(4):523–540.

Mosch, B., V. Hagena, S. Herpertz, and M. Diers. 2023. Brain morphometric changes in fibromyalgia and the impact of psychometric and clinical factors: A volumetric and diffusion-tensor imaging study. *Arthritis Research & Therapy* 25(1):81.

Mueller, C., J. C. Lin, S. Sheriff, A. A. Maudsley, and J. W. Younger. 2020. Evidence of widespread metabolite abnormalities in myalgic encephalomyelitis/chronic fatigue syndrome: Assessment with whole-brain magnetic resonance spectroscopy. *Brain Imaging and Behavior* 14(2):562–572.

Nagy-Szakal, D., B. L. Williams, N. Mishra, X. Che, B. Lee, L. Bateman, N. G. Klimas, A. L. Komaroff, S. Levine, J. G. Montoya, D. L. Peterson, D. Ramanan, K. Jain, M. L. Eddy, M. Hornig, and W. I. Lipkin. 2017. Fecal metagenomic profiles in subgroups of patients with myalgic encephalomyelitis/chronic fatigue syndrome. *Microbiome* 5(1):44.

Nakatomi, Y., K. Mizuno, A. Ishii, Y. Wada, M. Tanaka, S. Tazawa, K. Onoe, S. Fukuda, J. Kawabe, K. Takahashi, Y. Kataoka, S. Shiomi, K. Yamaguti, M. Inaba, H. Kuratsune, and Y. Watanabe. 2014. Neuroinflammation in patients with chronic fatigue syndrome/myalgic encephalomyelitis: An [11]C-(R)-PK11195 PET study. *Journal of Nuclear Medicine* 55(6):945–950.

NICE (National Institute for Health and Care Excellence). 2020. *COVID-19 rapid guideline: Managing the long-term effects of COVID-19*. London, UK: NICE.

NICE. 2021. *Myalgic encephalomyelitis (or encephalopathy)/chronic fatigue syndrome: Diagnosis and management.* London, UK: NICE.

Nunes, J. M., D. B. Kell, and E. Pretorius. 2023. Cardiovascular and haematological pathology in myalgic encephalomyelitis/chronic fatigue syndrome (ME/CFS): A role for viruses. *Blood Reviews* 60:101075.

O'Dowd, H., P. Gladwell, C. A. Rogers, S. Hollinghurst, and A. Gregory. 2006. Cognitive behavioural therapy in chronic fatigue syndrome: A randomised controlled trial of an outpatient group programme. *Health Technology Assessment (Winchester, England)* 10(37): 1–121.

Ojo-Amaize, E. A., E. J. Conley, and J. B. Peter. 1994. Decreased natural killer cell activity is associated with severity of chronic fatigue immune dysfunction syndrome. *Clinical Infectious Diseases* 18 (Suppl 1):S157–S159.

Oliveira, C. R., L. A. Jason, D. Unutmaz, L. Bateman, and S. D. Vernon. 2023. Improvement of long COVID symptoms over one year. *Frontiers in Medicine* 9:1065620.

Pairo-Castineira, E., S. Clohisey, L. Klaric, A. D. Bretherick, K. Rawlik, D. Pasko, S. Walker, N. Parkinson, M. H. Fourman, C. D. Russell, J. Furniss, A. Richmond, E. Gountouna, N. Wrobel, D. Harrison, B. Wang, Y. Wu, A. Meynert, F. Griffiths, W. Oosthuyzen, A. Kousathanas, L. Moutsianas, Z. Yang, R. Zhai, C. Zheng, G. Grimes, R. Beale, J. Millar, B. Shih, S. Keating, M. Zechner, C. Haley, D. J. Porteous, C. Hayward, J. Yang, J. Knight, C. Summers, M. Shankar-Hari, P. Klenerman, L. Turtle, A. Ho, S. C. Moore, C. Hinds, P. Horby, A. Nichol, D. Maslove, L. Ling, D. McAuley, H. Montgomery, T. Walsh, A. C. Pereira, A. Renieri, X. Shen, C. P. Ponting, A. Fawkes, A. Tenesa, M. Caulfield, R. Scott, K. Rowan, L. Murphy, P. J. M. Openshaw, M. G. Semple, A. Law, V. Vitart, J. F. Wilson, and J. K. Baillie. 2021. Genetic mechanisms of critical illness in COVID-19. *Nature* 591(7848):92–98.

Patell, R., T. Bogue, A. Koshy, P. Bindal, M. Merrill, W. C. Aird, K. A. Bauer, and J. I. Zwicker. 2020. Postdischarge thrombosis and hemorrhage in patients with COVID-19. *Blood* 136(11):1342–1346.

Pendergrast, T., A. Brown, M. Sunnquist, R. Jantke, J. L. Newton, E. B. Strand, and L. A. Jason. 2016. Housebound versus nonhousebound patients with myalgic encephalomyelitis and chronic fatigue syndrome. *Chronic Illness* 12(4):292–307.

Plaut, S. 2023. "Long COVID-19" and viral "fibromyalgia-ness": Suggesting a mechanistic role for fascial myofibroblasts (Nineveh, the shadow is in the fascia). *Frontiers Medicine (Lausanne)* 10:952278.

Pliszka, A. G. 2022. Modafinil: A review and its potential use in the treatment of long COVID fatigue and neurocognitive deficits. *American Journal of Psychiatry Residents' Journal* 17(4):5–7.

Prompetchara, E., C. Ketloy, and T. Palaga. 2020. Immune responses in COVID-19 and potential vaccines: Lessons learned from SARS and MERS epidemic. *Asian Pacific Journal of Allergy and Immunology* 38(1):1–9.

Puri, B. K., S. J. Counsell, R. Zaman, J. Main, A. G. Collins, J. V. Hajnal, and N. J. Davey. 2002. Relative increase in choline in the occipital cortex in chronic fatigue syndrome. *Acta Psychiatrica Scandinavica* 106(3):224–226.

Ram-Mohan, N., D. Kim, A. J. Rogers, C. A. Blish, K. C. Nadeau, A. L. Blomkalns, and S. Yang. 2022. Association between SARS-CoV-2 RNAemia and postacute sequelae of COVID-19. *Open Forum Infectious Diseases* 9(2):ofab646.

Randall, D. C., F. H. Cafferty, J. M. Shneerson, I. E. Smith, M. B. Llewelyn, and S. E. File. 2005. Chronic treatment with modafinil may not be beneficial in patients with chronic fatigue syndrome. *Journal of Psychopharmacology (Oxford, England)* 19(6):647–660.

Raveendran, A. V., R. Jayadevan, and S. Sashidharan. 2021. Long COVID: An overview. *Diabetes & Metabolic Syndrome* 15(3):869–875.

Rivas, J. L., T. Palencia, G. Fernández, and M. García. 2018. Association of T and NK cell phenotype with the diagnosis of myalgic encephalomyelitis/chronic fatigue syndrome (ME/CFS). *Frontiers in Immunology* 9:1028.

Roberts, L. N., M. B. Whyte, L. Georgiou, G. Giron, J. Czuprynska, C. Rea, B. Vadher, R. K. Patel, E. Gee, and R. Arya. 2020. Postdischarge venous thromboembolism following hospital admission with COVID-19. *Blood* 136(11):1347–1350.

Rodriguez-Perez, A. I., C. M. Labandeira, M. A. Pedrosa, R. Valenzuela, J. A. Suarez-Quintanilla, M. Cortes-Ayaso, P. Mayán-Conesa, and J. L. Labandeira-Garcia. 2021. Autoantibodies against ACE2 and angiotensin type-1 receptors increase severity of COVID-19. *Journal of Autoimmunity* 122:102683.

Rowe, P. C., R. A. Underhill, K. J. Friedman, A. Gurwitt, M. S. Medow, M. S. Schwartz, N. Speight, J. M. Stewart, R. Vallings, and K. S. Rowe. 2017. Myalgic encephalomyelitis/chronic fatigue syndrome diagnosis and management in young people: A primer. *Frontiers in Pediatrics* 5:121.

Ruscitti, P., F. Ursini, and Y. Shoenfeld. 2023. Ferritin and myalgic encephalomyelitis/chronic fatigue syndrome in post COVID-19, an unexpected facet of the hyperferritinemic syndrome? *Journal of Psychosomatic Research* 169:111231.

Russell, I. J., H. Vaeroy, M. Javors, and F. Nyberg. 1992. Cerebrospinal fluid biogenic amine metabolites in fibromyalgia/fibrositis syndrome and rheumatoid arthritis. *Arthritis & Rheumatology* 35(5):550–556.

Sarzi-Puttini, P., V. Giorgi, D. Marotto, and F. Atzeni. 2020. Fibromyalgia: An update on clinical characteristics, aetiopathogenesis and treatment. *Nature Reviews Rheumatology* 16(11):645–660.

Sasso, E. M., K. Muraki, N. Eaton-Fitch, P. Smith, O. L. Lesslar, G. Deed, and S. Marshall-Gradisnik. 2022. Transient receptor potential melastatin 3 dysfunction in post COVID-19 condition and myalgic encephalomyelitis/chronic fatigue syndrome patients. *Molecular Medicine* 28(1):98.

Sathyamoorthy, M., M. Verduzco-Gutierrez, S. Varanasi, R. Ward, J. Spertus, and S. Shah. 2022. Enhanced external counterpulsation for management of symptoms associated with long COVID. *American Heart Journal Plus: Cardiology Research and Practice* 13:100105.

Schaefer, C. P., E. H. Adams, M. Udall, E. T. Masters, R. M. Mann, S. R. Daniel, H. J. McElroy, J. C. Cappelleri, A. G. Clair, M. Hopps, R. Staud, P. Mease, and S. L. Silverman. 2016. Fibromyalgia outcomes over time: Results from a prospective observational study in the United States. *Open Rheumatology Journal* 10(1):109–121.

Scherbakov, N., M. Szklarski, J. Hartwig, F. Sotzny, S. Lorenz, A. Meyer, P. Grabowski, W. Doehner, and C. Scheibenbogen. 2020. Peripheral endothelial dysfunction in myalgic encephalomyelitis/chronic fatigue syndrome. *ESC Heart Failure* 7(3):1064–1071.

Shungu, D. C., N. Weiduschat, J. W. Murrough, X. Mao, S. Pillemer, J. P. Dyke, M. S. Medow, B. H. Natelson, J. M. Stewart, and S. J. Mathew. 2012. Increased ventricular lactate in chronic fatigue syndrome. III. Relationships to cortical glutathione and clinical symptoms implicate oxidative stress in disorder pathophysiology. *NMR in Biomedicine* 25(9):1073–1087.

Smith, M. E. B., E. Haney, M. McDonagh, M. Pappas, M. Daeges, N. Wasson, R. Fu, and H. D. Nelson. 2015. Treatment of myalgic encephalomyelitis/chronic fatigue syndrome: A systematic review for a national institutes of health pathways to prevention workshop. *Annals of Internal Medicine* 162(12):841–850.

Solomon, L., and W. C. Reeves. 2004. Factors influencing the diagnosis of chronic fatigue syndrome. *Archives of Internal Medicine* 164(20):2241–2245.

Srikanth, S., J. R. Boulos, T. Dover, L. Boccuto, and D. Dean. 2023. Identification and diagnosis of long COVID-19: A scoping review. *Progress in Biophysics and Molecular Biology* 182:1–7.

Strayer, D. R., D. Young, and W. M. Mitchell. 2020. Effect of disease duration in a randomized phase III trial of rintatolimod, an immune modulator for myalgic encephalomyelitis/chronic fatigue syndrome. *PLoS ONE* 15(10):e0240403.

Su, Y., D. Yuan, D. G. Chen, R. H. Ng, K. Wang, J. Choi, S. Li, S. Hong, R. Zhang, J. Xie, S. A. Kornilov, K. Scherler, A. J. Pavlovitch-Bedzyk, S. Dong, C. Lausted, I. Lee, S. Fallen, C. L. Dai, P. Baloni, B. Smith, V. R. Duvvuri, K. G. Anderson, J. Li, F. Yang, C. J. Duncombe, D. J. McCulloch, C. Rostomily, P. Troisch, J. Zhou, S. Mackay, Q. DeGottardi, D. H. May, R. Taniguchi, R. M. Gittelman, M. Klinger, T. M. Snyder, R. Roper, G. Wojciechowska, K. Murray, R. Edmark, S. Evans, L. Jones, Y. Zhou, L. Rowen, R. Liu, W. Chour, H. A. Algren, W. R. Berrington, J. A. Wallick, R. A. Cochran, M. E. Micikas, the ISB-Swedish COVID-19 Biobanking Unit, T. Wrin, C. J. Petropoulos, H. R. Cole, T. D. Fischer, W. Wei, D. S. B. Hoon, N. D. Price, N. Subramanian, J. A. Hill, J. Hadlock, A. T. Magis, A. Ribas, L. L. Lanier, S. D. Boyd, J. A. Bluestone, H. Chu, L. Hood, R. Gottardo, P. D. Greenberg, M. M. Davis, J. D. Goldman, and J. R. Heath. 2022. Multiple early factors anticipate post-acute COVID-19 sequelae. *Cell* 185(5):881–895.e20.

Sukocheva, O. A., R. Maksoud, N. M. Beeraka, S. V. Madhunapantula, M. Sinelnikov, V. N. Nikolenko, M. E. Neganova, S. G. Klochkov, M. Amjad Kamal, D. R. Staines, and S. Marshall-Gradisnik. 2021. Analysis of post COVID-19 condition and its overlap with myalgic encephalomyelitis/chronic fatigue syndrome. *Journal of Advanced Research* 40:179–196.

Sweetman, E., T. Kleffmann, C. Edgar, M. de Lange, R. Vallings, and W. Tate. 2020. A SWATH-MS analysis of myalgic encephalomyelitis/chronic fatigue syndrome peripheral blood mononuclear cell proteomes reveals mitochondrial dysfunction. *Journal of Translational Medicine* 18(1):365.

Tate, W., M. Walker, E. Sweetman, A. Helliwell, K. Peppercorn, C. Edgar, A. Blair, and A. Chatterjee. 2022. Molecular mechanisms of neuroinflammation in ME/CFS and long COVID to sustain disease and promote relapses. *Frontiers in Neurology* 13:877772.

Tay, M. Z., C. M. Poh, L. Rénia, P. A. MacAry, and L. F. P. Ng. 2020. The trinity of COVID-19: Immunity, inflammation and intervention. *Nature Reviews Immunology* 20(6):363–374.

Thapaliya, K., S. Marshall-Gradisnik, D. Staines, and L. Barnden. 2020. Mapping of pathological change in chronic fatigue syndrome using the ratio of T1- and T2-weighted MRI scans. *NeuroImage: Clinical* 28:102366.

Thapaliya, K., S. Marshall-Gradisnik, D. Staines, J. Su, and L. Barnden. 2022. Alteration of cortical volume and thickness in myalgic encephalomyelitis/chronic fatigue syndrome. *Frontiers in Neuroscience* 16:848730.

Thibord, F., M. V. Chan, M.-H. Chen, and A. D. Johnson. 2022. A year of COVID-19 GWAS results from the GRASP portal reveals potential genetic risk factors. *Human Genetics and Genomics Advances* 3(2):100095.

Tian, Y., K.-Y. Sun, T.-Q. Meng, Z. Ye, S.-M. Guo, Z.-M. Li, C.-L. Xiong, Y. Yin, H.-G. Li, and L.-Q. Zhou. 2021. Gut microbiota may not be fully restored in recovered COVID-19 patients after 3-month recovery. *Frontiers in Nutrition* 8:638825.

Tidmore, T., L. Jason, L. Chapo-Kroger, S. So, A. Brown, and M. Silverman. 2015. Lack of knowledgeable healthcare access for patients with neuro-endocrine-immune diseases. *Frontiers in Clinical Medicine* 2:46–54.

Tomaszewski Farias, S., D. Mungas, D. J. Harvey, A. Simmons, B. R. Reed, and C. Decarli. 2011. The measurement of everyday cognition: Development and validation of a short form of the Everyday Cognition scales. *Alzheimer's & Dementia* 7(6):593–601.

Tomo, S., M. Banerjee, S. Karli, P. Purohit, P. Mitra, P. Sharma, M. K. Garg, and B. Kumar. 2022. Assessment of DHEAS, cortisol, and DHEAS/cortisol ratio in patients with COVID-19: A pilot study. *Hormones (Athens, Greece)* 21(3):515–518.

Torjesen, I. 2020. NICE cautions against using graded exercise therapy for patients recovering from COVID-19. *BMJ (Clinical Research Edition)* 370:m2912.

Tuller, D., and M. Vink. 2023. Graded exercise therapy and cognitive behavior therapy do not improve employment outcomes in ME/CFS. *Work* 74(4):1235–1239.

Twisk, F. N. M., and M. Maes. 2009. A review on cognitive behavorial therapy (CBT) and graded exercise therapy (GET) in myalgic encephalomyelitis (ME)/chronic fatigue syndrome (CFS): CBT/GET is not only ineffective and not evidence-based, but also potentially harmful for many patients with ME/CFS. *Neuroendocrinology Letters* 30(3):284–299.

Twomey, R., J. DeMars, K. Franklin, S. N. Culos-Reed, J. Weatherald, and J. G. Wrightson. 2022. Chronic fatigue and postexertional malaise in people living with long COVID: An observational study. *Physical Therapy* 102(4):pzac005.

Urhan, E., Z. Karaca, G. K. Unuvar, K. Gundogan, and K. Unluhizarci. 2022. Investigation of pituitary functions after acute coronavirus disease 2019. *Endocrine Journal* 69(6):649–658.

Ursini, F., J. Ciaffi, L. Mancarella, L. Lisi, V. Brusi, C. Cavallari, M. D'Onghia, A. Mari, E. Borlandelli, J. F. Cordella, M. L. Regina, P. Viola, P. Ruscitti, M. Miceli, R. D. Giorgio, N. Baldini, C. Borghi, A. Gasbarrini, A. Iagnocco, R. Giacomelli, C. Faldini, M. P. Landini, and R. Meliconi. 2021. Fibromyalgia: A new facet of the post-COVID-19 syndrome spectrum? Results from a web-based survey. *RMD Open* 7(3):e001735.

Vahratian, A., J.-M. S. Lin, J. Bertolli, and E. R. Unger. 2023. Myalgic encephalomyelitis/chronic fatigue syndrome in adults: United States, 2021-2022. *NCHS Data Briefs* 488:1–8.

van Campen, C. L. M. C., P. C. Rowe, and F. C. Visser. 2022. Orthostatic symptoms and reductions in cerebral blood flow in long-haul COVID-19 patients: Similarities with myalgic encephalomyelitis/chronic fatigue syndrome. *Medicina* 58(1):28.

Varga, Z., A. J. Flammer, P. Steiger, M. Haberecker, R. Andermatt, A. S. Zinkernagel, M. R. Mehra, R. A. Schuepbach, F. Ruschitzka, and H. Moch. 2020. Endothelial cell infection and endotheliitis in COVID-19. *The Lancet* 395(10234):1417–1418.

Vella, L. A., J. R. Giles, A. E. Baxter, D. A. Oldridge, C. Diorio, L. Kuri-Cervantes, C. Alanio, M. B. Pampena, J. E. Wu, Z. Chen, Y. J. Huang, E. M. Anderson, S. Gouma, K. O. McNerney, J. Chase, C. Burudpakdee, J. H. Lee, S. A. Apostolidis, A. C. Huang, D. Mathew, O. Kuthuru, E. C. Goodwin, M. E. Weirick, M. J. Bolton, C. P. Arevalo, A. Ramos, C. J. Jasen, P. E. Conrey, S. Sayed, H. M. Giannini, K. D'Andrea, the UPenn COVID Processing Unit, N. J. Meyer, E. M. Behrens, H. Bassiri, S. E. Hensley, S. E. Henrickson, D. T. Teachey, M. R. Betts, and E. J. Wherry. 2021. Deep immune profiling of MIS-C demonstrates marked but transient immune activation compared with adult and pediatric COVID-19. *Science Immunology* 6(57):eabf7570.

Vojdani, A., E. Vojdani, E. Saidara, and M. Maes. 2023. Persistent SARS-CoV-2 infection, EBV, HHV-6 and other factors may contribute to inflammation and autoimmunity in long COVID. *Viruses* 15(2):400.

Wallukat, G., B. Hohberger, K. Wenzel, J. Fürst, S. Schulze-Rothe, A. Wallukat, A.-S. Hönicke, and J. Müller. 2021. Functional autoantibodies against G-protein coupled receptors in patients with persistent long-COVID-19 symptoms. *Journal of Translational Autoimmunity* 4:100100.

Weerahandi, H., K. A. Hochman, E. Simon, C. Blaum, J. Chodosh, E. Duan, K. Garry, T. Kahan, S. L. Karmen-Tuohy, H. C. Karpel, F. Mendoza, A. M. Prete, L. Quintana, J. Rutishauser, L. Santos Martinez, K. Shah, S. Sharma, E. Simon, A. Z. Stirniman, and L. I. Horwitz. 2021. Post-discharge health status and symptoms in patients with severe COVID-19. *Journal of General Internal Medicine* 36(3):738–745.

Weigel, B., N. Eaton-Fitch, R. Passmore, H. Cabanas, D. Staines, and S. Marshall-Gradisnik. 2022 Gastrointestinal symptoms, dietary habits, and the effect on health-related quality of life among Australian myalgic encephalomyelitis/chronic fatigue syndrome patients: A cross-sectional study. *Quality of Life Research* 29(6):1521–1531.

Weigel, B., N. Eaton-Fitch, K. Thapaliya, S. Marshall-Gradisnik. 2023. Symptom presentation and quality of life are comparable in myalgic encephalomyelitis/chronic fatigue syndrome and post COVID-19 condition. *Population Medicine* 5(Supplement):A372

Wessely, S. 1995. The epidemiology of chronic fatigue syndrome. *Epidemiologic Reviews* 17(1):139–151.

Whiteside, T. L., and D. Friberg. 1998. Natural killer cells and natural killer cell activity in chronic fatigue syndrome. *American Journal of Medicine* 105(3A):27S-34S.

WHO (World Health Organization). 2020. *Clinical management of COVID-19.* https://www.who.int/teams/health-care-readiness/covid-19 (accessed February 26, 2024).

Wirth, K. J., and M. Löhn. 2023. Myalgic encephalomyelitis/chronic fatigue syndrome (ME/CFS) and comorbidities: Linked by vascular pathomechanisms and vasoactive mediators? *Medicina* 59(5):978.

Wolfe, F., J. Anderson, D. Harkness, R. M. Bennett, X. J. Caro, D. L. Goldenberg, I. J. Russell, and M. B. Yunus. 1997. Health status and disease severity in fibromyalgia. Results of a six-center longitudinal study. *Arthritis & Rheumatology* 40(9):1571–1579.

Wong, T. L., and D. J. Weitzer. 2021. Long COVID and myalgic encephalomyelitis/chronic fatigue syndrome (ME/CFS)—A systemic review and comparison of clinical presentation and symptomatology. *Medicina* 57(5):418.

Worm-Smeitink, M., S. Nikolaus, K. Goldsmith, J. Wiborg, S. Ali, H. Knoop, and T. Chalder. 2016. Cognitive behaviour therapy for chronic fatigue syndrome: Differences in treatment outcome between a tertiary treatment centre in the United Kingdom and the Netherlands. *Journal of Psychosomatic Research* 87:43–49.

Wu, E., A. Mahdi, J. Nickander, J. Bruchfeld, L. Mellbin, K. Haugaa, M. Ståhlberg, and L. Desta. 2023. Enhanced external counterpulsation for management of postacute sequelae of SARS-CoV-2 associated microvascular angina and fatigue: An interventional pilot study. *Cardiology Research and Practice* 2023:6687803.

Xie, Y., and Z. Al-Aly. 2022. Risks and burdens of incident diabetes in long COVID: A cohort study. *The Lancet Diabetes & Endocrinology* 10(5):311–321.

Xiong, R., C. Gunter, E. Fleming, S. D. Vernon, L. Bateman, D. Unutmaz, and J. Oh. 2023. Multi-'omics of gut microbiome-host interactions in short- and long-term myalgic encephalomyelitis/chronic fatigue syndrome patients. *Cell Host Microbe* 31(2):273–287. e275.

Xu, E., Y. Xie, and Z. Al-Aly. 2023a. Risks and burdens of incident dyslipidaemia in long COVID: A cohort study. *The Lancet Diabetes & Endocrinology* 11(2):120–128.

Xu, S.-W., I. Ilyas, and J.-P. Weng. 2023b. Endothelial dysfunction in COVID-19: An overview of evidence, biomarkers, mechanisms and potential therapies. *Acta Pharmacologica Sinica* 44(4):695–709.

Yamamoto, Y., Y. Otsuka, K. Tokumasu, N. Sunada, Y. Nakano, H. Honda, Y. Sakurada, T. Hasegawa, H. Hagiya, and F. Otsuka. 2023. Utility of serum ferritin for predicting myalgic encephalomyelitis/chronic fatigue syndrome in patients with long COVID. *Journal of Clinical Medicine* 12(14):4737.

Yelin, D., C. D. Moschopoulos, I. Margalit, E. Gkrania-Klotsas, F. Landi, J.-P. Stahl, and D. Yahav. 2022. ESCMID rapid guidelines for assessment and management of long COVID. *Clinical Microbiology and Infection* 28(7):955–972.

Yeoh, Y. K., T. Zuo, G. C.-Y. Lui, F. Zhang, Q. Liu, A. Y. Li, A. C. Chung, C. P. Cheung, E. Y. Tso, K. S. Fung, V. Chan, L. Ling, G. Joynt, D. S.-C. Hui, K. M. Chow, S. S. S. Ng, T. C.-M. Li, R. W. Ng, T. C. Yip, G. L.-H. Wong, F. K. Chan, C. K. Wong, P. K. Chan, and S. C. Ng. 2021. Gut microbiota composition reflects disease severity and dysfunctional immune responses in patients with COVID-19. *Gut* 70(4):698–706.

6

Overall Conclusions

This chapter presents nine conclusions derived by the committee from evidence presented throughout the report. This chapter does not include references. Citations to support the text and conclusions herein are provided in previous chapters of the report.

DIAGNOSIS OF LONG COVID

Long COVID is associated with a wide range of new or worsening health conditions and encompasses more than 200 symptoms involving nearly every organ system. There currently are no consensus-based diagnostic criteria for the condition; criteria for diagnosis are evolving as experience and research findings develop. Diagnosis of Long COVID is generally based on a known or presumed history of acute SARS-CoV-2 infection (as indicated by a positive viral test or patient self-report; as of this writing, no diagnostic test for Long COVID is available), the presence of Long COVID health effects and symptoms, and consideration of other conditions and etiologies that could be causing the symptoms.

Testing to diagnose acute SARS-CoV-2 infection, as well as testing capacity and behaviors, has changed dramatically over the course of the COVID-19 pandemic. Testing was constrained during the early phase of the pandemic, although it subsequently became increasingly available, and the introduction of at-home testing meant that many people may not have reported their positive results to health care systems. As a result of these two drivers, many individuals infected with SARS-CoV-2 never received formal

215

documentation of their diagnosis. Sole reliance on a documented history of SARS-CoV-2 infection when diagnosing Long COVID will miss these individuals. Therefore, the presence of signs and symptoms and self-reported prior infection are generally considered sufficient to establish a diagnosis of SARS-CoV-2 infection. Continued research on and discussion of Long COVID will help inform a case definition and standardized diagnosis.

Based on its review of the literature, the committee reached the following conclusion:

1. *Long COVID is a complex chronic condition caused by SARS-CoV-2 infection that affects multiple body systems. Because of wide variability in testing practices over the course of the pandemic, many people experiencing Long COVID have not received a formal diagnosis of prior SARS-CoV-2 infection. A positive test for SARS-CoV-2 is not necessary to consider a diagnosis of Long COVID.*

EPIDEMIOLOGY

Long COVID can impact people across the lifespan, from children to older adults, as well as across sex, gender, racial, ethnic, and other demographic groups. Women are twice as likely as men to experience Long COVID. Population surveys suggest that in 2022 the overall prevalence of Long COVID was around 3.4 percent in U.S. adults and 0.5 percent in children. Estimates of the prevalence of specific long-term health effects of SARS-CoV-2 vary in the literature. This variation reflects the dynamic nature of the pandemic itself, as the virus has evolved and spawned many variants and subvariants (likely with different propensities to cause Long COVID), as well as the introduction of vaccines and treatments for acute infection (e.g., antivirals, steroids), both of which have been shown to reduce the risk of long-term health effects. Variation in incidence and prevalence estimates also stem from the heterogeneity of study designs, including choice of control groups, methods used to account for the effect of baseline health, specification of outcomes, and other methodological differences.

In addition, the broad multisystem nature of Long COVID and the fact that the associated health effects are expressed differently by age group and sex and by baseline health compound the challenge of identifying and quantifying affected populations. Symptoms of SARS-CoV-2 infection range in severity from mild to severe, and the literature suggests that the severity of acute SARS-CoV-2 infection is a risk factor for Long COVID. For example, a large Scottish population-based study found that 5 percent of those with mild infection had not recovered at least 6 months following infection, compared with 16 percent of those who required hospitalization—a ratio of approximately 1:3.

Based on its review of the literature, the committee reached the following conclusion:

2. *The risk of Long COVID increases with the severity of acute infection. By the committee's best estimate, people whose infection was sufficiently severe to necessitate hospitalization are 2–3 times more likely to experience Long COVID than are those who were not hospitalized, and among those who were hospitalized, individuals requiring life support in the intensive care unit may be twice as likely to experience Long COVID. However, people with mild disease can also develop Long COVID, and given the much higher number of people with mild versus severe disease, they make up the great majority of people with Long COVID.*

HEALTH EFFECTS

Long COVID is associated with hundreds of symptoms and new or worsening health effects that manifest in many different body systems. In keeping with the three domains of functioning in the *International Classification of Functioning, Disability and Health* model of disability, health effects experienced in Long COVID may manifest as impairments in body structures and physical and psychological functions, with resulting activity limitations and restrictions on participation. Evidence on clustering of the post-acute and long-term health effects of SARS-CoV-2 infection remains inconsistent across studies. Consensus is needed on terms, definitions, and methodological approaches for generating better-quality and more consistent evidence.

Based on its review of the literature, the committee reached the following conclusion:

3. *Long COVID is associated with a wide range of new or worsening health conditions impacting multiple organ systems. Long COVID can cause more than 200 symptoms and affects each person differently. Attempts to cluster symptoms have yielded heterogeneous results.*

FUNCTIONAL IMPACT AND RISK FACTORS

Some of the symptoms and health effects associated with Long COVID can be severe enough to interfere with an individual's day-to-day functioning, including participation in work and school activities. Functional disability associated with Long COVID has been characterized as the inability to return to work, poor quality of life, diminished ability to perform activities of daily living, decreased physical and cognitive function, and overall disability.

The severity of acute COVID-19 is a major risk factor for poor functional outcomes, but even people with mild initial illness can experience long-term functional impairments. Increased number and severity of long-term symptoms correlate with decreased quality of life, physical functioning, and ability to work or perform in school. Other risk factors for poor functional outcomes include female sex, lack of vaccination against SARS-CoV-2, baseline disability or comorbidities, and smoking.

There is some overlap between SSA's current Listing of Impairments (Listings) and health effects associated with Long COVID, such as impaired lung and heart function. However, it is likely that most individuals with Long COVID applying for Social Security disability benefits will do so based on health effects not covered in the Listings. Three frequently reported health effects that can significantly interfere with the ability to perform work or school activities and may not be captured in the SSA Listings are chronic fatigue and post-exertional malaise, post-COVID-19 cognitive impairment, and autonomic dysfunction, all of which can be difficult to assess clinically in terms of their severity and effects on a person's functioning.

Based on its review of the literature, the committee reached the following conclusion:

4. *Long COVID can result in the inability to return to work (or school for children and adolescents), poor quality of life, diminished ability to perform activities of daily living, and decreased physical and cognitive function for 6 months to 2 years or longer after the resolution of acute infection with SARS-CoV-2. Increased number and severity of long-term health effects correlates with decreased quality of life, physical and mental functioning, and ability to participate in work and school. Health effects that may not be captured in SSA's Listing of Impairments yet may significantly affect an individual's ability to participate in work or school include, but are not limited to, post-exertional malaise and chronic fatigue, post-COVID-19 cognitive impairment, and autonomic dysfunction.*

LONG COVID IN CHILDREN AND ADOLESCENTS

While there are various definitions of children, adolescents, and young people, for the purposes of this report, "children" or "pediatrics" refers to the entire pediatric age range and "adolescents" to children at the older end of the spectrum (i.e., ages ~11 to 18 years). Even though most children experience mild acute COVID-19 illness, they can experience Long COVID regardless of the severity of their acute infection. As with adults, they may experience health effects across many body systems. Commonly reported symptoms include fatigue, weakness, headache, sleep disturbance, muscle and joint pain, respiratory problems, palpitations, altered sense of smell or taste, dizziness, and dysautonomia. Although pediatric presentations and intervention options may overlap with those in adults—particularly among adolescents, who may be more likely than children to mimic the adult presentation and trajectory—pediatric management of Long COVID entails specific considerations related to developmental age and/or disabilities and history gathering. In general, children have fewer preexisting chronic health conditions compared with adults; thus, Long COVID may represent a substantial change from their baseline, particularly for those who were previously healthy.

Limited data are available on long-term outcomes in children. Some youth with persistent symptoms experience difficulties that affect their quality of life and result in increased school absences, as well as decreased participation and performance in school, sports, and other activities. Risk factors for the development of Long COVID include acute-phase hospitalization, preexisting comorbidity, and infection with pre-Omicron variants. Most children with Long COVID recover slowly over time, but not all. In one prospective cohort study of 1,243 children (ages 4–10) with Long COVID, for example, 48 percent remained symptomatic at 6 months, 13 percent at 12 months, and 5 percent at 18 months after infection. Importantly, severity of symptoms and functional impairment from Long COVID symptoms were not correlated with traditional clinical testing (e.g., lung ultrasound, standard systolic and diastolic function on echocardiogram).

It is important to note that in pediatrics, because of typical development, the baseline for performance of skills is constantly changing, especially among young children. This can make deviations in their performance during Long COVID challenging to assess, and there may be a delay in recognition of any deviations (e.g., lack of developing a skill at the appropriate age). Additionally, the duration of symptoms (e.g., 1 or 3 months) can feel very different to and have a greater impact on children compared with adults. Currently, there is a dearth of prospective and cross-sectional studies on the prevalence, risk factors, and time course and pattern of Long COVID in children. More research is needed to identify the long-term functional implications of Long COVID in children, because information from adult studies may not be directly applicable to the pediatric population.

Based on its review of the literature, the committee reached the following conclusion:

5. *Although the large majority of children recover fully from SARS-CoV-2 infection, some develop Long COVID and experience persistent or intermittent symptoms that can reduce their quality of life and result in increased school absences as well as decreased participation and performance in school, sports, and other activities. Overall, the trajectory*

for recovery is better among children compared with adults. More research is needed to understand the long-term functional implications of Long COVID in children, as information from adult studies may not be directly applicable.

DISEASE MANAGEMENT

Currently there are no Food and Drug Administration (FDA)–approved drugs or disease-modifying treatments for Long COVID. As with other complex multisystem conditions, management of Long COVID relies on techniques for controlling symptoms and improving functional ability, such as pacing (i.e., balancing periods of activity and rest in daily life), mobility support, social support, diet modulation, pharmacological treatment of secondary health effects, cognitive-behavioral therapy, and rehabilitation. Management often requires a multidisciplinary team. Because of the multisystem nature of the condition, different approaches may be needed to address the variety of clinical presentations and environmental factors (e.g., living situation, work requirements, family support) among individuals. Numerous randomized controlled trials are currently being undertaken to determine the efficacy of a number of identified pharmacological agents; however, limited data have been published, and trials are yet to be finalized.

Based on its review of the literature, the committee reached the following conclusion:

6. *There currently is no curative treatment for Long COVID itself. Management of the condition is based on current knowledge about treating the associated health effects and other sequelae. As with other complex multisystem chronic conditions, treatment focuses on symptom management and optimization of function and quality of life.*

DISEASE COURSE AND PROGNOSIS

Recovery from Long COVID varies among individuals, and data on recovery trajectories are rapidly evolving. Initial data suggest that people with persistent Long COVID symptoms generally improve over time, although preliminary studies suggest that recovery can plateau 6–12 months after acute infection. Studies have shown that only 18–22 percent of those who have persistent symptoms at 5–6 months following infection have fully recovered by 1 year. Among those who do not improve, most remain stable, but some worsen. More information on recovery trajectories at 1 year or longer may become available in the next few years. Rehabilitation and symptom management, including pacing, may improve function in some people with Long COVID, regardless of the severity of disease or duration of symptoms, although the benefits are greater for those who are younger and who have had Long COVID for a shorter period of time.

Based on its review of the literature, the committee reached the following conclusion:

7. *Recovery from Long COVID varies among individuals, and data on recovery trajectories are rapidly evolving. There is some evidence that many people with persistent Long COVID symptoms at 3 months following acute infection, including children and adolescents, have improved by 12 months. Data for durations longer than 12 months are limited, but preliminary data suggest that recovery may plateau or progress at a slower rate after 12 months.*

HEALTH EQUITY

The burden of seeking care and finding adequate services for Long COVID is challenging and can impact the potential for recovery. Patients with Long COVID may encounter skepticism about their symptoms when they present in medical settings, which discourages care seeking. This is particularly true for individuals disadvantaged by their social or economic status, geographic location, or environment, and can result in preventable disparities in the burden of disease and opportunities to achieve optimal health. Disadvantaged groups include members of some racial and ethnic minorities, people with disabilities, women, LGBTQI+ (lesbian, gay, bisexual, transgender, queer, intersex, or other) individuals, people with limited English proficiency, and others.

Individuals with Long COVID have increased health care utilization and financial burden, which may be exacerbated if they are unable to work to gain income and or receive health insurance coverage. Members of disadvantaged groups, especially early in the pandemic, were more likely to contract SARS-CoV-2, more likely to be hospitalized with acute COVID-19, more likely to have adverse clinical outcomes, and less likely to be vaccinated, potentially increasing their risk of developing Long COVID. In addition, these groups are more likely to be uninsured or underinsured. Even for those with insurance coverage, some of the services that have been shown to improve function may not be covered by their benefits. Moreover, the availability of specialized Long COVID services is limited, and capacity does not match the demand for rehabilitation specialists. Limited transportation, distance from clinics, and the inability to take time away from work or school are known barriers to care. The availability issue is particularly problematic for individuals living in medically underserved areas.

Information about COVID is rapidly evolving, and this dynamic nature of the science may contribute to some patient hesitancy regarding prophylactic and therapeutic management for acute infection or Long COVID. Low levels of health literacy may also place some individuals at increased risk for misinformation, which may prevent them from fully taking advantage of health care resources to protect and improve their health. Low health literacy may also impact individual self-management of the symptoms and conditions associated with Long COVID.

Based on its review of the literature, the committee reached the following conclusion:

8. *Social determinants of health, such as socioeconomic status, geographic location, health literacy, and race and ethnicity, affect access to health care. With respect to acute SARS-CoV-2 infection and Long COVID, adverse social determinants of health have contributed to disparities in access to SARS-CoV-2 testing; vaccination; and therapeutics, including treatments for acute infection and specialized rehabilitation clinics for Long COVID. In addition, the demand for specialty care exceeds capacity, resulting in waitlists for the receipt of services.*

SIMILAR CHRONIC CONDITIONS

Long COVID shares many features with other complex multisystem conditions, including myalgic encephalomyelitis/chronic fatigue syndrome (ME/CFS), fibromyalgia, and postural orthostatic tachycardia syndrome (POTS). The mechanism of action for infection-associated chronic illnesses remains unclear, and further investigation is needed. Current theories regarding potential mechanisms of action include viral persistence, immune dysregulation (including cytokine dysregulation or mast cell activation), neurological disturbances (e.g., neuroinflammation), cardiovascular damage (e.g., endothelial dysfunction, coagulation issues, orthostatic intolerance), gastrointestinal dysfunction (e.g., secondary to gut microbiome dysbiosis), metabolic issues (energy insufficiency, reactive oxygen species production, mitochrondrial dysfunction), and genetic variations.

Currently, there are no specific laboratory-based diagnostic tests for Long COVID or ME/CFS, and diagnosis involves consideration of other potential causes of the symptoms. In general, Long COVID (especially that which does not meet criteria for ME/CFS) has a better prognosis than ME/CFS. Some manifestations of Long COVID are similar to those of ME/CFS, and like ME/CFS, Long COVID appears to be a chronic illness, with few patients achieving full remission. Studies comparing Long COVID and ME/CFS have several limitations, however. Because Long COVID is a new disease, study participants are usually newly diagnosed, while ME/CFS study participants often have had the condition for longer and so are less likely to improve. Moreover, the definition of ME/CFS requires that symptoms be ongoing for 6 months or more, whereas the duration criteria for Long COVID vary in the literature from 2 to 6 months, making the two conditions difficult to compare.

Based on its review of the literature, the committee reached the following conclusion:

9. *Complex, infection-associated chronic conditions affecting multiple body systems are not new, and Long COVID shares many features with such conditions as myalgic encephalomyelitis/chronic fatigue syndrome, fibromyalgia, and postural orthostatic tachycardia syndrome. Current theories about the pathophysiology of these conditions include immune dysregulation, neurological disturbances, cardiovascular damage, gastrointestinal dysfunction, metabolic issues, and mitochondrial dysfunction. More research is needed to understand the natural history and management of complex multisystem chronic conditions, including Long COVID.*

Appendix A

Public Meeting Agendas

**COMMITTEE ON THE LONG-TERM HEALTH EFFECTS
STEMMING FROM COVID-19 AND IMPLICATIONS
FOR THE SOCIAL SECURITY ADMINSTRATION**

The Keck Center, 500 Fifth Street, NW
Washington, DC 20001

MEETING 1

**JANUARY 26, 2023
VIRTUAL**

3:05 p.m. **Welcome and Introductions**
Paul Volberding, Committee Chair
*Steve Rollins, Acting Associate Commissioner, U.S. Social
Security Administration (SSA)*

3:15 p.m. **Social Security Administration Overview**
*Vincent Nibali, Policy Analyst, Office of Medical Policy &
Office of Disability Policy*
- Provide an overview of SSA and its mission/goals/processes
- Explanation of interest in Long COVID and how it
applies to their work
- Explanation of the Statement of Task and key elements of
interest to SSA

3:40 p.m.	**Questions and Discussion**
	Committee Members and SSA Staff
4:30 p.m.	**Adjourn Public Session**

The Keck Center, 500 Fifth Street, NW
Washington, DC 20001

MEETING 2

FEBRUARY 12, 2023
KECK 100

1:00 p.m.	**Welcome**
	Paul Volberding, Committee Chair
1:05 p.m.	**Long COVID: Overview of the course of disease and demographics**
	David Putrino, Director of Rehabilitation Innovation, Icahn School of Medicine at Mount Sinai
2:00 p.m.	**Current practices in defining and diagnosing Long COVID**
	Avindra Nath, Director, Translational Neuroscience Center at National Institute of Neurological Disorders and Stroke
3:00 p.m.	**Adjourn Public Session**

University of California, San Francisco Medical Center at Mission Bay
550 16th Street, San Francisco, CA

MEETING 3

MAY 9, 2023
MISSION HALL, ROOM 2105

12:00 p.m.	**Welcome and Opening Remarks**
	Paul Volberding, Committee Chair
12:05 p.m.	**Immunology of Long COVID**
	Akiko Iwasaki, Sterling Professor of Immunobiology and Professor of Dermatology and of Molecular, Cellular, and Developmental Biology and of Epidemiology (Microbial Diseases) at Yale School of Medicine; Investigator, Howard Hughes Medical Institute

12:45 p.m.   **Long COVID and ME/CFS share both symptoms and underlying biological abnormalities**
Anthony Komaroff, Steven P. Simcox/Patrick A. Clifford/ James H. Higby Professor of Medicine at Harvard Medical School, Senior physician at Brigham and Women's Hospital in Boston

1:30 p.m.   **BREAK**

1:45 p.m.   **Epigenetic Diagnosis and the Human "Flight Data Recorder"**
Eric Van Gieson, Senior Advisor at The Conafay Group, Chief Executive Officer at Severn Innovations

2:30 p.m.   **Closing Remarks**
Paul Volberding, Committee Chair

2:35 p.m.   **Adjourn Public Session**

The National Academy of Sciences
2101 Constitution Ave NW
Washington, DC 20418

MEETING 4

JULY 24, 2023
NAS BOARD ROOM

9:30 a.m.   **Welcome and Opening Remarks**
Paul Volberding, Committee Chair

9:35 a.m.   **Patient experience and follow-up**
Lucas Denault, Long COVID Patient
Karin Denault, Parent and Caregiver

10:00 a.m.   **Long COVID in children and adolescents**
Alexandra Yonts, Director, Post-COVID Program and Infectious Diseases Specialist, Children's National Hospital

10:45 a.m.   **Underserved populations and Long COVID**
Angela Meriquez Vázquez, MSW, Long COVID Patient and Policy Director, The Children's Partnership

11:30 a.m.   **Presentation to NASEM Committee on the Long-Term Health Effects Stemming from COVID-19 and Implications for the Social Security Administration**
Robert Holman, Medical Director, District of Columbia Fire and Emergency Medical Services Department

12:15 p.m.   **Closing Remarks**
Paul Volberding, Committee Chair

12:20 p.m.   **Adjourn Public Session**

Appendix B

Literature Search Strategies

Long-Term Health Effects Stemming from COVID-19 and Implications for the Social Security Administration—Function Literature Search

Date of Search: 6/12/2023
Request: Functional changes due to Long COVID
Search Parameters:
Date: 2020—Present
Geographic Focus: All
Language: English
Databases: PubMed, Embase (Ovid) and Scopus
Article Type: Prospective cohort studies. If not many, include cross-sectional studies

Database Searches:

PubMed

("Post-Acute COVID-19 Syndrome"[Mesh] or Post-Acute-COVID-19-Syndrome[tiab] or Post-Acute-COVID-19-Syndromes[tiab] or Long-Haul-COVID-19[tiab] or COVID-19-Long-Haul[tiab] or Long-Haul-COVID-19[tiab] or Post-Acute-COVID-19-Syndrome[tiab] or Long-COVID[tiab] or Post-Acute-Sequelae-of-SARS-CoV-2-Infection[tiab] or Post-Acute-Sequelae-of-SARS-CoV-2-Infection[tiab] or Post-COVID-Conditions[tiab] or Post-COVID-Conditions[tiab] or Post-COVID-Condition[tiab] or Long-Haul-COVID[tiab] or COVID-Long-Haul[tiab] or Long-Haul-COVID[tiab] or long-covid[tiab] or pediatric-long-covid[tiab] or pediatric-PASC[tiab] or COVID-19/ complications[Mesh]) AND (Employment[Mesh] or Unemployment[Mesh] or Quality of Life[Mesh] or "Functional Status"[Mesh] or "Disability Evaluation"[Mesh] or "International Classification of Functioning, Disability and Health"[Mesh] or "Return to Work"[Mesh] or "Return to School"[Mesh] or "Occupational Health"[Mesh] or functional[tiab] or employment[tiab] or unemployment[tiab] or life quality[tiab] or "quality of life"[tiab] or return to work[tiab] or return to school[tiab] or trajectory recovery[tiab]) AND ("Prospective Studies"[Mesh] or prospective study[tiab] or prospective studies[tiab] or prospective cohort[tiab] or "Cross-Sectional Studies"[Mesh] or cross-sectional[tiab])

Language: English

Results: 262 results

Embase (Ovid)

Embase <1980 to 2023 Week 23>		
1	*coronavirus disease 2019/co [Complication]	314
2	long covid/ or (Post-Acute-COVID-19-Syndrome or COVID-19-Syndrome-Post-Acute or Post-Acute-COVID-19-Syndromes or Long-Haul-COVID-19 or COVID-19-Long-Haul or Long-Haul-COVID-19 or Post-Acute-COVID-19-Syndrome or Post-Acute-COVID-19-Syndrome or Long-COVID or Post-Acute-Sequelae-of-SARS-CoV-2-Infection or Post-Acute-Sequelae-of-SARS-CoV-2-Infection or Post-COVID-Conditions or Post-COVID-Conditions or Post-COVID-Condition or Long-Haul-COVID or COVID-Long-Haul or Long-Haul-COVID or long-covid or chronic-COVID-syndrome or chronic-COVID-19 or COVID-long-hauler or COVID-19-long-hauler or long-haul-COVID or long-hauler-COVID or post-COVID-19-fatigue or post-COVID-19-neurological-syndrome or post-COVID-19-syndrome or post-COVID-fatigue or post-COVID-impairment or post-COVID-syndrome or post-acute-COVID-syndrome or post-acute-COVID-19 or post-acute-COVID-19-fatigue or post-acute-COVID-19-neurological-syndrome or pediatric-long-covid or pediatric-PASC or long-covid-in-children or ((late-sequelae or long-term-sequelae) adj4 covid)).ti,ab,kw.	6377
3	1 or 2	6685
4	exp employment/ or exp unemployment/ or exp functional status/ or exp functional assessment/ or exp disability assessment/ or exp return to work/ or exp return to school/ or exp "quality of life"/ or exp occupational health/ or (employment or unemployment or functional or disability-assessment* or disability-evaluation* or return-to-school or return-to-work or life-quality or quality-of-life or occupational-health or trajectory-recovery).ti,ab,kw.	3011277
5	3 and 4	1422

6	exp prospective study/ or (prospective-stud* or prospective cohort). ti,ab,kw.	1014974
7	5 and 6	201
8	limit 7 to English language	196
9	exp cross-sectional study/ or cross-sectional.ti,ab,kw.	805834
10	5 and 9	162
11	limit 10 to English language	161

Scopus:

TITLE-ABS-KEY((Post-Acute-COVID-19-Syndrome or COVID-19-Syndrome-Post-Acute or Post-Acute-COVID-19-Syndromes or Long-Haul-COVID-19 or COVID-19-Long-Haul or Long-Haul-COVID-19 or Post-Acute-COVID-19-Syndrome or Post-Acute-COVID-19-Syndrome or Long-COVID or Post-Acute-Sequelae-of-SARS-CoV-2-Infection or Post-Acute-Sequelae-of-SARS-CoV-2-Infection or Post-COVID-Conditions or Post-COVID-Conditions or Post-COVID-Condition or Long-Haul-COVID or COVID-Long-Haul or Long-Haul-COVID or long-covid or chronic-COVID-syndrome or chronic-COVID-19 or COVID-long-hauler or COVID-19-long-hauler or long-haul-COVID or long-hauler-COVID or post-COVID-19-fatigue or post-COVID-19-neurological-syndrome or post-COVID-19-syndrome or post-COVID-fatigue or post-COVID-impairment or post-COVID-syndrome or post-acute-COVID-syndrome or post-acute-COVID-19 or post-acute-COVID-19-fatigue or post-acute-COVID-19-neurological-syndrome or pediatric-long-covid or pediatric-PASC or long-covid-in-children) AND (employment or unemployment or functional or disability-assessment* or disability-evaluation* or return-to-school or return-to-work or life-quality or quality-of-life or occupational-health or trajectory-recovery) AND (cross-section* or prospective-stud* or prospective-cohort*))

Language: English

Results: 274

6/13/23—Title Screening

196 papers included

Inclusion and Exclusion Criteria:
- Inclusion:
  - prospective cohort
  - exposure: covid

- o   outcomes: function, disability, quality of life
- o   follow-up: 6 months +
- o   population: children and working-age adults
- Exclusion:
  - o   ICU outcomes with short-term followup
  - o   pharmaceutical safety and treatment efficacy
  - o   elderly/geriatric population
  - o   in-hospital complications
- Included as potentially relevant:
  - o   ICU/intubation/ventilation outcomes with 6+ month followup
  - o   Shorter followup but relevant functional outcomes
  - o   Long covid in patients with specific conditions
  - o   Changes in function after rehab

6/20/23—Final Papers Included in Report Divided into Categories After Abstract Screening:
Children: 7
Hospital: 57
ICU: 13
Non-hospital: 51
Rehab: 14

Long-Term Health Effects Stemming from COVID-19 and Implications for the Social Security Administration—Health Effects Literature Search

Date of search: June 14, 2023
Search Parameters:
Date: 2020—Present
Geographic Focus: All
Language: English
Databases: PubMed, Embase (Ovid) and Scopus
Article Type: Exclude case studies—focus on large cohort studies

Database Searches:

PubMed

("Post-Acute COVID-19 Syndrome"[Mesh] or Post-Acute-COVID-19-Syndrome[tiab] or Post-Acute-COVID-19-Syndromes[tiab] or Long-Haul-COVID-19[tiab] or COVID-19-Long-Haul[tiab] or Long-Haul-COVID-19 [tiab] or Post-Acute-COVID-19-Syndrome[tiab] or Long-COVID[tiab] or Post-Acute-Sequelae-of-SARS-CoV-2-Infection[tiab] or Post-Acute-Sequelae-of-SARS-CoV-2-Infection[tiab] or Post-COVID-Conditions[tiab] or Post-COVID-Conditions[tiab] or Post-COVID-Condition[tiab] or Long-Haul-COVID[tiab] or COVID-Long-Haul[tiab] or Long-Haul-COVID[tiab] or long-covid[tiab] or pediatric-long-covid[tiab] or pediatric-PASC[tiab] or COVID-19/complications[Mesh]) AND (symptom*[tiab] or outcome*[tiab] or clinical-feature*[tiab]) AND (persist*[tiab] or clinical-sequelae[tiab] or evolution[tiab]) AND ("Cohort Studies"[Mesh] or cohort*[tiab] or retrospective stud*[tiab] or multicenter stud*[tiab]) NOT "Case Reports" [Publication Type]

Language: English

Results: *556*

Embase (Ovid)

Embase {1980 to 2023 Week 23}		
1	*coronavirus disease 2019/co [Complication]	314
2	long covid/ or (Post-Acute-COVID-19-Syndrome or COVID-19-Syndrome-Post-Acute or Post-Acute-COVID-19-Syndromes or Long-Haul-COVID-19 or COVID-19-Long-Haul or Long-Haul-COVID-19 or Post-Acute-COVID-19-Syndrome or Post-Acute-COVID-19-Syndrome or Long-COVID or Post-Acute-Sequelae-of-SARS-CoV-2-Infection or Post-Acute-Sequelae-of-SARS-CoV-2-Infection or Post-COVID-Conditions or Post-COVID-Conditions or Post-COVID-Condition or Long-Haul-COVID or COVID-Long-Haul or Long-Haul-COVID or long-covid or chronic-COVID-syndrome or chronic-COVID-19 or COVID-long-hauler or COVID-19-long-hauler or long-haul-COVID or long-hauler-COVID or post-COVID-19-fatigue or post-COVID-19-neurological-syndrome or post-COVID-19-syndrome or post-COVID-fatigue or post-COVID-impairment or post-COVID-syndrome or post-acute-COVID-syndrome or post-acute-COVID-19 or post-acute-COVID-19-fatigue or post-acute-COVID-19-neurological-syndrome or pediatric-long-covid or pediatric-PASC or long-covid-in-children or ((late-sequelae or long-term-sequelae) adj4 covid)).ti,ab,kw.	6377
3	1 or 2	6685
4	(symptom* or outcome* or clinical-feature* or condition*).ti,ab,kw.	7813432
5	(persist* or clinical-sequelae or evolution).ti,ab,kw.	1230131
6	exp cohort analysis/ or cohort*.ti,ab,kw.	1678149
7	exp case study/	99189
8	3 and 4 and 5 and 6	495
9	8 not 7	491
10	limit 9 to English language	489

Scopus:

TITLE-ABS-KEY((Post-Acute-COVID-19-Syndrome or COVID-19-Syndrome-Post-Acute or Post-Acute-COVID-19-Syndromes or Long-Haul-COVID-19 or COVID-19-Long-Haul or Long-Haul-COVID-19 or Post-Acute-COVID-19-Syndrome or Post-Acute-COVID-19-Syndrome or Long-COVID or Post-Acute-Sequelae-of-SARS-CoV-2-Infection or Post-Acute-Sequelae-of-SARS-CoV-2-Infection or Post-COVID-Conditions or Post-COVID-Conditions or Post-COVID-Condition or Long-Haul-COVID or COVID-Long-Haul or Long-Haul-COVID or long-covid or chronic-COVID-syndrome or chronic-COVID-19 or COVID-long-hauler or COVID-19-long-hauler or long-haul-COVID or long-hauler-COVID or post-COVID-19-fatigue or post-COVID-19-neurological-syndrome or post-COVID-19-syndrome or post-COVID-fatigue or post-COVID-impairment or post-COVID-syndrome or post-acute-COVID-syndrome or post-acute-COVID-19 or post-acute-COVID-19-fatigue or post-acute-COVID-19-neurological-syndrome or pediatric-long-covid or pediatric-PASC or long-covid-in-children) AND (symptom* or outcome* or clinical-feature* or condition*) AND (persist* or evolution or clinical-sequelae) AND (cohort*))

Language: English

Results: 358

Appendix C

Biographical Sketches of Committee Members

Paul A. Volberding, M.D. (*Chair*), is a retired professor of medicine and previous director of the AIDS Research Institute at the University of California, San Francisco. Trained in medical oncology, he became involved in the early AIDS epidemic in San Francisco and has experience in clinical and translational research in antiviral therapeutics. Dr. Volberding is a member of the National Academy of Medicine, a fellow of the American Association for the Advancement of Science, a master of the American College of Physicians, and a fellow of the Infectious Diseases Society of America. He is editor-in-chief of the *Journal of Acquired Immune Deficiency Syndromes* and *Current HIV/AIDS Reports*. Dr. Volberding currently serves on the National Academies of Sciences, Engineering, and Medicine's Standing Committee of Medical and Vocational Experts for the Social Security Administration's Disability Programs and has chaired numerous National Academies committees, including several for the Social Security Administration, most recently, the Committee on Selected Heritable Disorders of Connective Tissue and Disability. He received his medical degree from the University of Minnesota and completed his residency at the University of Utah in internal medicine and his fellowship in medical oncology at the University of California, San Francisco.

Ziyad Al-Aly, M.D., is director of the Clinical Epidemiology Center and Chief of Research and Education Service at the U.S. Department of Veterans Affairs (VA) St. Louis Healthcare System. He is a clinical epidemiologist at Washington University in St. Louis. He led work that provided the first systematic characterization of the post-acute sequelae of SARS-CoV 2 infection and, subsequently, the characterization of the increased risks of cardiovascular disease, neurologic disorders, diabetes, and kidney disease following SARS-CoV-2 infection. His lab also produced evidence characterizing the effects of vaccines on Long COVID, the health consequences of repeated infections with SARS-CoV-2, and the effect of antivirals on the short- and long-term outcomes of SARS-CoV-2 infection. His research interests include pharmacoepidemiology, environmental epidemiology, global health, and most recently short- and long-term effects of COVID-19 on health outcomes. In his work on COVID-19, Dr. Al-Aly regularly interacts with pharmaceutical companies in an uncompensated capacity, including ongoing, informal discussions with Pfizer about the VA's work on antivirals and Long COVID and previous ad hoc paid consultations for Gilead and Tonix. His work is published in several major journals, highly cited, and frequently featured in scientific and mainstream media outlets. Dr. Al-Aly serves on the editorial board of several major journals. He has also testified before the U.S. Senate as an expert witness on Long COVID. Dr. Al-Aly obtained his medical degree from the American University of Beirut and completed his postgraduate medical education at St. Louis University and Washington University in St. Louis.

Jacqueline Becker, Ph.D., is a licensed clinical neuropsychologist, assistant professor of medicine, and researcher in the Division of General Internal Medicine at the Icahn School of Medicine at Mount Sinai. Dr. Becker is multiple principal investigator of the National Institutes of Health's (NIH's) RECOVER-Neuro, a multisite randomized controlled trial to treat cognitive dysfunction post COVID-19. She is principal investigator of an Alzheimer's Association/National Academy of Neuropsychology award investigating the neuropsychological effects of COVID-19 in older adults from populations with health disparities. She is co-investigator of various Long COVID initiatives, such as an Agency for Healthcare Research and Quality–sponsored project integrating primary and Long COVID care to improve outcomes for minoritized adults in New York City and a NIH/National Institute of Neurological Disorders and Stroke award to identify the long-term neurological effects of COVID-19 using 7 Tesla multimodal neuroimaging. Dr. Becker is co-chair of the International Neuropsychological Society's NeuroCOVID-19 SIG [special interest group], joining efforts to harmonize global data on post-COVID cognitive sequelae. Her research focuses on the bidirectional impact of cognitive impairment in chronic medical diseases, particularly in underserved minority populations. She completed her doctoral training at Fordham University in New York, her residency at Harvard Medical School/Massachusetts General Hospital, and then a 2-year clinical neuropsychology postdoctoral fellowship in the Department of Neurology at Northwell Health.

Alfred O. Berg, M.D., M.P.H., is professor and chair emeritus of the Department of Family Medicine at the University of Washington in Seattle. He has served on many national expert panels to assess evidence and provide clinical guidance, including serving as chair of the U.S. Preventive Services Task Force and committees convened by the Agency for Healthcare Research and Quality, the U.S. Centers for Disease Control and Prevention, the National Institutes of Health, the Patient-Centered Outcomes Research Institute, and the American Medical Association. Dr. Berg was elected to the National Academy of Medicine in 1996 and has participated in more than a dozen committees convened by the National Academies of Sciences, Engineering, and Medicine, including serving as chair of committees on post-traumatic stress disorder, formaldehyde toxicity, genetic testing, and standards for systematic reviews. He has also served on the Board of Population Health, and as reviewer, monitor, and coordinator for the National Research Council. Dr. Berg received the Thomas W. Johnson Award for career contributions to family medicine education from the American Academy of Family Physicians; the F. Marian Bishop Leadership Award from the Society of Teachers of Family Medicine Foundation; and the Curtis Hames Research Award, family medicine's highest research honor. He earned his medical degree at Washington University in St. Louis and his master of public health at the University of Washington in Seattle.

Andrew B. Bindman, M.D., is executive vice president and chief medical officer for Kaiser Permanente. He is also Kaiser Permanente's executive sponsor for the Kaiser Permanente Bernard J. Tyson School of Medicine. Dr. Bindman served as director of the Agency for Healthcare Research and Quality in 2016–2017. Prior to joining Kaiser Permanente, he spent more than 30 years on the faculty at the University of California, San Francisco (UCSF), where he practiced and taught clinical medicine while conducting research on health access and outcomes that resulted in more than 200 published scientific articles. Dr. Bindman is an elected member of the National Academy of Medicine, where he serves on the Board for Health Care Services and chairs a series of workshops on diagnostic excellence. He is a board-certified general internist, and he completed his residency in internal medicine at UCSF. He was Robert Wood Johnson Foundation Clinical Scholar at Stanford University. Dr. Bindman is a graduate of Harvard College and the Mount Sinai School of Medicine.

Aluko A. Hope, M.D., M.S.C.E., is associate professor in the Department of Medicine at Oregon Health & Science University (OHSU), where he works as an intensivist in the Medical Intensive Care Unit and serves as medical director of OHSU's Long COVID program. Previously, Dr. Hope worked for 11 years at Albert Einstein College of Medicine, where he was founding director of the COVID-19 Recovery Engagement clinic. His research, which receives funding from the National Heart, Lung, and Blood Institute, seeks to improve the long-term outcomes of adult survivors of acute illnesses such as pneumonia, acute respiratory distress syndrome, and sepsis. His postgraduate training was in primary care internal medicine at Columbia University Medical Center, followed by training in pulmonary and critical care medicine at Mount Sinai Hospital and Montefiore Medical Center, with a focus on integrating palliative care and geriatric principles into the critical care setting. As a graduate of the Montefiore-Einstein Certificate Program in Bioethics and Medical Humanities, Dr. Hope has also developed and facilitated postgraduate courses to teach empathic communication skills to learners at all levels. He graduated from Vassar College with a B.A. in biology and Hispanic studies and earned his medical degree and master's degree in clinical epidemiology from the University of Pennsylvania School of Medicine.

Leora I. Horwitz, M.D., is director of the Center for Healthcare Innovation and Delivery Science at New York University (NYU) Langone Health, director of the Division of Healthcare Delivery Science in the Department of Population Health at NYU School of Medicine, tenured professor of population health and of medicine, and a practicing internist. Dr. Horwitz was on faculty at Yale University for 7 years before moving to NYU in 2014. Her work focuses on improving the safety and quality of health care delivery. She is currently co–principal investigator of the Clinical Science Core for the National Institutes of Health's RECOVER Initiative to study post-acute sequelae of SARS-CoV-2, responsible for the adult cohort study, from which publications on Long COVID are forthcoming. Dr. Horwitz also conducts federally funded research on value in health care; has developed quality measures for the Centers for Medicare & Medicaid Services; and co-directs a T32 training program in population health and health care delivery. She was named an emerging leader by the National Academy of Medicine and is an elected fellow of the American Society of Clinical Investigation. Dr. Horwitz received her undergraduate degree in social studies from Harvard and her medical degree from Harvard Medical School. She then completed residency and chief residency in internal medicine at Mount Sinai Hospital in New York and the Robert Wood Johnson Clinical Scholars Program at Yale University.

Clarion E. Johnson, M.D., is vice chair of the Yale School of Public Health and is a national associate of the National Research Council. Formerly, he was global medical director at ExxonMobil. Dr. Johnson is on the advisory board at the Center for Work, Health, & Well-being and the Harvard T. H. Chan School of Public Health. He is board-certified in internal medicine, cardiology, and occupational medicine. In 2012, Dr. Johnson received the Society of Petroleum Engineers Award for Health, Safety, Security, Environment and Social Responsibility. He is also the recipient of a French Army Medal for the antimalaria project Tetrapole. Dr. Johnson is a member of the National Academies of Sciences, Engineering, and Medicine Standing Committee of Medical and Vocational Experts for the Social Security Administration's Disability Programs and has served on a number of National Academies committees, including as co-chair of the planning committee for Public–Private Partnership Responses to COVID-19 and Future Pandemics: A Workshop and co-chair of the Forum on Public–Private Partnerships for Global Health and Safety. He is a graduate of Sarah Lawrence College and has received an Outstanding Alumni Award.

Barbara L. Kornblau, J.D., O.T.R./L., FAOTA, DASPE, CCM, CDMS, is a retired professor and program director of Idaho State University's Occupational Therapy Program. She has served as a consultant on disability access and disability employment and policy issues for the American Association on Health and Disability, the United Spinal Association, and the Coalition for Disability Health Equity. As an occupational therapist, Dr. Kornblau has consulted with employers, developers, and local governments on Americans with Disabilities Act (ADA) accessibility. As an attorney, she has litigated cases under ADA, in employment discrimination, state and local government services, and health care services. Dr. Kornblau is past president of the American Occupational Therapy Association and a former Robert Wood Johnson Health Policy fellow in the U.S. Senate, where she worked on disability issues. She has also served as a government relations and health policy consultant to Special Olympics International. She is recognized as an expert in disability policy, return-to-work issues, assistive technology, and reasonable accommodations under the ADA and the Rehabilitation Act. Dr. Kornblau previously served on two National Academies' committees for the Social Security Administration, including the Committee on Selected Heritable Disorders of Connective Tissue and Disability. She received a J.D. from the University of Miami and an occupational therapy degree from the University of Wisconsin–Madison.

Joao Pedro Matias Lopes, M.D., is assistant professor at Case Western Reserve University and an attending physician in the Division of Allergy, Immunology, and Rheumatology at University Hospitals (UH) Rainbow and Babies Hospital, UH Cleveland Medical Center, in Cleveland, Ohio. His primary clinical and research interest is in immunology, particularly in the area of inborn errors of immunity, including participation in projects to identify the impact of COVID-19 infection in patients with inborn errors of immunity and the pathogenesis of prolonged COVID-19 symptoms.

Dr. Lopes earned his medical degree from Nova Medical School in Lisbon, Portugal, and then completed an internal medicine residency at University Hospitals, Case Western Reserve University, followed by an allergy and immunology fellowship at the Icahn School of Medicine at Mount Sinai in New York City.

Laura A. Malone, M.D., Ph.D., is pediatric neurologist and director of the Pediatric Post COVID-19 Rehabilitation Clinic at the Kennedy Krieger Institute in Baltimore, Maryland. She is also a physician scientist in the Center for Movement Studies and assistant professor of neurology and physical medicine and rehabilitation at The Johns Hopkins University School of Medicine. Dr. Malone addresses the pediatric neurology needs of children with post-acute/Long COVID syndromes and is actively engaged in research to improve outcomes for children after COVID-19. Her research interests also include neurorehabilitation and improving outcomes after neurological injury. Dr. Malone has contributed to national and international programs and guidance regarding pediatric Long COVID, including serving as lead author on the American Academy of Physical Medicine and Rehabilitation's Post-Acute Sequelae of SARS-CoV-2 (PASC) Infection Collaborative guidance statement on the assessment and treatment of PASC in children and adolescents. She has also served on the expert panel for the World Health Organization's Post COVID-19 Condition Case Definition for Children and Young People and on the planning committee for Long-Term Health Effects Stemming from COVID-19 and Implications for the Social Security Administration workshop organized by the National Academies of Sciences, Engineering, and Medicine. Dr. Malone is a member of the International Pediatric Rehabilitation Collaborative, the Child Neurology Society, and numerous other professional societies related to neurological rehabilitation. Dr. Malone has a Ph.D. in biomedical engineering from The Johns Hopkins University School of Medicine, where she studied gait rehabilitation and motor control after brain injury. She earned her medical degree from The University of North Carolina at Chapel Hill and completed her residency in pediatrics and pediatric neurology at The Johns Hopkins Hospital.

Louise Elaine Vaz, M.D., M.P.H., is associate professor of pediatrics in the Department of Infectious Diseases at Oregon Health & Science University. She is also medical director of complex outpatient antibiotic therapy, allowing children to transition from hospital to home to complete their antibiotics for severe infections. Dr. Vaz maintains memberships with the Infectious Diseases Society of America and the Pediatric Infectious Diseases Society. Her research is in optimization of care transitions and the effect of disparities and social vulnerability on health outcomes. Dr. Vaz has taken care of acute COVID, multisystem inflammatory syndrome in children, as well as Long COVID pediatric patients. In late 2020, she led efforts to create a multidisciplinary clinic to care for children with Long COVID in Oregon and southwest Washington state. From January 2021 to May 2022, Dr. Vaz saw children in a joint visit with Long COVID pediatric physical therapists and led a dynamic team that included multiple subspecialists in nearly every pediatric subspecialty to help address the diverse effects of Long COVID in children. In May 2022, she transitioned out of the clinical role and focused efforts on large education initiatives to clinicians, school administrators, and nurses. In 2021, Dr. Vaz was invited to co-chair the American Academy of Physical Medicine and Rehabilitation (AAPM&R) national workgroup on pediatric Long COVID and is coauthor on the AAPM&R's Post-Acute Sequelae of SARS-CoV-2 (PASC) Infection Collaborative guidance statement on the assessment and treatment of PASC in children and adolescents. Dr. Vaz graduated from Vanderbilt School of Medicine and completed her residency in pediatrics at the Seattle Children's Hospital/University of Washington. She completed dual pediatric infectious disease and health services research fellowships at Boston Children's Hospital and holds a master's degree in clinical effectiveness from the Harvard School of Public Health.

Monica Verduzco-Gutierrez, M.D., is an academic physiatrist and professor and chair of the Department of Rehabilitation Medicine at the Joe R. and Teresa Lozano Long School of Medicine at The University of Texas Health Science Center at San Antonio. She also is currently clinical chief of physical medicine and rehabilitation at the University Hospital System and medical director of critical illness recovery and neurorehabilitation at Warm Springs Rehabilitation Hospitals in San Antonio. Previously, Dr. Verduzco-Gutierrez served as medical director of the Brain Injury and Stroke Program at TIRR Memorial Hermann in Houston, Texas. Her area of clinical expertise is traumatic brain injury, stroke rehabilitation, interventional spasticity management, and now post-acute sequelae of SARS-CoV-2. She is currently directing a COVID-19 recovery clinic, the first in South Texas, which aligns with her mission to increase access to interdisciplinary care, optimize function, and improve quality of life for survivors with Long COVID. She is a co–principal investigator at one of the National Institutes of Health's RECOVER Initiative sites and received an Agency for Healthcare Research and Quality grant to expand access to Long COVID care. Dr. Verduzco-Gutierrez is coauthor on all eight of the current published guidance statements by the American Academy of Physical Medicine and Rehabilitation's (AAPM&R's) Multi-Disciplinary Post-Acute Sequelae of SARS-CoV-2 Infection Collaborative. She is also associate editor of the *American Journal of PM&R*. Dr. Verduzco-Gutierrez has current consultancies with AbbVie, Merz, Ipsen, Revance, and Piramal, related to her work in interventional spasticity management, and a past consultancy with ReNeuron and Medtronic. She previously had a consultancy with Moderna for education on vaccinations and with Pfizer related to her work in migraines. She also is an uncompensated consultant to AstraZeneca, addressing outcomes data for patients with cancer and immunodeficiencies and with GSK addressing outcomes of persons with meningococcal disease. Dr. Verduzco-Gutierrez has testified twice before Congress on issues pertaining to Long COVID. She has received the Top 25 Women in Healthcare Award from the National Diversity Council and Healthcare Diversity Council and the Distinguished Member Award from AAPM&R.

Sarah Wulf Hanson, Ph.D., M.P.H., is lead research scientist of global health metrics at the Institute for Health Metrics and Evaluation at the University of Washington in Seattle. She has more than a decade of experience estimating the burden of disease for several diseases, conditions, and risk factors in the Global Burden of Disease (GBD) study. In her current role, she is working to estimate the health burden of Long COVID and to improve GBD methods and stability of nonfatal burden estimates over time. Dr. Wulf Hanson received a B.S. in bioengineering from Rice University and both an M.P.H. and Ph.D. in global health metrics from the University of Washington in Seattle.